Biochemical Actions of Hormones


Volume XI

# Contributors

EYTAN R. BARNEA

P. MICHAEL CONN

MICHAEL P. CZECH

MARY K. DAHMER

EUGENE R. DeSOMBRE

WILLIAM L. DUAX

RICHARD H. EBRIGHT

GEOFFREY L. GREENE

JANE F. GRIFFIN

JOSEPH F. GRIPPO

SVEN HAMMARSTRÖM

JOSÉ A. HEDO

PAUL R. HOUSLEY

C. RONALD KAHN

MASATO KASUGA

JERZY K. KULSKI

NEIL J. MacLUSKY

JOAN MASSAGUÉ

FREDERICK NAFTOLIN

KEVIN R. NICHOLAS

WILLIAM B. PRATT

HENRI ROCHEFORT

DOUGLAS C. ROHRER

LAKSHMANAN SANKARAN

JONATHAN R. SEALS

ROBERT A. STEINBERG

YALE J. TOPPER

CHARLES M. WEEKS

BRUCE WESTLEY

KIN-TAK YU

# Biochemical Actions of Hormones

Edited by GERALD LITWACK

*Fels Research Institute*
*Health Sciences Center*
*Temple University, School of Medicine*
*Philadelphia, Pennsylvania*

## VOLUME XI

1984

ACADEMIC PRESS, INC.
(Harcourt Brace Jovanovich, Publishers)

Orlando   San Diego   San Francisco   New York   London
Toronto   Montreal   Sydney   Tokyo   São Paulo

ACADEMIC PRESS, INC.
Orlando, Florida 32887


*United Kingdom Edition published by*
ACADEMIC PRESS, INC. (LONDON) LTD.
24/28 Oval Road, London NW1 7DX


Library of Congress Cataloging in Publication Data
Main entry under title:

Biochemical actions of hormones.

  Includes bibliographies.
  1. Hormones--Collected works.  2. Hormones.
3. Physiology.  I. Litwack, Gerald, ed.  II. Axelrod,
Julius, Date.  [DNLM: 1. Hormones--Physiology.
WK 102 B615]
QP571.B56    574.19'27    70-107567
ISBN 0–12–452811–2  (v. 11)


PRINTED IN THE UNITED STATES OF AMERICA

84 85 86 87      9 8 7 6 5 4 3 2 1

# Contents

## 1.  The Leukotrienes

### Sven Hammarström

## 2.  Molecular Approaches to the Study of Cyclic AMP Action

### Robert A. Steinberg

## 3.  Molecular Mechanism of Gonadotropin Releasing Hormone Action

### P. Michael Conn

4.   **Mechanisms of Biological Signaling by the Insulin Receptor**

*Michael P. Czech, Joan Massagué, Jonathan R. Seals, and Kin-Tak Yu*

5.   **Antibodies to the Insulin Receptor: Studies of Receptor Structure and Function**

*C. Ronald Kahn, José A. Hedo, and Masato Kasuga*

6.   **Insulin Biology from the Perspective of Studies on Mammary Gland Development**

*Yale J. Topper, Kevin R. Nicholas, Lakshmanan Sankaran, and Jerzy K. Kulski*

7. **Steroid Hormone Action Interpreted from X-Ray Crystallographic Studies**

  *William L. Duax, Jane F. Griffin, Douglas C. Rohrer, Charles M. Weeks, and Richard H. Ebright*

8. **Application of Immunochemical Techniques to the Analysis of Estrogen Receptor Structure and Function**

  *Geoffrey L. Greene*

9. **Role of the Estrogen Receptor in Estrogen-Responsive Mammalian Cells**

  *Henri Rochefort and Bruce Westley*

## 10. Catechol Estrogens

### Eytan R. Barnea, Neil J. MacLusky, and Frederick Naftolin

## 11. Peroxidase: A Marker for Estrogen Expression

### Eugene R. DeSombre

## 12. Inactivation, Activation, and Stabilization of Glucocorticoid Receptors

### Paul R. Housley, Joseph F. Grippo, Mary K. Dahmer, and William B. Pratt

# Contributors

*Numbers in parentheses indicate the pages on which the authors' contributions begin.*

Eytan R. Barnea (267), Department of Obstetrics and Gynecology, Yale University School of Medicine, New Haven, Connecticut 06510

P. Michael Conn (67), Department of Pharmacology, Duke University Medical Center, Durham, North Carolina 27710

Michael P. Czech (93), Department of Biochemistry, University of Massachusetts Medical School, Worcester, Massachusetts 01605

Mary K. Dahmer (347), Department of Pharmacology, The University of Michigan School of Medicine, Ann Arbor, Michigan 48109

Eugene R. DeSombre (309), Ben May Laboratory for Cancer Research, The University of Chicago, Chicago, Illinois 60637

William L. Duax (187), Molecular Biophysics Department, Medical Foundation of Buffalo, Inc., Buffalo, New York 14203

Richard H. Ebright (187), Department of Microbiology and Molecular Genetics, Harvard Medical School, Boston, Massachusetts 02115

Geoffrey L. Greene (207), Ben May Laboratory for Cancer Research, The University of Chicago, Chicago, Illinois 60637

Jane F. Griffin (187), Molecular Biophysics Department, Medical Foundation of Buffalo, Inc., Buffalo, New York 14203

Joseph F. Grippo (347), Department of Pharmacology, The University of Michigan School of Medicine, Ann Arbor, Michigan 48109

Sven Hammarström (1), Department of Physiological Chemistry, Karolinska Institute, Stockholm S-104 01, Sweden

José A. Hedo* (127), Diabetes Branch, National Institute of Arthritis, Diabetes, and Digestive and Kidney Diseases, National Institutes of Health, Bethesda, Maryland 20205

Paul R. Housley (347), Department of Pharmacology, The University of Michigan School of Medicine, Ann Arbor, Michigan 48109

C. Ronald Kahn (127), Research Division, Joslin Diabetes Center, and Department of Medicine, Brigham and Women's Hospital, Harvard Medical School, Boston, Massachusetts 02115

Masato Kasuga† (127), Research Division, Joslin Diabetes Center, and Department of Medicine, Brigham and Women's Hospital, Harvard Medical School, Boston, Massachusetts 02215

Jerzy K. Kulski** (163), Laboratory of Biochemistry and Metabolism, National Institute of Arthritis, Diabetes, and Digestive and Kidney Diseases, National Institutes of Health, Bethesda, Maryland 20205

Neil J. MacLusky (267), Department of Obstetrics and Gynecology, Yale University School of Medicine, New Haven, Connecticut 06510

Joan Massagué (93), Department of Biochemistry, University of Massachusetts Medical School, Worcester, Massachusetts 01605

Frederick Naftolin (267), Department of Obstetrics and Gynecology, Yale University School of Medicine, New Haven, Connecticut 06510

Kevin R. Nicholas‡ (163), Laboratory of Biochemistry and Metabolism, National Institute of Arthritis, Diabetes, and Digestive and Kidney Diseases, National Institutes of Health, Bethesda, Maryland 20205

*Present address: Department of Experimental Endocrinology, Universidad Autónoma de Madrid, Clínica Puerta de Hierro, San Martín de Porres, 4, Madrid-35, Spain

†Present address: The Third Department of Internal Medicine, Faculty of Medicine, University of Tokyo, 7-3-1 Hongo, Bunkyo-ku, Tokyo, Japan 113

**Present address: Department of Microbiology, University of Western Australia, The Queen Elizabeth II Medical Centre, Nedlands, Western Australia 6009, Australia

‡Present address: Division of Wildlife and Rangelands Research, CSIRO, P.O. Box 84, Lyneham, Canberra, ACT 2602, Australia

William B. Pratt (347), Department of Pharmacology, The University of Michigan School of Medicine, Ann Arbor, Michigan 48109

Henri Rochefort (241), Unité d'Endocrinologie Cellulaire et Moléculaire, U 148 INSERM, Montpellier, France

Douglas C. Rohrer (187), Molecular Biophysics Department, Medical Foundation of Buffalo, Inc., Buffalo, New York 14203

Lakshmanan Sankaran (163), Laboratory of Biochemistry and Metabolism, National Institute of Arthritis, Diabetes, and Digestive and Kidney Diseases, National Institutes of Health, Bethesda, Maryland 20205

Jonathan R. Seals (93), Department of Biochemistry, University of Massachusetts Medical School, Worcester, Massachusetts 01605

Robert A. Steinberg (25), The Biological Sciences Group, The University of Connecticut, Storrs, Connecticut 06268

Yale J. Topper (163), Laboratory of Biochemistry and Metabolism, National Institute of Arthritis, Diabetes, and Digestive and Kidney Diseases, National Institutes of Health, Bethesda, Maryland 20205

Charles M. Weeks (187), Molecular Biophysics Department, Medical Foundation of Buffalo, Inc., Buffalo, New York 14203

Bruce Westley (241), Unité d'Endocrinologie Cellulaire et Moléculaire, U 148 INSERM, Montpellier, France

Kin-Tak Yu (93), Department of Biochemistry, University of Massachusetts Medical School, Worcester, Massachusetts 01605

# Preface

Volume XI of this treatise continues in the tradition set by previous volumes. The arrangement of chapters conforms to that generated before to set forth contributions dealing with general aspects first and then to proceed to more focused subjects. In the latter category, chapters on polypeptide hormones appear first, followed by discussions of the steroid hormones.

In this volume, the more general subjects are exemplified by reviews on the leukotrienes by S. Hammarström, on the actions of cyclic AMP by R. Steinberg, and on the molecular actions of the gonadotropin releasing hormone by P. M. Conn.

Next come the more detailed contributions on polypeptide hormones. Two chapters summarizing the most recent results on the topic of insulin actions derive from the laboratories of M. Czech and C. R. Kahn. Y. J. Topper's laboratory reviews the role of insulin in mammary gland development.

The last series of chapters on steroid hormones includes X-ray crystallographic analysis of steroidal structures and the import from these studies on steroid–receptor interactions from the laboratory of W. L. Duax and R. H. Ebright and their collaborators. G. L. Greene summarizes recent work on the analysis of the estrogen receptor with monoclonal antibodies. The estrogen receptor is also the topic of the three succeeding chapters: on the role of the receptor in responsive mammalian cells from H. Rochefort's laboratory, on the catechol estrogens from F. Naftolin's laboratory, and on the use of peroxidase as a marker of estrogen action by E. R. DeSombre. The final chapter deals with the activation and stabilization of the glucocorticoid receptor by W. B. Pratt's group.

Future volumes in this treatise will contain chapters aimed at service to endocrinology and related fields in terms of summarizing recent advances in the general field of hormone action and providing extensive coverage. Readers are encouraged to make suggestions to the editor directly concerning areas that they sense should be reviewed more frequently.

Gerald Litwack

# CHAPTER 1

# The Leukotrienes

*Sven Hammarström*

Department of Physiological Chemistry
Karolinska Institute
Stockholm, Sweden

## I. STRUCTURES AND BIOSYNTHESIS

### A. DISCOVERY

The leukotrienes were discovered as a smooth muscle stimulating factor released into perfusates from dog lungs during treatment with cobra venom (Feldberg and Kellaway, 1938). The same or a similar factor was formed by perfused guinea pig lungs from animals sensitized to egg albumin during challenge with antigen (Kellaway and Trethewie, 1940). Histamine, which

BIOCHEMICAL ACTIONS OF HORMONES, VOL. XI

was also released in these experiments, induced rapid, shortlasting contractions of isolated guinea pig jejunum, whereas the new factor [called slow reacting substance (SRS) by Kellaway and Trethewie, 1940] induced contractions with a slow onset and of prolonged duration. Brocklehurst (1960) extended the name for immunologically released SRS to "slow reacting substance of anaphylaxis" (SRS-A). This designation was used until 1979 when the chemical structure of SRS-A was reported and the term "leukotriene" was adopted as a trivial name for the new class of compounds (Murphy *et al.*, 1979).

A great deal of interest in SRS-A followed after observations by Brocklehurst (1960) that exposure of lung tissue from asthmatic patients to pollen induced formation of SRS-A. SRS-A was also produced during allergen-induced contractions of bronchial rings from these patients. Moreover, human bronchial smooth muscle was very sensitive to SRS-A obtained from guinea pig lung (Brocklehurst, 1962). These results and the observations that immunoglobulin E or human atopic sera could be used to sensitize monkey lung fragments *in vitro* to form SRS-A in response to antigen challenge (Ishizaka *et al.*, 1970) suggested that SRS-A mediates the bronchospasm in human asthma and anaphylaxis (reviewed by Austen, 1978). In addition to the airway, smooth muscle stimulating activity SRS-A also enhanced permeability of blood vessels in guinea pig skin (Orange and Austen, 1969). The latter effect may contribute to the development of symptoms in asthma and immunological tissue injuries.

## B. PRELIMINARY CHARACTERIZATION

The task of chemical characterization of SRS-A attracted the interests of several groups of investigators for a number of years. Early experiments indicated that the factor was soluble in water, 80% methanol, or 80% ethanol but not in acetone, chloroform, and chloroform–methanol mixtures (Chakravarty, 1959; Brocklehurst, 1962; Änggård *et al.*, 1963). The solubility of SRS-A in diethyl ether was enhanced by acidification to pH 2–3, suggesting the presence of acidic groups in the molecule. Additional studies were performed with SRS formed by cat paws during perfusions with compound 48/80. Treatment of partially purified SRS with $N,N'$-carbodi-$p$-tolylimide, phenyl isocyanate, iodinemonobromide, potassium permanganate, or acetic anhydride abolished or reduced the biological activity (Strandberg and Uvnäs, 1971). Based on these results, the authors suggested that SRS is an unsaturated carboxylic acid containing hydroxyl groups. A more efficient purification procedure for SRS-A from human lung or rat peritoneal cavity consisted of ethanol precipitation of proteins, mild alkaline hydrolysis of phospholipids, desalting Amberlite XAD-2 chromatography, and fractiona-tion on silicic acid chromatography (Orange *et al.*, 1973). The purified mate-rials were analyzed by Sephadex LH-20 chromatography, polyacrylamide gel electrophoresis, and ultraviolet spectroscopy. The results suggested that SRS-A was a low-molecular-weight compound (MW, 350–450) with an iso-electric point of 4.7 and was absorbing ultraviolet light in the regions 210–240 and 250–300 nm. Gas chromatographic analyses showed that the purified preparations of SRS-A were contaminated with a number of saturat-ed and unsaturated fatty acids. Observations that limpet and snail arylsul-fatases inactivated SRS-A and the analyses by spark source mass spectrome-try showing increased abundance of phosphorus, sulfur, and potassium in biologically active samples of SRS-A compared to controls led to a suggestion that SRS-A might contain a sulfate ester group (Orange *et al.*, 1974).

Bach and Brashler (1974, 1978) observed that a calcium ionophore (A 23187) stimulated the formation of SRS-A by rat peritoneal cells. Orange and Chang (1975) and Orange and Moore (1976) reported that cysteine enhanced the immunologic release of SRS-A. Using cultured rat basophilic leukemia cells, Jakschik *et al.* (1977) reported that arachidonic acid further stimulated ionophore A 23187-induced SRS formation and that the acetylenic analog of arachidonic acid (5,8,11,14-eicosatetraenoic acid) had the opposite effect. The latter compound inhibits prostaglandin endoperoxide synthase, which converts arachidonic acid to prostaglandin $H_2$ and platelet lipoxygenase, which forms a 12-hydroperoxy-5,8,10,14-eicosatetraenoic acid from arach-idonic acid. Indomethacin, a selective inhibitor of the former enzyme, had no effect on SRS formation. Jakschik *et al.* (1977) also reported that radioac-tivity from $^{14}C$ or tritium-labeled arachidonic acid comigrated with SRS activity on two-dimensional thin-layer chromatography and on DEAE-cel-lulose column chromatography. They suggested that SRS was a metabolite of arachidonic acid metabolism, possibly formed by a lipoxygenase pathway. Other reports, however (e.g., Bach *et al.*, 1977), show that indomethacin and other prostaglandin synthesis inhibitors prevent formation of SRS. This illustrates the problem of using inhibitors, which may have multiple effects, to investigate biochemical pathways.

## C. Structure of Leukotriene $C_4$

The results described above provided the starting point for recent work involving the complete characterization of SRS-A and the proposal of a path-way for its biosynthesis (Murphy *et al.*, 1979; Hammarström *et al.*, 1979, 1980). Since mast cells produce SRS-A (see Orange and Austen, 1969), a mast cell tumor was tried as a new system that might give larger amounts of

SRS-A. Murine mastocytoma cells (>$10^8$ cells per mouse) were harvested after 2 weeks of intraperitoneal propagation. After lysing erythrocytes (when present) with $NH_4Cl$ the remaining cells were incubated with L-cysteine, ionophore A 23187, and arachidonic acid. A modification of the purification scheme for SRS-A described by Orange *et al.* (1973) was combined with two steps of reverse phase high-performance liquid chromatography (HPLC). Together, these techniques yielded chemically pure SRS in appreciable amounts (e.g., 100 μg per 5·$10^9$ cells). The ultraviolet (UV) spectrum of this compound (Fig. 1) resembled spectra of 9-*cis*-11,13-*trans*-octadecatrienoic acid (Crombie and Jacklin, 1957) and 8,15-dihydroperoxy-5,9,11,13-eicosatetraenoic acid (Bild *et al.*, 1977). It was, however, shifted ca. 10 nm bathochromically compared to the latter spectra, suggesting that the SRS molecule had a conjugated triene with an allylic sulfur substituent (Koch, 1949).

Initially, incubations were performed with $^{35}$S-labeled cysteine and tritium-labeled arachidonic acid. After stimulating the cells with ionophore A 23187 and purifying the SRS, the HPLC chromatogram shown in Fig. 2 was obtained. The distributions of $^3$H, $^{35}$S, and SRS activity on guinea pig ileum were determined in fractions collected during the chromatography. The results showed that tritium from arachidonic acid and $^{35}$S from cysteine were incorporated into the biologically active, UV-absorbing SRS. Additional experiments performed with [3-$^3$H] and [U-$^{14}$C]cysteine indicated that the entire amino acid (not just sulfur) was converted to SRS. Analyses with fluorescamine furthermore showed one free amino group per molecule. These results suggested that the SRS molecule from mastocytoma cells was a metabolite of arachidonic acid that had three conjugated double bonds with a cysteine-containing substituent linked via the sulfhydryl group to one of the allylic positions in relation to the triene. Based on this preliminary structure,

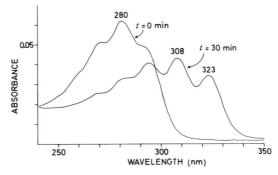

Fig. 1. UV spectrum of a slow reacting substance (SRS) from murine mastocytoma cells before and after 30 minutes of incubation with soybean lipoxygenase.

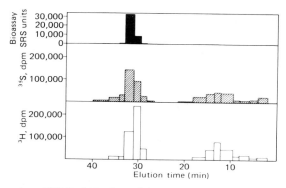

FIG. 2. Reverse phase HPLC of SRS formed during an incubation of mastocytoma cells with [35]S-labeled cysteine and [3]H₈-labeled arachidonic acid. Fractions collected during the chromatography were assayed for SRS biological activity, [35]S-radioactivity and [3]H-radioactivity. [From Murphy *et al.* (1979).]

methods for chemical degradation of the molecule were chosen. To determine the positions of double bonds, SRS biosynthesized from [5,6,8,9,11, 12,14,15-[3]H₈]arachidonic acid was subjected to ozonolysis. The ozonide was reduced with NaBH₄ in order to preserve the tritium label at the double bonds. A product formed after these reactions was identified as [[3]H]l-hexanol by gas liquid chromatography and HPLC. Since it was derived from the methyl end of the fatty acid, the formation of this product showed that a double bond was present at the n-6 position (corresponding to the $\Delta^{14}$ position of a 20-carbon fatty acid). At about this time, a report describing inactivation of SRS-A by soybean lipoxygenase was published (Sirois, 1979). The lipoxygenase converts unsaturated acids with cis double bonds at the n-6 and n-9 positions to hydroperoxy derivatives. It seemed likely that the inactivation of SRS-A was due to a reaction at the n-6 double bond. The SRS molecule isolated from mastocytoma cells was treated with soybean lipoxygenase and the UV spectrum was recorded before (Fig. 1, $t = 0$ minutes) and after 30 minutes of incubation at room temperature (Fig. 1, $t = 30$ minutes). The UV spectrum changed during this treatment and the absorbance maximum appeared at 308 nm after the reaction. This indicated that the triene in SRS had been converted to a conjugated tetraene with an allylic sulfur substituent. Based on previous information on the substrate specificity and the structures of the products formed by soybean lipoxygenase, the inactivation product was probably a 6-sulfidocysteinyl derivative of 15-hydroperoxy-7,9,11,13-eicosatetraenoic acid* and the untreated SRS molecule was probably a 6-sulfidocysteinyl derivative of 7,9,11,14-eicosatetraenoic

*This compound has now been isolated and characterized (Örning and Hammarström, 1983).

acid. To obtain further information on the structures of the fatty acid and the amino acid parts of the molecule, SRS formed from tritium-labeled arachidonic acid was reduced with Raney nickel catalyst. This treatment was expected to eliminate sulfur by cleavage of two C-S bonds in the molecule. The fatty acid part was extracted with diethyl ether, esterified with diazomethane and purified by silicic acid chromatography. It was eluted in a more polar eluate than normal fatty acid methyl esters and was therefore subjected to trimethylsilylation prior to analyses by gas liquid radiochromatography and by gas liquid chromatography–mass spectrometry. The radioactive product was identified as 5-hydroxyeicosanoic acid by these techniques. The results demonstrated that the 20 carbon atoms of arachidonic acid had been incorporated and suggested that the SRS contained a hydroxyl group at C-5. The expected desulfurization product of cysteine (alanine) could not be identified in the aqueous phase after the reduction with Raney nickel. The SRS molecule was therefore hydrolyzed with HCl and amino acid analyses performed. These showed about 0.4 mol of half-cystine, 1 mol of glycine, and 1 mol of glutamic acid per mol of SRS-triene absorption ($\epsilon^{280}$ : 40,000). Terminal residues were determined by the Dansyl method and hydrazinolysis. The sequence of the tripeptide substituent was glutamylcysteinylglycine. The bond between the aminoterminal glutamic acid and cysteine was resistant to Edman degradation but susceptible to hydrolysis by γ-glutamyl transpeptidase (see below), indicating that the tripetide was γ-glutamylcysteinylglycine (glutathione). Thus, the complete structure of the SRS molecule was 5-hydroxy-6-S-glutathionyl-7,9,11,14-eicosatetraenoic acid (Fig. 3). This compound was named "leukotriene" because of the presence of a conjugated triene and since SRS is formed by leukocytes and related cells. A letter "C" and a subscript 4 were added to indicate the nature of the substituents and the total number of double bonds.

Leukotriene $C_4$ (Fig. 3) has four asymmetric carbon atoms, two of which are in the peptide part, and four double bonds. To determine the stereochemistry at these centers, methods were developed for the chemical synthesis of several stereoisomers of leukotriene $C_4$ (Corey et al., 1980).

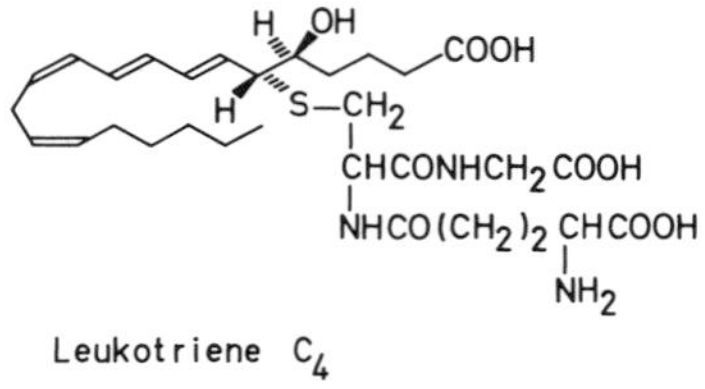

Leukotriene $C_4$

FIG. 3. Structure of the SRS from mastocytoma cells (leukotriene $C_4$).

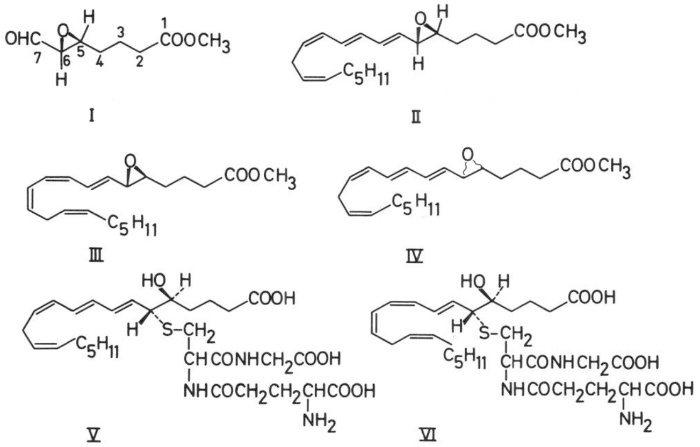

FIG. 4. Structures of intermediates (I–IV) and products in chemical syntheses of leukotriene C$_4$ (V) and a stereoisomer of this compound.

Some intermediates and products of these syntheses are shown in Fig. 4. An optically active aldehyde ester (I) was obtained from D-ribose after conversion to the 5,7-dibenzoyl-6-tosyl derivative of 5,6,7-trihydroxyheptanoic acid methyl ester. Two chain extensions of I, according to methods by Wollenberg and Wittig, respectively, provided methyl *trans*-5(S), 6(S)-oxido-7, 9-*trans*-11,14-*cis*-eicosatetraenoate (II). The corresponding mixture of racemic cis and trans epoxides (IV) had been synthesized before (Corey *et al.*, 1979). Treatment of epoxides II and IV in methanol containing triethylamine with glutathione yielded 5(S)-hydroxy-6(R)-S-glutathionyl-7,9-*trans*-11,14-*cis*-eicosatetraenoic acid (V) from II and the same product plus three stereoisomers of V [the 5(S),6(R)-,5(S),6(S)- and 5 (R),6(R)-isomers] from IV. These products were compared by HPLC, bioassay, and UV spectroscopy with leukotriene C$_4$ isolated from mastocytoma cells (Hammarström *et al.*, 1980). The three 5,6-stereoisomers of V could be distinguished from leukotriene C$_4$ by HPLC and by their lower myotropic activity on guinea pig ileum. The 5(S),6(R)-7,9-*trans*-11,14-*cis*-isomer (V) cochromatographed with leukotriene C$_4$ on reverse phase HPLC and had the same smooth muscle contractile potency as the natural compound. The 9-*cis* isomer of II (III, Fig. 4) was synthesized from I by 2-carbon silylimine and Wittig chain extensions. Epoxide III was converted to the glutathione conjugate VI (9-*cis* leukotriene C$_4$), which had a longer retention time on reverse-phase HPLC than leukotriene C$_4$. The results indicated that the stereochemistry of natural leukotriene C$_4$ was identical to that of compound V in Fig. 4.

A product similar to leukotriene C$_4$ and eluting somewhat later on HPLC

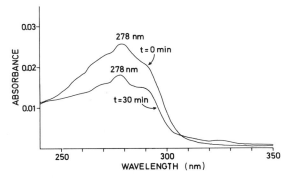

FIG. 5. UV spectrum of a second component of the SRS from mastocytoma cells (11-*trans*-leukotriene $C_4$) before and 30 minutes after addition of soybean lipoxygenase.

was also formed by mastocytoma cells. This product appeared in about 25% of the amounts of leukotriene $C_4$ and had an absorbance maximum at 278 nm (Fig. 5) compared to the absorbance maximum of leukotriene $C_4$ at 280 nm. A similar difference in UV spectra had been reported for 9,11,13-*trans*-octadecatrienoic acid ($\lambda_{max}$ : 268 nm) compared to 9-*cis*-11,13-*trans*-octadecatrienoic acid ($\lambda_{max}$ : 270 nm; Crombie and Jacklin 1957). This suggested that the second product from mastocytoma cells contained an all *trans* triene (Fig. 6). Further evidence for this structure was the lack of conversion to a conjugated tetraene product by soybean lipoxygenase (cf. Fig. 5). This enzyme requires that both of the double bonds at n-6 and n-9 have cis geometry. Chemical synthesis of 11-*trans* leukotriene $C_4$ confirmed that the second component of SRS from mastocytoma cells had this structure (Clark *et al.*, 1980).

## D. STRUCTURE OF LEUKOTRIENE $D_4$

Jakschik *et al.* (1977) used rat basophilic leukemia cells to generate a slow reacting substance. This SRS was related to leukotriene $C_4$ because the fatty

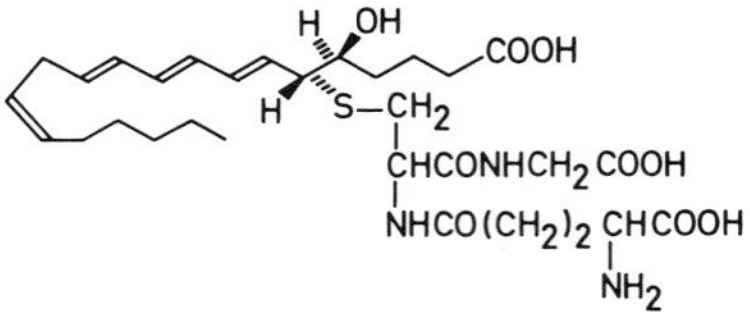

FIG. 6. Structure of the second component of the SRS from mastocytoma cells (11-*trans*-leukotriene $C_4$).

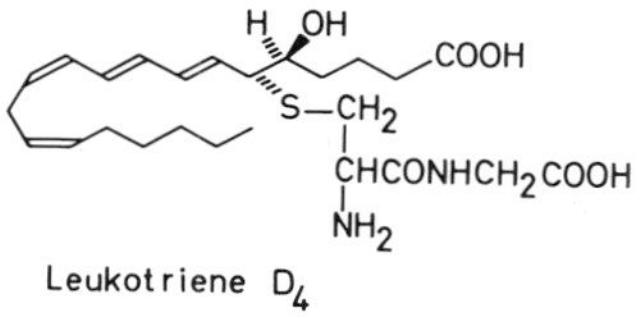

Leukotriene $D_4$

FIG. 7. Structure of SRS from rat basophilic leukemia cells (leukotriene $D_4$).

acid parts were identical and the peptide substituent was identified as cys-teinylglycine (Örning *et al.*, 1980; see Fig. 7). This product is formed from leukotriene $C_4$ in a reaction catalyzed by the enzyme γ-glutamyl transpep-tidase (Örning and Hammarström, 1980). The trivial name of this compound is leukotriene $D_4$.

Leukotrienes $C_4$ and $D_4$ have subsequently been identified as the biolog-ically active constituents of SRS (–A) isolated from other animal cells or tissues (Bach *et al.*, 1980a,b; Lewis *et al.*, 1980; Houglum *et al.*, 1980; Morris *et al.*, 1980a,b).

## E. BIOSYNTHESIS

A key intermediate in the chemical synthesis of leukotriene $C_4$ is *trans*-5(S),6(S)-oxido-7,9-*trans*-11,14-*cis*-eicosatetraenoic acid (Corey *et al.*, 1980). This epoxide was postulated as an intermediate in the biosynthesis of leuko-triene $C_4$ (Murphy *et al.*, 1979) and in the biosynthesis of 5(S),12(R)-di-hydroxy-6,8,10,14-eicosatetraenoic acid (Borgeat and Samuelsson, 1979a,b). The intermediate in leukocytes was detected by a reaction with alcohols, which yielded 5-hydroxy-12-alkoxy-6,8,10,14-eicosatetraenoic acids. Using this trapping procedure, the half-life of the intermediate in 50% aqueous acetone solution was determined as 4 minutes at 37° and pH 7.4. The inter-mediate was rapidly hydrolyzed by lowering of the pH to 1. 5(S), 12(R)-Dihydroxy-6,8,10,14-eicosatetraenoic acid and 5,6-oxido-7,9,11,14-eicosatetraenoic acid were named leukotrienes B and A (later $B_4$ and $A_4$), respectively (Samuelsson *et al.*, 1979).

Evidence that leukotriene $A_4$ is an intermediate in the biosynthesis of leukotriene $C_4$ has been obtained by alcohol trapping (Hammarström and Samuelsson, 1980) and enzymatic conversion of synthetic, unlabeled epox-ide to leukotriene $C_4$ (Rådmark *et al.*, 1980a). The synthetic epoxide was also enzymatically transformed to leukotriene $B_4$ (Rådmark *et al.*, 1980b). These transformations are shown in Fig. 8.

A common feature among leukotrienes $A_4$, $B_4$, and $C_4$ is the presence of a

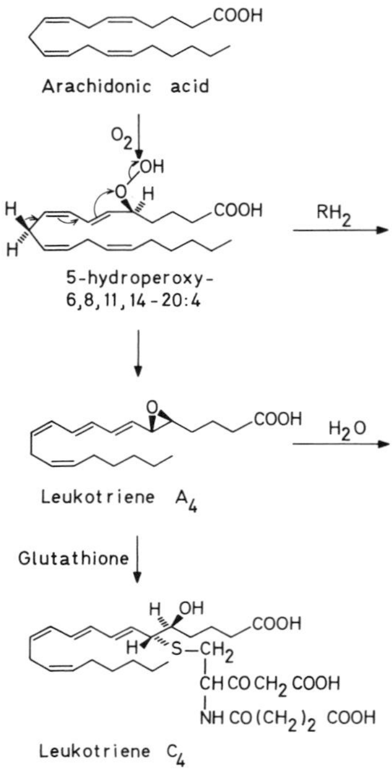

FIG. 8. Biosynthesis of leukotrienes from arachidonic acid.

5(S)-oxygen substituent. Labeling experiments with $^{18}O_2$ showed that this oxygen in leukotriene $B_4$ is derived from molecular oxygen (Borgeat and Samuelsson, 1979a). The same was true for 5(S)-hydroperoxy-6,8,11,14-eicosatetraenoic acid, another product of arachidonic acid metabolism in polymorphonuclear leukocytes. (The $^{18}O$ label was demonstrated in 5(S)-hydroxy-6,8,11,14-eicosatetraenoic acid, which is formed by peroxidase reduction of the hydroperoxy acid.)

Evidence that 5(S)-hydroperoxy-6,8,11,14,17-eicosapentaenoic acid is an intermediate in the conversion of 5,8,11,14,17-eicosapentaenoic acid to leukotriene $C_5$ (cf. below) was obtained from experiments in which [1 $^{14}C,10D_S$-$^3H$] and [1-$^{14}C$, $10L_R$-$^3H$]5,8,11,14,17-eicosapentaenoic acids were incubated with mastocytoma cells (Hammarström, 1983). Determinations of the $^3H/^{14}C$ ratios of leukotriene $C_5$ and 5-hydroxy-6,8,11,14,17-eicosapentaenoic acid formed in these experiments demonstrated that the $10D_S$-tritium was stereospecifically lost during the biosynthesis of leukotriene $C_5$. The 5-hydroxyeicosapentaenoic acid formed from the $10D_S$-isomer but not from the $10L_R$-isomer of the tritium-labeled precursor acid was markedly enriched in tritium. This was interpreted as being due to a primary kinetic isotope effect (cf. Northrop, 1981). The results indicate that the substrate for the elimination of hydrogen at C-10 during leukotriene $C_5$ biosynthesis is 5-hydroperoxy-6,8,11,14,17-eicosapentaenoic acid (Hammarström, 1983).

As mentioned above, several unsaturated fatty acids besides arachidonic acid can be converted to leukotrienes. Leukotriene $C_5$ (Hammarström, 1980) differs structurally from leukotriene $C_4$ by the presence of an additional double bond at the $\Delta^{17}$ position. Two isomers of eicosatrienoic acid are also transformed to leukotrienes: 5,8,11-eicosatrienoic acid gives rise to leukotriene $C_3$ and 11-*trans* leukotriene $C_3$ (Hammarström, 1981a), which differ from the corresponding four-series leukotrienes by the lack of a double bond at the $\Delta^{14}$ position: 8,11,14-eicosatrienoic acid is converted to a glutathione containing leukotriene that has a hydroxyl group at C-8, a peptide substituent at C-9, and a triene at the $\Delta^{10,12,14}$ position. This product (8,9-leukotriene $C_3$, a positional isomer of leukotriene $C_3$) is probably formed after oxygenation of the acid at C-8. Evidence has also been obtained that positional isomers of leukotrienes may be formed from arachidonic acid, following lipoxygenase reactions at C-15 (Lundberg *et al.*, 1981; Jubiz *et al.*, 1981; Maas *et al.*, 1981; Turk *et al.*, 1982) and C-12 (Samuelsson, 1983).

## II. BIOLOGICAL ACTIONS

### A. Respiratory Effects

Because of the proposed mediator role of SRS-A in asthma, the effects of leukotrienes on airway smooth muscles were among the first to be investigated using chemically pure compounds with known structures. Early experiments (Hedqvist *et al.*, 1980) showed that leukotrienes $C_4$ and $D_4$ induced contractions of guinea pig trachea and lung parenchymal strips (Fig. 9). The responses of the lung strips, which are primarily due to contractions of smooth muscles of the small airways, occurred at leukotriene concentrations 100 times lower than that necessary for contractions of spirally cut trachea. Leukotriene $C_4$ given intravenously to anesthetized guinea pigs raised the insufflation pressure. The dose required to double the pressure was 120 pmol of leukotriene $C_4$. Histamine also increased the insufflation pressure but the dose required to double the pressure was 14,000 pmol.

Some species differences in airway responses to leukotrienes have been reported: rabbit (Hedqvist *et al.*, 1980) and rat airways (Krell *et al.*, 1981) did

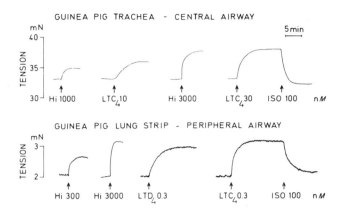

FIG. 9. Myotropic effects of histamine (Hi) and leukotrienes (LT) $C_4$ and $D_4$ on trachea and lung parenchyma from guinea pigs. [From Hedqvist *et al.* (1980).]

not respond to leukotrienes $C_4$ and $D_4$, whereas monkey (Smedegård *et al.*, 1982), guinea pig (Hedqvist *et al.*, 1980), and human airways (Dahlén *et al.*, 1980; Hanna *et al.*, 1981; Holroyde *et al.*, 1981a,b; Jones *et al.*, 1982) were very sensitive.

Synthetic leukotriene analogs have been used to investigate structure-activity relations on guinea pig lung parenchymal strips (Drazen *et al.*, 1981). The relative contractile activities of 9,10,11,12,14,15-hexahydro-leukotrienes $C_4$ and $D_4$, compared to leukotrienes $C_4$ and $D_4$, were 20% and 2%, respectively. The corresponding values for 7-*cis* hexahydroleukotrienes $C_4$ and $D_4$ isomers were 6% and 3%, respectively. 5-Dehydroxy-hexahydroleukotriene $D_4$ was inactive on lung strips. Leukotrienes $C_3$ and $D_3$ had relative activities (compared to leukotrienes $C_4$ and $D_4$) of 19% and 66%, respectively. Other investigators have reported that leukotrienes $C_3$ and $C_4$ are equipotent on guinea pig lung parenchymal strips (Dahlén *et al.*, 1983a; Fig. 10). Some positional isomers of leukotrienes $C_4$ and $D_4$ were analyzed as racemic *erythro*- and *threo*-diastereoisomers (11,12-leukotrienes $C_4$ and $D_4$, and 5,12-leukotriene $C_4$), whereas 14,15-leukotrienes $C_4$ and $D_4$ and 8,9-leukotriene $D_4$ were analyzed as single isomers. The more potent diastereoisomers of 11,12-leukotrienes $C_4$ and $D_4$ were 6 and 20 times more potent than 14,15-leukotrienes $C_4$ and $D_4$, respectively. Neither 8,9-leukotriene $D_4$ nor 5,12-leukotriene $C_4$ contracted the guinea pig lung strips (Drazen *et al.*, 1981). Dahlén *et al.* (1983a) have reported that 8,9-leukotriene $C_3$ is approximately as potent as leukotriene $C_4$ on lung strips (Fig. 10).

The effects of structural variations in the polar parts of leukotriene $D_4$ have been investigated by Lewis *et al.* (1981). The results showed that the arachidonyl carboxyl group could be converted to an amide without loss of contractile activity on guinea pig lung parenchyma. Conversion of the carboxyl group of glycine to an amide, however, reduced the contractile activity 10-fold and when both carboxyl groups in leukotriene $D_4$ were derivatized, the activity was less than 1% of that of leukotriene $D_4$. Elimination or acetylation of the amino group reduced the potency to 5% and 3%, respectively, compared to leukotriene $D_4$. Substitution of the glycine residue for D- or L-alanine reduced the activity to 10%, whereas analogs containing proline, glutamic acid, or valine instead of glycine had 3%, 2%, and 0.8% of the contractile activity of leukotriene $D_4$. If the cysteine residue was replaced with L-homocysteine, the corresponding analog had 26% of the activity of leukotriene $D_4$. The D-penicillamine analog was inactive and the 5-epi-, the 6-epi-, and the D-cysteine isomers of leukotriene $D_4$ were, respectively, 4%, 4%, and 11% as active as the natural isomer.

Respiratory effects of leukotriene $C_4$ have also been investigated *in vivo* in anesthetized *Macaca irus* monkeys (Smedegård *et al.*, 1982). Administration of 20 nmol leukotriene $C_4$ as aerosol increased the transpulmonary pressure by 180%. In contrast, 30 nmol leukotriene $C_4$ injected via a catheter into the right atrium of the heart produced a smaller effect (66% increase). Thus, aerosol administration was four times more effective than systemic administration even without considering that only a fraction of the nebulized leukotriene was taken up by the lungs. The results are consistent with rapid metabolism and elimination of leukotriene C from the circulation, which

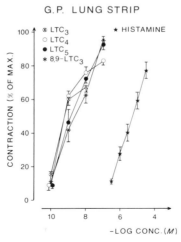

FIG. 10. Dose-response curves (noncumulative) for leukotrienes (LT) $C_3$, $C_4$, $C_5$, and 8,9-$C_3$ on guinea pig lung parenchymal strips. [From Dahlén *et al.* (1983a).]

take place following systemic administration (Hammarström, 1982). The effects of leukotriene $C_4$ on transpulmonary pressure were mainly due to decreased pulmonary dynamic compliance; the effects on pulmonary resistance were minimal. This is compatible with a greater sensitivity of peripheral compared to central airways in the guinea pig, as mentioned above (see Fig. 9).

## B. CARDIOVASCULAR EFFECTS

It has been reported that leukotrienes induce biological responses in microvessels, larger blood vessels, and in the heart.

Increased vascular permeability was observed after injection of leukotrienes $C_4$ and $D_4$ (0.1 pmol) in the skin of guinea pigs pretreated with Evans blue (Hedqvist et al., 1980). In addition to this effect, leukotriene $C_4$ (but not leukotriene $D_4$) induced cutaneous vasoconstriction (Drazen et al., 1980). Purified SRS-A (leukotriene $D_4$) also induced accumulation of radioactivity in guinea pig skin in animals preinjected with $^{131}$I-labeled albumin (Williams and Piper, 1980). The permeability stimulating effects of leukotrienes have been investigated in greater detail by intravital microscopy of the microcirculation in the cheek pouch of golden hamsters, Mesocricetus auratus (Dahlén et al., 1981). Addition of leukotriene $C_4$ or $D_4$ to buffer surrounding the pouch of animals preinjected with fluorescein isothiocyanate-conjugated (FITC) dextran led to constriction of arterioles and terminal arterioles (Fig. 11a and b). This response lasted for a few minutes and was followed by leakage of FITC dextran from postcapillary venules (Fig. 11c). Leakage, determined as the number of leakage spots per square centimeter, was greater for a given concentration of leukotriene $C_4$ than for leukotriene $D_4$, with a difference in potency of about fivefold.

Leukotrienes $C_4$ and $D_4$ also induced contractions of isolated pulmonary arteries from guinea pigs but were less potent agonists than on trachea or lung parenchymal strips (Hand et al., 1981). Weak responsiveness of rabbit pulmonary artery and vein and portal vein was observed by Kito et al. (1981). These authors also reported that rabbit coronary arteries were more sensitive than the vessels just mentioned and that renal artery and vein, mesenteric artery, and thoracic aorta from rabbits were not contracted by these substances.

Leukotrienes $C_4$, $D_4$, and $E_4$ (a metabolite of leukotriene $D_4$, formed by elimination of glycine; see Fig. 12) had negative inotropic effects on isolated guinea pig hearts and reduced the coronary flow rate. Leukotriene $D_4$ was most potent, followed by leukotrienes $C_4$ and $E_4$ (Burke et al., 1982). The decreased contraction force of the hearts was not caused by the reduced coronary flow. Human myocardium (electrically paced) responded with re-

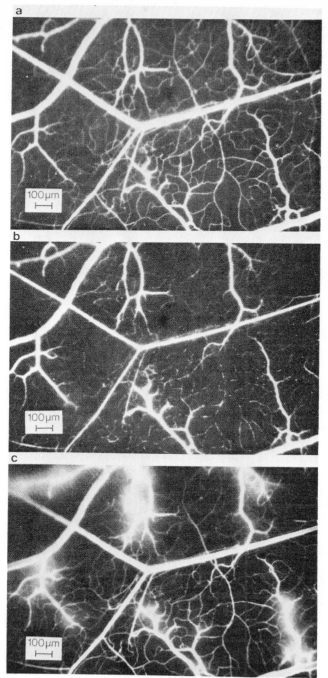

Fig. 11. Effects of leukotriene $D_4$ (4 n$M$) on hamster cheek pouch microvasculature ($\times$ 42). Light areas represent fluorescence from FITC dextran. (a) Before administration. The straight Y-shaped vessel traversing the field is an arteriole and the more tortuous vessels are venules. (b) One minute after administration of leukotriene $D_4$. (c) Five minutes after administration of leukotriene $D_4$. [From Dahlén *et al.* (1981).]

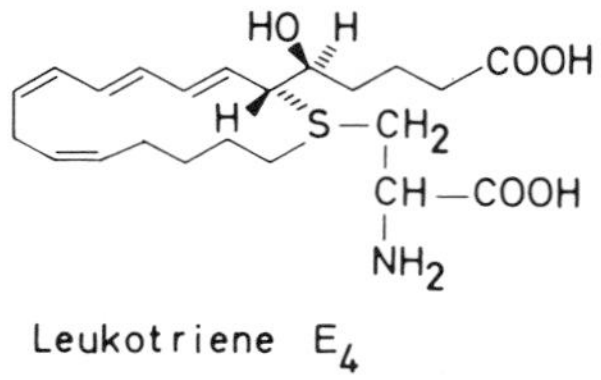

Leukotriene $E_4$

FIG. 12. Structure of a metabolite of leukotriene $D_4$ formed by elimination of glycine (leukotriene $E_4$).

duced contractile force, and the relative potencies of leukotrienes $C_4$, $D_4$, and $E_4$ were similar to those observed using spontaneously beating guinea pig hearts (Burke et al., 1982). Letts and Piper (1982) reported that leukotriene $C_4$ was more potent than leukotriene $D_4$ in reducing coronary blood flow of isolated guinea pig hearts and that leukotriene $D_4$ gave a larger reduction in contractile force than leukotriene $C_4$. Terashita et al. (1981) observed that leukotrienes $C_4$ and $D_4$ were equipotent in reducing guinea pig heart contractile force and coronary blood flow and that both compounds stimulated formation of 6-ketoprostaglandin $F_{1\alpha}$.

When administered to anesthetized monkeys, leukotriene $C_4$ influenced both respiration and cardiovascular dynamics (Smedegård et al., 1982). The cardiovascular effects were more pronounced after systemic as compared with aerosol administration: A rapid, transient increase of the mean arterial pressure was followed by prolonged hypotension. Similar changes were observed for pressures recorded in the pulmonary artery and the right and left atria. The initial pressor response was probably caused by the vasoconstrictor effects of leukotriene $C_4$, and the hypotension probably reflects the negative inotropic effect of leukotriene $C_4$ (see above) since cardiac output was reduced (35%) during this period. A decreased plasma volume, indicated by a 10% increase in hematocrit, was probably caused by peripheral leakage of plasma proteins. This may also have contributed to the hypotension.

## C. Gastrointestinal Effects

In contrast to guinea pig lung parenchymal strips on which the contractile effects of leukotrienes $C_4$, $D_4$, and $E_4$ could not be distinguished (Dahlén et al., 1983a), isolated guinea pig ileum segments submerged in buffer containing 1 $\mu M$ atropine and 1 $\mu M$ mepyramine responded quite differently to these compounds. Leukotriene $D_4$ induced a more rapid contraction than leukotriene $C_4$ and was 3 to 10 times more potent (Örning et al., 1980). A

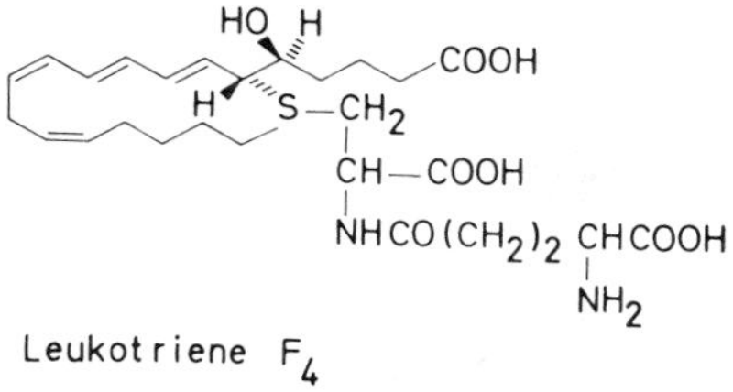

HO  H

S—CH$_2$

CH—COOH

NHCO(CH$_2$)$_2$  CHCOOH

NH$_2$

Leukotriene F$_4$

FIG. 13. Structure of a metabolite of leukotriene E$_4$ formed by addition of glutamic acid (leukotriene F$_4$).

similar rapid contraction was induced by leukotriene E$_4$ which, however, was about 100 times less potent than leukotriene D$_4$ (Bernström and Hammarström, 1981). Leukotriene F$_4$, a further metabolite of leukotriene E$_4$, formed by transpeptidation (Bernström and Hammarström, 1982; Anderson *et al.*, 1982) was about 1000-fold less potent than leukotriene D$_4$. This compound differs structurally from leukotriene C$_4$ by the absence of a glycine residue (Fig. 13).

The 11-*trans* isomer of leukotriene C$_4$ was somewhat less potent than leukotriene C$_4$ on guinea pig ileum segments (Fig. 14) and lung parenchymal strips (Dahlén *et al.*, 1983a). In contrast, no appreciable difference was observed between leukotriene E$_4$ and 11-*trans* leukotriene E$_4$ on either ileum (Bernström and Hammarström, 1981) or lung parenchyma (Dahlén *et al.*, 1983a). Geometrical isomerism at the $\Delta^{11}$ double bond was more important for activity for leukotrienes of the three series compared to the four series; thus 11-*trans* leukotriene C$_3$ was 3–20 times less potent than leukotriene C$_3$ on guinea pig ileum, whereas leukotrienes C$_3$ and D$_3$ were equipotent with leukotrienes C$_4$ and D$_4$ (Hammarström, 1981a). Leukotriene C$_3$ was also nearly as potent as leukotriene C$_4$ on guinea pig lung parenchyma (Dahlén *et al.*, 1983a; Fig. 10), whereas leukotriene C$_5$ was less potent than

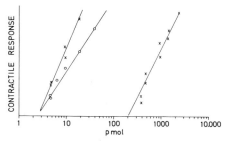

FIG. 14. Dose-response curves (cumulative) for leukotrienes C$_4$ (x–x, to the left), 11-*trans* C$_4$ (O–O) and histamine (the x–x curve to the right) on guinea pig ileum.

leukotriene $C_4$ on both guinea pig ileum (Hammarström, 1980) and guinea pig lung parenchyma (Dahlén et al., 1983a; Fig. 10).

Several of the synthetic leukotriene analogs used to investigate structure–activity relations on lung parenchymal strips were also used for similar experiments on guinea pig ileum (Drazen et al., 1981; Lewis et al., 1981). Large differences in the sensitivity of these tissues to leukotriene analogs were reported: the relative potency of 9,10,11,12,14,15-hexahydroleukotriene $C_4$ compared to leukotriene $C_4$ was twice as high and the relative potency of the corresponding leukotriene $D_4$ analog compared to leukotriene $D_4$ was four times lower on guinea pig ileum versus guinea pig lung strips and the activities of 7-cis hexahydroleukotrienes $C_4$ and $D_4$ were six times higher and four times lower, respectively, on ileum compared to lung parenchyma. Leukotriene $D_4$ monoamide (at C-1 of the arachidonyl part) was four times less potent than leukotriene $D_4$ on ileum but equipotent with leukotriene $D_4$ on lung parenchyma. The relative potency of the leukotriene $D_4$ analog containing D-alanine instead of glycine was three times higher on ileum than on lung parenchyma, whereas the corresponding L-alanine analog was half as active on ileum as on lung strips. Similarly, the relative potency of the leukotriene $D_4$ diastereoisomer containing D-cysteine was five times lower on ileum than on lung, whereas desamino leukotriene $D_4$ had four times higher relative potency on ileum compared to lung. The results suggest that the specificity of ileum leukotriene receptors is different from that of lung leukotriene receptors. Based on these data it seems difficult, however, to draw general conclusions regarding what parts of the molecule are important for binding to one or the other receptor. In another investigation on the actions of leukotriene $D_4$ stereoisomers on lung and ileum (Baker et al., 1981), 5(R),6(S)-leukotriene $D_4$ had a relative potency compared to leukotriene $D_4$ (which has the 5(S),6(R)-configuration) of 1% on ileum and 0.1% on lung parenchyma. The corresponding values for 9-cis leukotriene $D_4$, 11-trans leukotriene $D_4$, and 9-cis-11-trans leukotriene $D_4$ were 39%, 10%, and 50% on ileum and 15%, 10%, and 50% on lung strips.

Species variability regarding the sensitivity of gastrointestinal smooth muscles to leukotrienes has been observed: Thus, rat duodenum and ileum did not respond to leukotrienes $C_4$ and $D_4$, whereas guinea pig ileum was very responsive (cf. above). Rat stomach and colon also responded to these leukotrienes (Goldenberg and Subers, 1982) as did guinea pig stomach (Francis and Goadby, 1981).

The biochemical mechanisms of leukotriene-induced contractions of longitudinal smooth muscles from guinea pig ileum appeared to be similar to that of other agonists acting on the same preparation, namely stimulation of $Ca^{2+}$ influx, which triggers the mechanical response (Findlay et al., 1981). The stimulation of $Ca^{2+}$ influx is probably secondary to interaction of leukotrienes with a specific receptor. The dissociation constant for this interaction may be unusually low in view of the long duration of leukotriene-induced responses compared to responses induced by other agonists.

## D. Stimulation of Prostaglandin Synthesis

Crude preparations of SRS-A were previously shown to stimulate the release of prostaglandin-like materials and thromboxane $A_2$ from perfused guinea pig lung (Engineer et al., 1978). Following the characterization of leukotrienes $C_4$ and $D_4$, several groups have shown that these compounds stimulate prostaglandin formation in guinea pig lung (Piper and Samhoun, 1981; Folco et al., 1981; Ziljstra et al., 1981; Vargaftig et al., 1981; Weichman et al., 1982). These leukotrienes also induce prostaglandin and thromboxane synthesis in rat peritoneal macrophages (Feuerstein et al., 1981).

The importance of prostaglandin and thromboxane biosynthesis for the contractile effects of leukotrienes has been investigated by Dahlén et al. (1983b). They observed that leukotrienes $B_4$ and $C_4$ induce synthesis of thromboxane $A_2$ in guinea pig lung strips. This was accompanied by mechanical responses. Leukotriene $C_4$ was ca. 100 times more potent than leukotriene $B_4$ in inducing contractions. Contractions induced by leukotriene $B_4$ were prevented if the tissue was pretreated with an inhibitor of prostaglandin synthesis. No effect of such inhibitors was observed for contractions elicited by leukotriene $C_4$. If the lung strips were perifused instead of submerged in an organ bath, the sensitivity to leukotriene $C_4$ decreased to the same level as observed for leukotriene $B_4$ and the responses were prevented by prostaglandin synthesis inhibitors. This suggests that leukotriene $C_4$ stimulates prostaglandin synthesis and smooth muscle contractions by independent mechanisms. Leukotriene $B_4$ shares the ability to induce prostaglandin formation but lacks the direct myotropic action that is a characteristic property of the cysteinyl containing leukotrienes.

## E. Actions of Leukotriene $B_4$

In addition to stimulating prostaglandin synthesis, leukotriene $B_4$ exerts various effects on leukocytes, i.e., the induction of leukocyte adhesion to endothelial cells in venules of the hamster cheek pouch (Dahlén et al., 1981), stimulation of chemotaxis and chemokinesis of human polymorphonuclear leukocytes in vitro (Ford-Hutchinson et al., 1980; Palmblad et al., 1981), and induction of degranulation and release of lysosomal enzymes from human leukocytes (Hafström et al., 1981; Feinmark et al., 1981). The secretory actions of leukotriene $B_4$ depended partly on cytochalasin B and were enhanced by extracellular $Ca^{2+}$ (Hafström *et al.*, 1981; Showell *et al.*, 1982). Leukotriene $B_4$ also induced $Ca^{2+}$ mobilization in leukocytes (Sha'afi *et al.*, 1981) and acted as a calcium ionophore in liposomes (Serhan *et al.*, 1982). The effects on calcium movements may explain the prostaglandin stimulating activity of leukotrienes since calcium ionophores stimulate prostaglandin formation by activating enzymes that release arachidonic acid from cellular phospholipids.

## F. Other Effects

Palmer *et al.* (1981) have reported that leukotriene $D_4$ (but not leukotriene $B_4$) induces prolonged excitation of rat cerebellar purkinje neurons. Webb *et al.* (1982) have suggested that leukotrienes $D_4$ and $E_4$ (in femtomolar concentrations) reduced thymidine incorporation into DNA in phytohemagglutinin-stimulated mouse spleen cells. Leukotriene $B_4$ (but not leukotriene $D_4$) was reported to induce suppressor T lymphocytes in human peripheral blood lymphocytes at femtomolar concentration of leukotriene (Rola-Pleszczynski *et al.*, 1982).

## ACKNOWLEDGMENTS

Work from the author's laboratory was supported by grants from the Swedish Medical Research Council (projects 03X-5914, 03X-6526, and 03P-6396).

## REFERENCES

Anderson, M. E., Allison, R. D., and Meister, A. (1982). Proc. Natl. Acad. Sci. U.S.A. **79**, 1088–1091.
Änggård, E., Bergquist, U., Johansson, K., Thon, I. L., and Uvnäs, B. (1963). *Acta Physiol. Scand.* **59**, 97–110.
Austen, K. F. (1978). *J. Immunol.* **121**, 793–805.
Bach, M. K., and Brashler, J. R. (1974). *J. Immunol.* **113**, 2040–2044.
Bach, M. K., and Brashler, J. R. (1978). *Life Sci.* **23**, 2119–2126.
Bach, M. K., Brashler, J. R., and Gorman, R. R. (1977). *Prostaglandins* **14**, 21–38.
Bach, M. K., Brashler, J. R., Hammarström, S., and Samuelsson, B. (1980a). *J. Immunol.* **125**, 115–117.
Bach, M. K., Brashler, J. R., Hammarström, S., and Samuelsson, B. (1980b). *Biochem. Biophys. Res. Commun.* **93**, 1121–1126.
Baker, S. R., Boot, J. R., Jamiesson, W. B., Osborne, D. J., and Sweatman, W. J. F. (1981). *Biochem. Biophys. Res. Commun.* **103**, 1258–1264.

Bernström, K., and Hammarström, S. (1981). *J. Biol. Chem.* **256**, 9579–9582.
Bernström, K., and Hammarström, S. (1982). *Biochem. Biophys. Res. Commun.* **109**, 800–804.
Bild, G. S., Ramadoss, C. S., Lim, S., and Axelrod, B. (1977). *Biochem. Biophys. Res. Commun.* **74**, 949–954.
Borgeat, P., and Samuelsson, B. (1979a). *Proc. Natl. Acad. Sci. U.S.A.* **76**, 3213–3217.
Borgeat, P. and Samuelsson, B. (1979b). *J. Biol. Chem.* **254**, 7865–7869.
Brocklehurst, W. E. (1960). *J. Physiol. (London)* **151**, 416–435.
Brocklehurst, W. E. (1962). *In* "Progress in Allergy" (P. Kallos and B. H. Waksman, eds.), Vol. 6, pp. 539–558. Karger, Basel.
Burke, J. A., Levi, R., Guo, Z.-G., and Corey, E. J. (1982). *J. Pharmacol. Exp. Ther.* **122**, 235–241.
Chakravarty, N. (1959). *Acta Physiol. Scand.* **46**, 298–313.
Clark, D. A., Goto, G., Marfat, A., Corey, E. J., Hammarström, S., and Samuelsson, B. (1980). *Biochem. Biophys. Res. Commun.* **94**, 1133–1139.
Corey, E. J., Arai, Y., and Mioskowski, C. (1979). *J. Am. Chem. Soc.* **101**, 6748–6749.
Corey, E. J., Clark, D. A., Goto, G., Marfat, A., Mioskowski, C., Samuelsson, B., and Hammarström, S. (1980). *J. Am. Chem. Soc.* **102**, 1436–1439.
Crombie, L., and Jacklin, A. G. (1957). *J. Chem. Soc.* 1632–1646.
Dahlén, S. E., Hedqvist, P., Hammarström, S., and Samuelsson, B. (1980). *Nature (London)* **288**, 484–486.
Dahlén, S. E., Björk, J., Hedqvist, P., Arfors, K. E., Hammarström, S., Lindgren, J. Å, and Samuelsson, B. (1981). *Proc. Natl. Acad. Sci. U.S.A.* **78**, 3887–3891.
Dahlén, S. E., Hedqvist, P., and Hammarström, S. (1983a). *Eur. J. Pharmacol.* **86**, 207–215.
Dahlén, S. E., Hedqvist, P., Westlund, P., Granström, E., Hammarström, S., Lindgren, J. Å., and Rådmark, O. (1983b). *Acta Physiol. Scand.*, **118**, 393–403.
Drazen, J. M., Austen, K. F., Lewis, R. A., Clark, D. A., Goto, G., Marfat, A., and Corey, E. J. (1980). *Proc. Natl. Acad. Sci. U.S.A.* **77**, 4354–4358.
Drazen, J. M., Lewis, R. A., Austen, K. F., Toda, M., Brion, F., Marfat, A., and Corey, E. J. (1981). *Proc. Natl. Acad. Sci. U.S.A.* **78**, 3195–3198.
Engineer, D. M., Morris, H. R., Piper, P. J., and Sirois, P. (1978). *Br. J. Pharmacol.* **64**, 211–218.
Feinmark, S. J., Lindgren, J. Å., Claesson, H. E., Malmsten, C., and Samuelsson, B. (1981). *FEBS Lett.* **136**, 141–144.
Feldberg, W., and Kellaway, C. H. (1938). *J. Physiol. (London)* **94**, 187–226.
Feuerstein, N., Foegh, M., and Ramwell, P. W. (1981). *Br. J. Pharmacol.* **72**, 389–391.
Findlay, S. R., Lichtenstein, L. M., Siegel, H., and Triggle, D. J. (1981). *J. Immunol.* **126**, 1728–1730.
Folco, G., Hansson, G., and Granström, E. (1981). *Biochem. Pharmacol.* **30**, 2491–2493.
Ford-Hutchinson, A. W., Bray, M. A., Doig, M. V., Shipley, M. E., and Smith, M. J. H. (1980). *Nature (London)* **286**, 264–265.
Francis, H. P., and Goadby, P. (1981). *Br. J. Pharmacol.* **74**, 926P.
Goldenberg, M. M., and Subers, E. M. (1982). *Eur. J. Pharmacol.* **78**, 463–466.
Hafström, I., Palmblad, J., Malmsten, C., Rådmark, O., and Samuelsson, B. (1981). *FEBS Lett.* **130**, 146–148.
Hammarström, S. (1980). *J. Biol. Chem.* **255**, 7093–7094.
Hammarström, S. (1981a). *J. Biol. Chem.* **256**, 2275–2279.
Hammarström, S. (1981b). *J. Biol. Chem.* **256**, 7712–7714.
Hammarström, S. (1982). *In* "Advances in Prostaglandin, Thromboxane and Leukotriene Research" (B. Samuelsson and R. Paoletti, eds.), Vol. 9, pp. 83–101. Raven Press, New York.
Hammarström, S. (1983). *J. Biol. Chem.* **258**, 1427–1430.

Hammarström, S., and Samuelsson, B. (1980). *FEBS Lett.* **122**, 83–86.

Hammarström, S., Murphy, R. C., Samuelsson, B., Clark, D. A., Mioskowski, C., and Corey, E. J. (1979). *Biochem. Biophys. Res. Commun.* **91**, 1266–1272.

Hammarström, S., Samuelsson, B., Clark, D. A., Goto, G., Marfat, A., Mioskowski, C., and Corey, E. J. (1980). *Biochem. Biophys. Res. Commun.* **92**, 946–953.

Hand, J. M., Will, J. A., and Buckner, C. K. (1981). *Eur. J. Pharmacol.* **76**, 439–442.

Hanna, C. J., Bach, M. K., Parc, P. D., and Schellenberg, R. R. (1981). *Nature (London)* **290**, 343–344.

Hedqvist, P., Dahlén, S. E., Gustafsson, L., Hammarström, S., and Samuelsson, B. (1980). *Acta Physiol. Scand.* **110**, 331–333.

Holroyde, M. C., Altounyan, R. E. C., Cole, M., Dixon, M., and Elliot, E. V. (1981a) *Lancet*, July 4, 17–18.

Holroyde, M. C., Altounyan, R. E. C., Cole, M., Dixon, M., and Elliot, E. V. (1981b). *Agents and Actions* **11**, 573–574.

Houglum, J., Pai, J.-K., Atrache, V., Sok, D.-E., and Sih, C. J. (1980). *Proc. Natl. Acad. Sci. U.S.A.* **77**, 5688–5692.

Ishizaka, T., Ishizaka, K., Orange, R. P., and Austen, K. F. (1970). *J. Immunol.* **104**, 335–343.

Jakschik, B. A., Falkenhein, S., and Parker, C. W. (1977). *Proc. Natl. Acad. Sci. U.S.A.* **74**, 4577–4581.

Jones, T. R., Davis, C., and Daniel, E. E. (1982). *Can. J. Physiol. Pharmacol.* **60**, 638–643.

Jubiz, W., Rådmark, O., Lindgren, J. Å., Malmsten, C., and Samuelsson, B. (1981). *Biochem. Biophys. Res. Commun.* **99**, 976–986.

Kellaway, C. H., and Trethewie, E. R. (1940). *Q. J. Exp. Physiol. Cogn. Med. Sci.* **30**, 121–145.

Kito, G., Okuda, H., Ohkawa, S., Terao, S., and Kikuchi, K. (1981). *Life Sci.* **29**, 1325–1332.

Koch, H. P. (1949). *J. Chem. Soc.* 387–394.

Krell, R. D., Osborn, R., Vickery, L., Falcone, K., O'Donnell, M., Gleason, J., Kinzig, C., and Bryan, D. (1981). *Prostaglandins* **22**, 387–409.

Letts, L. G., and Piper, P. J. (1982). *Br. J. Pharmacol.* **76**, 169–176.

Lewis, R. A., Austen, K. F., Drazen, J. M., Clark, D. A., Marfat, A., and Corey, E. J. (1980). *Proc. Natl. Acad. Sci. U.S.A.* **77**, 3710–3714.

Lewis, R. A., Drazen, J. M., Austen, K. F., Toda, M., Brion, F., Marfat, A., and Corey, E. J. (1981). *Proc. Natl. Acad. Sci. U.S.A.* **78**, 4579–4583.

Lundberg, U., Rådmark, O., Malmsten, C., and Samuelsson, B. (1981). *FEBS Lett.* **126**, 127–132.

Maas, R. L., Brash, A. R., and Oates, J. A. (1981). *Proc. Natl. Acad. Sci. U.S.A.* **78**, 5523–5527.

Morris, H. R., Taylor, G. W., Piper, P. J., Samhoun, M. N., and Tippins, J. R. (1980a). *Prostaglandins* **19**, 185–201.

Morris, H. R., Taylor, G. W., Piper, P. J., and Tippins, J. R. (1980b). *Nature (London)* **285**, 104–106.

Murphy, R. C., Hammarström, S., and Samuelsson, B. (1979). *Proc. Natl. Acad. Sci. U.S.A.* **76**, 4275–4279.

Northrop, D. B. (1981). *Ann. Rev. Biochem.* **50**, 103–131.

Orange, R. P., and Austen, K. F. (1969). *Adv. Immunol.* **10**, 105–144.

Orange, R. P., and Chang, P. L. (1975). *J. Immunol.* **115**, 1072–1075.

Orange, R. P., and Moore, E. G. (1976). *J. Immunol.* **116**, 392–397.

Orange, R. P., Murphy, R. C., Karnovsky, M. L., and Austen, K. F. (1973). *J. Immunol.* **110**, 760–770.

Orange, R. P., Murphy, R. C., and Austen, K. F. (1974). *J. Immunol.* **113**, 316–322.

Örning, L., and Hammarström, S. (1980). *J. Biol. Chem.* **255**, 8023–8026.

Örning, L., and Hammarström, S. (1983). *FEBS Lett.* **153**, 253–256.

Örning, L., Hammarström, S., and Samuelsson, B. (1980). *Proc. Natl. Acad. Sci. U.S.A.* **77**, 2014–2017.

Palmblad, J., Malmsten, C., Udén, A. M., Rådmark, O., Engstedt, L., and Samuelsson, B. (1981). *Blood* **58**, 658–661.

Palmer, M. R., Mathews, W. R., Hoffer, B. J., and Murphy, R. C. (1981). *J. Pharmacol. Exp. Ther.* **219**, 91–96.

Piper, P. J., and Samhoun, M. N. (1981). *Prostaglandins* **21**, 793–803.

Rådmark, O., Malmsten, C., and Samuelsson, B. (1980a). *Biochem. Biophys. Res. Commun.* **96**, 1679–1687.

Rådmark, O., Malmsten, C., Samuelsson, B., Clark, D. A., Goto, G., Marfat, A., and Corey, E. J. (1980b). *Biochem. Biophys. Res. Commun.* **92**, 954–961.

Rola-Pleszczynski, M., Borgeat, P., and Sirois, P. (1982). *Biochem. Biophys. Res. Commun.* **108**, 1531–1537.

Samuelsson, B. (1983). In "Advances in Prostaglandin, Thromboxane and Leukotriene Research" (B. Samuelsson, R. Paoletti, and P. Ramwell , eds.), Vol. 11, pp. 1–26. Raven Press, New York.

Samuelsson, B., and Hammarström, S. (1980). *Prostaglandins* **19**, 645–648.

Samuelsson, B., Borgeat, P., Murphy, R. C., and Hammarström, S. (1979). *Prostoglandins* **17**, 785–787.

Serhan, C. N., Fridovich, J., Goetzl, E. J., Dunham, P. B., Weissmann, G. (1982). *J. Biol. Chem.* **257**, 4746–4752.

Sha'afi, R. I., Molski, T. F. P., Borgeat, P., Naccache, P. H. (1981). *Biochem. Biophys. Res. Commun.* **103**, 766–773.

Showell, H. J., Naccache, P. H., Borgeat, P., Picard, S., Vallerand, P., Becker, E., and Sha'afi, R. (1982). *J. Immunol.* **128**, 811–816.

Sirois, P. (1979). *Prostaglandins* **17**, 395–404.

Smedegård, G., Hedqvist, P., Dahlén, S. E., Revenäs, B., Hammarström, S., and Sammuelsson, B. (1982). *Nature (London)* **295**, 327–329.

Strandberg, K., and Uvnäs, B. (1971). *Acta Physiol. Scand.* **82**, 358–374.

Terashita, Z.-I., Fukui, H., Hirata, M., Terao, S., Ohkawa, S., Nishikawa, K., and Kikuchi, S. (1981). *Eur. J. Pharmacol.* **73**, 357–361.

Turk, J., Maas, R. L., Brash, A. R., Roberts, L. J., and Oates, J. A. (1982). *J. Biol. Chem.* **257**, 7068–7076.

Vargaftig, B. B., Lefort, J., and Murphy, R. C. (1981). *Eur. J. Pharmacol.* **72**, 417–418.

Webb, D. R., Nowowiejski, I., Healy, C., and Rogers, T. J. (1982). *Biochem. Biophys. Res. Commun.* **104**, 1617–1622.

Weichman, B. M., Muccitelli, R. M., Osborn, R. R., and Holden, D. A., Gleason, J. G., and Wasserman, M. A. (1982). *J. Pharmacol. Exp. Ther.* **222**, 202–208.

Williams, T. J., and Piper, P. J. (1980). *Prostaglandins* **19**, 779–789.

Ziljstra, F. J., Bonta, I. L., Adolfs, M. J. P., and Vincent, J. E. (1981). *Eur. J. Pharmacol.* **76**, 297–298.

# CHAPTER 2

# Molecular Approaches to the Study of Cyclic AMP Action*

*Robert A. Steinberg*

The Biological Sciences Group
The University of Connecticut
Storrs, Connecticut

*Abbreviations: cAMP, cyclic AMP; R, regulatory subunit of cAMP-dependent protein kinase; C, catalytic subunit of cAMP-dependent protein kinase; $R_I$ and $R_{II}$, regulatory subunits from protein kinase isozyme types I and II; $R_N$ and $R_P$, nonphosphorylated and phosphorylated forms of $R_I$; $Bt_2cAMP$, dibutyryl cAMP; BrdU, 8-bromodeoxyuridine; $kin^-$, kinase-negative; CHO, Chinese hamster ovary; MIX, methyl isobutylxanthine; BrcAMP, 8-bromo cAMP.

BIOCHEMICAL ACTIONS OF HORMONES, VOL. XI

*Robert A. Steinberg*

## I. INTRODUCTION

Since the discovery more than 25 years ago of a role for reversible protein phosphorylation in hormonal regulation of glycogen metabolism (Fischer and Krebs, 1955; Sutherland and Wosilait, 1955), the importance of protein phosphorylation in cellular regulation has gained increasing recognition. Protein phosphorylation has now been implicated in a broad array of regulatory phenomena (Cohen, 1980; Rosen and Krebs, 1981). These include the following: responses to hormones and factors acting through a variety of protein kinase systems; regulation of cell growth, shape, and motility; modulation of nervous function and muscle contraction; regulation of protein synthesis by hemin and double-stranded RNA; and tumorigenic transformation. Of the many systems employing protein phosphorylation in regulation, the most intensively studied has been effector-mediated elevation of intracellular cyclic AMP (cAMP) and concomitant activation of cAMP-dependent protein kinase. In addition to its own importance to diverse physiological processes, the cAMP response system has served as a model for investigations of other systems employing protein phosphorylation.

Figure 1 presents, in schematic form, a general model for hormonal regulation of cell function through cAMP elevation. This model emerged from studies of a number of hormonally regulated enzyme systems (reviewed in Robison *et al.*, 1971; Krebs, 1972). In response to interaction between hormones and cell surface receptors, the activity of a plasma membrane-associated adenylate cyclase is stimulated; intracellular accumulation of cAMP is

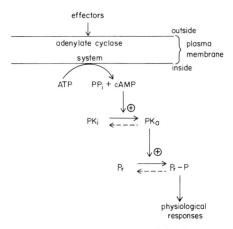

F IG. 1. Model for cAMP-dependent regulation of cellular functions. $PK_i$ and $PK_a$ represent inactive and active forms of cAMP-dependent protein kinase. Pr and Pr-P designate non-phosphorylated and phosphorylated forms of a representative substrate protein.

thereby enhanced. Elevation of cAMP causes activation of cAMP-dependent protein kinase, an enzyme that phosphorylates specific serine and threonine sites on target substrate proteins. Phosphorylation of substrate proteins alters their enzymatic functions and leads to a shift in the metabolic activities of the stimulated cell. In this model, effector selectivity is determined by the specificities of receptors on a given cell's surface, and the physiological response is determined by the particular target substrates for phosphorylation in a stimulated cell.

A number of recent observations, however, suggest that the actual cAMP response system is considerably more subtle. The response of adenylate cyclase to a particular effector can vary with the nature of receptors and coupling factors that mediate interactions between the effectors and cyclase (Lai *et al.*, 1982; Cooper, 1982). Compartmentalization of cAMP and cAMP-dependent protein kinase may allow selective phosphorylation of specific subsets of potential kinase substrates in response to specific effectors (reviewed in Hayes and Brunton, 1982). And, regulation of specific protein synthesis may be as important as substrate phosphorylation in determining a cell's response pattern to cAMP elevation (Jungmann and Russell, 1977; Steinberg, 1981).

Until quite recently, most studies of cAMP action have been of a strictly biochemical nature, using purified components to investigate the enzymology of phosphorylations and dephosphorylations under cAMP control (reviewed in Krebs, 1972; Rubin and Rosen, 1975; Nimmo and Cohen, 1977; Krebs and Beavo, 1979). As characterization of the enzymes involved in cAMP-dependent regulation has progressed, however, it has become apparent that detailed understanding of the regulation of cAMP action requires study of the dynamic aspects of cAMP-mediated responses in intact cells. Because of the experimental difficulties of working with whole animals, a variety of alternative systems have been employed, including organ cultures (Hayes *et al.*, 1979), cell suspensions or primary cell cultures (Moyle *et al.*, 1973; Witters *et al.*, 1979), and tissue-culture cell lines (reviewed in Gottesman, 1980). In progressing from the intact animal through organ culture and primary cell cultures to established cell lines, there is a significant gain in experimental manipulability, the cost of which is decreased fidelity to the *in vivo* situation. Nevertheless, many cultured cell lines retain the hormonal responsiveness of their tissue of origin (reviewed in Pollack, 1981). The advantages of cell lines for studies of physiological regulation include homogeneity of cell type, enhanced accessibility to pharmacological agents and radioactive tracer molecules, and relative ease of genetic manipulation.

In this chapter I will summarize research combining genetic, metabolic, and biochemical approaches for studying intracellular regulation of cAMP action. Results from these investigations in cultured cell systems comple-

ment results from more traditional biochemical investigations. I will emphasize recent studies in the S49 mouse lymphoma cell system both because the
genetics of cAMP regulation have been more thoroughly analyzed in this
than in any other cell system and because techniques used in these studies
should provide a foundation for research in other cell systems. Some aspects
of the genetic regulation of cAMP action in cultured cell lines have been
reviewed previously (Coffino *et al.*, 1976; Gottesman, 1980; Coffino, 1981). I
will refer only briefly to analysis of the adenylate cyclase system, since a
detailed review of this work has been presented elsewhere (Ross and Gilman, 1980). To provide a background for discussion of molecular approaches
to cAMP action, I will outline the current status of research on cAMP-
dependent protein kinases, the intracellular transducers for cAMP effects. I
will stress mechanisms that regulate kinase activation and aspects of kinase
structure relevant to the genetic studies to be presented subsequently.

## II. CYCLIC AMP-DEPENDENT PROTEIN KINASES

### A. DISTRIBUTION AND SUBUNIT COMPOSITION

Cyclic AMP-dependent protein kinases appear to be ubiquitous among
animal species and tissues (Kuo and Greengard, 1969; Langan, 1973). They
have also been found in cellular slime molds (Sampson, 1977) and in a variety
of fungi (reviewed in Pall, 1981). Where characterized, the animal and fungal
enzymes have been found to consist of regulatory (R) and catalytic (C) subunits in tetrameric holoenzymes with an R subunit dimer at the core (Krebs
and Beavo, 1979; Pall, 1981). Evolutionary conservation of these enzymes
transcends similarities in subunit composition: protein substrate specificities
of kinases from yeast and mammals are similar; fungal kinases are inhibited
by a heat-stable mammalian protein specific for inhibition of C subunit
activity; and functional kinase holoenzyme can be reconstituted from heterologous mixtures of R and C subunits from yeast and mammalian tissues
(reviewed in Pall, 1981).

Mammalian cAMP-dependent protein kinases all have C subunits with
very similar physical and functional properties (Nimmo and Cohen, 1977;
Zoller *et al.*, 1979; Schwoch *et al.*, 1980). DEAE-cellulose chromatography
reveals two classes of mammalian kinases that are designated as type I and
type II, on the basis of their order of elution with increasing ionic strength;
purified enzymes of the two classes differ in a number of functional parameters (reviewed in Rosen *et al.*, 1977; Walter and Greengard, 1981), and the

differences appear to be wholly attributable to differences in R subunits (Hofmann *et al.*, 1975; Zoller *et al.*, 1979). Mammalian cAMP-dependent protein kinases also exhibit additional diversity. Reports of separate soluble and membrane-associated compartments of kinase holoenzyme or R subunit (e.g., Rubin, 1979) suggest possibilities of posttranslational modifications or additional primary structure differences in kinase subunits. Immunological evidence suggests structural differences between $R_{II}$ subunits from muscle and from brain (Erlichman *et al.*, 1980). $R_{II}$ subunits in holoenzyme undergo autophosphorylation when incubated with MgATP (Erlichman *et al.*, 1974) and can be phosphorylated at a second site by casein kinase II (Carmichael *et al.*, 1982); both sites are phosphorylated *in vivo* (Rangel-Aldao *et al.*, 1979; Carmichael *et al.*, 1982). $R_I$ subunits do not undergo autophosphorylation *in vitro* (Hofmann *et al.*, 1975; Walter *et al.*, 1977) but can be phosphorylated by cGMP-dependent protein kinase at a site homologous to the site auto-phosphorylated in $R_{II}$ (Geahlen and Krebs, 1980a; Hashimoto *et al.*, 1981). $R_I$ does undergo phosphorylation *in vivo*, but it does so at another site (Steinberg *et al.*, 1977; Geahlen and Krebs, 1980b; Steinberg, 1983a). The complete amino acid sequences of C subunit and $R_{II}$ subunit from bovine heart have been published recently (Shoji *et al.*, 1981; Carr *et al.*, 1982; Takio *et al.*, 1982).

## B. Mechanism of Activation

Each R subunit monomer has two binding sites for cAMP as well as a site for binding C subunit (Corbin *et al.*, 1978; Weber and Hilz, 1979; Builder *et al.*, 1980a). The cAMP-binding sites are distinguishable by differences in dissociation rates of bound cAMP and by differences in relative affinities for analogs of cAMP (Rannels and Corbin, 1980; Rannels and Corbin, 1981; Kerlavage and Taylor, 1982). "Site 1" exhibits slow dissociation of cAMP and has a preference for C-8 modified derivatives of cAMP; "site 2" shows preferential binding of N-6 modified derivatives of cAMP and rapid dissociation of cAMP (Rannels and Corbin, 1980; Rannels and Corbin, 1981). Cyclic AMP is preferentially bound to site 1 in holoenzyme (Rannels and Corbin, 1981), but cAMP is bound to both sites with apparently equal affinities in purified R subunit (Rannels and Corbin, 1980). The cAMP-binding sites interact in a positively cooperative manner in holoenzyme such that C-8 modified cAMP derivatives enhance binding of N-6 modified derivatives and vice versa (Rannels and Corbin, 1981; Corbin *et al.*, 1982). Binding of cAMP causes structural changes in R that can be detected by changes in reactivity of cysteine residues (Armstrong and Kaiser, 1978) and by changes in circular dichroism (Smith *et al.*, 1981). These structural or conformational changes presumably contribute to both the cooperativity of cAMP binding and the activation of kinase holoenzyme. Kinase activation involves a concerted reaction, with intermediate $R_2C_2(cAMP)_{1-4}$ forms leading to the release of active C monomers from an $R_2(cAMP)_4$ complex (Jastorff *et al.*, 1979; Builder *et al.*, 1980b). In pure enzyme preparations, kinase activation correlates with binding of 4 mol of cAMP per mol of holoenzyme. Full activation has been reported at stoichiometries of 2 mol of effector per mol of holoenzyme using cAMP analogs specific to either site 1 or site 2 (Rannels and Corbin, 1981; Kerlavage and Taylor, 1982), but these reports have been challenged recently. Synergism in the effects of site 1- and site 2-directed analogs on kinase activation implicates both sites in activation (Robinson-Steiner and Corbin, 1983; Øgreid *et al.*, 1983). It is not known whether or not complete dissociation of C subunit is necessary for activation of kinase holoenzyme, but such an activation pathway is supported by two disparate sets of observations: R subunit is a competitive inhibitor of protein substrate binding to C subunit (Granot *et al.*, 1980a); and dissociation accompanies activation in cell-free systems (Rangel-Aldao and Rosen, 1976). Cyclic AMP alone does not efficiently dissociate kinases from at least two fungal species, but it is possible that further dissociation is promoted by interaction with substrate proteins (Moreno and Passeron, 1980; Trevillyan and Pall, 1982). The significance of R dimer interactions to kinase activation is not clear, but there is the possibility of cooperativity through such interactions (see also Section VI). In contrast to the activity of C subunit, the cAMP-binding and C subunit-inhibiting activities of R subunit survive treatment of the protein with urea or other chaotropic agents; this reversible denaturation provides a convenient method for preparing R subunit free of bound cAMP (Schwechheimer and Hofmann, 1977). Recent results, however, suggest that urea treatment causes subtle alterations in R subunit properties (Corbin and Rannels, 1981).

## C. Functional Domains of R Subunits

Proteolysis of native $R_I$ and $R_{II}$ subunits with endoproteases reveals a common structure consisting of two proteolytically resistant domains connected by a proteolytically sensitive "hinge" region (Corbin *et al.*, 1978; Potter and Taylor, 1979a; Weber and Hilz, 1979). The aminoterminal domain comprises about one fourth of R subunit and appears to be involved in R–R dimer interaction (Potter and Taylor, 1980); the carboxyterminal domain comprises about two-thirds of R subunit and contains the cAMP-binding sites (Potter and Taylor, 1979a). The hinge region contains sites for autophosphorylation of $R_{II}$ and cGMP-dependent kinase-mediated phosphorylation of $R_I$, which are a few residues carboxyterminal to arginine–arginine sequences that serve as major cleavage sites for trypsin (Potter and Taylor, 1979b; Hashimoto *et al.*, 1981). A carboxyterminal fragment generated by tryptic cleavage between these two arginine residues in $R_{II}$ is incapable of inactivating C subunit or of serving as a phosphate acceptor for C subunit-dependent phosphorylation; a fragment larger by two residues retains both of these R subunit activities (Takio *et al.*, 1982). These observations suggest that the trypsin-sensitive region of R subunit plays a critical role in interaction with C subunit. Such a rule is consistent with the extreme sensitivity of the C subunit-binding function of R to inhibition by the arginine-specific reagent 2,3-butanedione (Corbin *et al.*, 1978). Furthermore, C subunit protects the trypsin-sensitive region of R against cleavage in holoenzyme (Potter and Taylor, 1980), and phosphorylation of sites just carboxyterminal to the trypsin-sensitive arginine residues inhibits the C subunit-binding activity of R (Erlichman *et al.*, 1974; Granot *et al.*, 1980b; Geahlen *et al.*, 1981). Both $R_I$ and $R_{II}$ have very acidic regions to the carboxyterminal side of the region discussed above (Takio *et al.*, 1982; Steinberg, 1983a). Takio *et al.* (1982) have proposed that these acidic regions are also important for R–C interaction, since C subunit is very basic (especially in the region of its MgATP binding site), all known protein inhibitors of C are acidic, and basic proteins such as histones and protamines promote dissociation of kinase holoenzyme. The carboxyterminal cAMP-binding domain of $R_{II}$ subunit contains a long internal sequence homology, suggesting the occurrence of a tandem internal duplication in evolution of the $R_{II}$ gene (Takio *et al.*, 1982); such a duplication could explain the presence of two cAMP-binding sites in R subunits. A tyrosine residue at position 381 (of a total of 400 residues) in the $R_{II}$ sequence is the primary target for photoaffinity labeling with [$^{32}$P]8-azido-cAMP (Kerlavage and Taylor, 1980; Takio *et al.*, 1982), but it is not known whether or not this residue is actually contained within a cAMP-binding site.

## III. GENETIC APPROACHES TO STUDYING THE cAMP RESPONSE PATHWAY

Although the central role of cAMP-dependent protein kinase(s) in mediating physiological responses to cAMP elevation was inferred by the ubiquitous distribution of the enzyme and its ability to catalyze phosphorylation and concomitant activation or deactivation of several hormonally regulated enzymes (reviewed by Nimmo and Cohen, 1977; Krebs and Beavo, 1979), biochemical studies alone could not rule out the possibility of other mechanisms for cAMP action. Where complex physiological processes such as growth or phagocytosis were modulated, candidate substrates for cAMP-dependent phosphorylation were not available to test even the plausibility of kinase-mediated regulation. Furthermore, in addition to affecting protein phosphorylation, cAMP regulates specific mRNA expression in animal cells (Iynedjian and Hanson, 1977; Noguchi *et al.*, 1978; Kellems *et al.*, 1979; Brown and Papaconstantinou, 1979; Derda *et al.*, 1980). In light of the bacterial cAMP response system in which gene transcription is regulated by a cAMP-binding protein factor (reviewed in Rickenberg, 1974; Adhya and Garges, 1982), these cAMP effects on mRNA expression have led to speculation about possible kinase-independent mechanisms for cAMP regulation in animal cells (e.g., Friedman and Chambers, 1978).

Guided by the successes of molecular genetics in elucidating regulatory mechanisms in procaryotes, Tomkins and his co-workers initiated efforts to isolate animal-cell mutants carrying lesions in the cAMP response pathway. S49 mouse lymphoma cells were used in these studies because their cytolytic response to elevated cAMP provides a very strong selection for non-responsive variants (Daniel *et al.*, 1973). As illustrated in Fig. 2, a variety of pharmacological agents are available for manipulating metabolism of cAMP or for bypassing the cAMP generation system to activate cAMP-dependent protein kinase directly. This diversity of drugs has proven invaluable in the selection and characterization of mutants affected in different components of the cAMP response system. Four different lesions in the S49 cell adenylate cyclase complex have been characterized (Johnson *et al.*, 1979; Bourne *et al.*, 1982). Mutations affecting cAMP secretion and cAMP phosphodiesterase activities have also been described (Steinberg *et al.*, 1979; Brothers *et al.*, 1982). Most S49 cell variants resistant to the cAMP analog dibutyryl cAMP ($Bt_2cAMP$) carry lesions affecting cAMP-dependent protein kinase, which in S49 cells is almost entirely a type I enzyme (Steinberg *et al.*, 1978). These variants and their isolation will be described in detail in Section IV. In some cell systems, growth inhibition is elicited equally well by both cyclic and noncylic AMP derivatives using an adenylate cyclase-dependent pathway (Martin and Kowalchyk, 1981); as a result, both cyclase and kinase mutants are isolated in these systems as variants resistant to cAMP analogs (Rae *et al.*, 1979; Martin and Ronning, 1981). Mutations affecting adenylate cyclase and cAMP-dependent protein kinase also have been described in yeast, where cAMP is required for growth (reviewed in Thorner, 1982). Such mutations raise prospects for further dissection of the cAMP response system both by genetic manipulation of yeast genes and by introduction of mammalian genes to complement yeast gene functions.

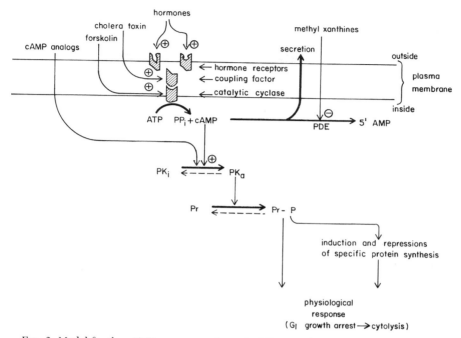

FIG. 2. Model for the cAMP response pathway in S49 mouse lymphoma cells emphasizing targets for pharmacological interventions. PK$_i$, PK$_a$, Pr, and Pr-P are used as in Fig. 1; PDE denotes cAMP phosphodiesterase. Inductions and repressions of specific protein synthesis are shown as consequences of specific protein phosphorylation, but such a mechanism has not been verified (Section VII).

Mutations affecting cAMP-dependent protein kinase have effectively established the importance of this enzyme in mediating cAMP action in S49 and a variety of other cultured cell lines (Insel *et al.*, 1975; Gottesman, 1980). The thrust of the studies described next has been to elucidate the molecular natures of these lesions and to understand how kinase mutations arising in a single step* could survive selection in diploid S49 cells (Lemaire and Coffino, 1977a; Francke and Gehring, 1980). This research has led into the areas of metabolic regulation of kinase subunit expression, structure-function relationships within kinase subunits, and intracellular responses to kinase activation. In consequence, it has provided new perspectives on the regulation of cAMP action.

*This is assumed from the spontaneous mutation frequency of about $2 \times 10^{-7}$ per cell per generation (Coffino *et al.*, 1975).

## IV.  MUTATIONS AFFECTING cAMP-DEPENDENT
## PROTEIN KINASE

### A.  Selection and Counterselection in S49 Mouse
### Lymphoma Cells

When exposed to analogs or inducers of intracellular cAMP, S49 cells are growth arrested in the $G_1$ (or postmitotic) phase of the cell cycle and, subsequent to growth arrest, undergo a time-dependent cytolytic response (reviewed by Coffino, 1981). The biochemical events causing cell death are not known, but it is possible to select mutant cells specifically deficient in the cytolytic response (Lemaire and Coffino, 1977b). $Bt_2cAMP$-arrested wild-type cells can be rescued from cytolysis if washed free of the drug and allowed to reenter the cell cycle before cytolysis has occurred. Mutants have been isolated that have wild-type levels of protein kinase but are growth arrested less efficiently than are wild-type cells (R. A. Steinberg and T. van Daalen Wetters, unpublished results); these cells escape cytolysis to about the extent that they escape growth arrest, suggesting that cytolysis is a secondary response to growth arrest rather than a direct response to cAMP-dependent kinase activation.

S49 cells grow in suspension cultures and form colonies in media solidified with agarose. "Feeder layers" of mouse embryo fibroblast cells were used to promote clonal growth in early mutant isolation experiments (Coffino *et al.*, 1975; Freidrich and Coffino, 1977). Feeder-independent cloning has been used in our most recent mutant isolations (R. A. Steinberg and C. S. Murphy, unpublished results). With $Bt_2cAMP$ as a selective agent, up to $2 \times 10^6$ wild-type S49 cells can be plated in a 6-cm diameter culture dish without adversely affecting the isolation of rare mutants (Friedrich and Coffino, 1977). An optimal concentration of $Bt_2cAMP$ for mutant selection is about 0.5 m$M$, and, when feeder cells are used, a cAMP phosphodiesterase inhibitor is also necessary to ensure efficient killing of sensitive cells. This difference in conditions required for efficient killing with and without feeder cells suggests that feeder cells metabolize $Bt_2cAMP$. Even with phosphodiesterase inhibitors, it is not clear that $Bt_2cAMP$ concentrations remain at toxic levels throughout the selection procedure. Differences in $Bt_2cAMP$ stability may explain why unstable $Bt_2cAMP$-resistant variants arise at relatively high frequencies in selections with feeder cells but seldom in selections without feeder cells (Section IV,B).

Until recently, genetic analysis of the S49 cell cAMP response system was hampered by an inability to select cAMP-sensitive revertants of cAMP-resistant mutants. T. van Daalen Wetters has remedied this situation by developing a counterselection procedure appropriate for such revertant isolations (van Daalen Wetters and Coffino, 1982). Populations of mutagenized or nonmutagenized cAMP-resistant cells are exposed successively to $Bt_2cAMP$ and 8-bromodeoxyuridine (BrdU), an analog of thymidine that is incorporated into DNA by replicating cells. Times of exposure to the two drugs are optimal for chasing any cAMP-sensitive cells out of S phase before BrdU addition and for ensuring that most cAMP-resistant cells traverse at least part of S phase in the presence of BrdU. Cells that have incorporated BrdU are killed by exposure to a photo-sensitizing dye and fluorescent light; cAMP-sensitive cells that have been spared BrdU incorporation by $Bt_2cAMP$-mediated growth arrest are rescued by removing the cAMP analog. For adequate enrichment of rare revertants, the procedure is repeated several times. Surviving cells are cloned in media containing hypoxanthine, aminopterin, and thymidine to select against cells enriched because of a deficiency in thymidine kinase.

Direct cloning in $Bt_2cAMP$ has yielded three categories of S49 cell variants with alterations in cAMP-dependent protein kinase: "$V_{max}$ mutants" have reduced levels of enzyme with normal cAMP activation parameters; "$K_a$ mutants" have normal or nearly normal levels of fully activated kinase but with increased apparent activation constants for cAMP; and "kinase-negative mutants" ($kin^-$ mutants) lack detectable cAMP-dependent protein kinase activity. In some previous reports, members of these three mutant classes have been designated type A for $V_{max}$, type B or D for $K_a$, and type C for $kin^-$ (Insel *et al.*, 1975; Hochman *et al.*, 1977; Friedrich and Coffino, 1977). Cyclic AMP-sensitive revertants have been isolated from both $K_a$ and $kin^-$ mutant cells (van Daalen Wetters and Coffino, 1982; T. van Daalen Wetters, personal communication).

## B. $V_{max}$ MUTANTS

Lesions causing $V_{max}$ phenotypes in S49 cells are not well understood; *a priori* such phenotypes might result from functional inactivation of a C subunit allele, structural mutations affecting C subunit activity, or mutations in a regulatory locus affecting C subunit expression. In an analysis of more than 100 $Bt_2cAMP$-resistant S49 cell clones, the distribution of variants among the three classes of kinase phenotypes varied with mutagenic treatment; $V_{max}$ cells comprised 25–100% of isolates from any mutagenized population (Friedrich and Coffino, 1977). On subsequent analysis, however, many of these variants no longer had kinase activities distinguishable from wild-type cells and were no longer resistant to $Bt_2cAMP$-mediated cytolysis (R. A. Steinberg and T. van Daalen Wetters, unpublished results). Two variants that had retained $V_{max}$ phenotypes were subcloned under nonselective conditions; subclones from each variant exhibited a wide range of endogenous kinase specific activities (R. A. Steinberg, unpublished results). These observations suggest that many $V_{max}$ variants result from unstable phenotypic suppression of cAMP-dependent protein kinase activity leading to mixed populations of cells with low and high levels of kinase expression. In recent experiments characterizing 130 $Bt_2$cAMP-resistant S49 subclones isolated without feeder cells, no $V_{max}$ variants were found (R. A. Steinberg and C. S. Murphy, unpublished results). S49 sublines with apparently stable $V_{max}$ phenotypes have been isolated recently as cAMP-sensitive revertants of a $kin^-$ mutant subline; these revertants exhibit cAMP sensitivities intermediate between those of wild-type and $kin^-$ mutant cells and roughly in proportion to endogenous kinase activities (T. van Daalen Wetters, personal communication). Whether or not S49 mutants with stable low expression of kinase can be isolated as cAMP analog-resistant clones has yet to be determined. Variants of Chinese hamster ovary (CHO) cells with $V_{max}$ phenotypes (described as kinase deficient) have been isolated and partially characterized; the "mutations" in these cells are recessive in hybrids between mutant and wild-type CHO cells and appear to cause decreased expression of C subunit activity (Gottesman *et al.*, 1980; Singh *et al.*, 1981). Information is not currently available on the stability of $V_{max}$ phenotypes among subclones of these CHO variants.

## C. $K_a$ MUTANTS

Figure 3 shows cAMP activation curves for protein kinase activities in extracts from wild-type S49 cells and from several $K_a$ mutant sublines. The shifts in apparent kinase activation constants range from about 5-fold to 20-fold. Figure 3 also illustrates the very small proportions of kinase with wild-type activation parameters in $K_a$ mutant cell extracts. Studies on DEAE-cellulose-fractionated extracts from $K_a$ mutant cells suggest that some, if not all, of the "wild-type" kinase in $K_a$ mutant extracts is contributed by a small amount of type II kinase (R. A. Steinberg, unpublished results). $K_a$ phenotypes result from structural lesions in kinase R subunit. This conclusion was suggested initially by studies in which subunits from wild-type and $K_a$ mutant kinases were separated and reconstituted into homologous and heterologous holoenzyme complexes; mutant properties correlated with the presence of mutant R subunit in the complexes (Hochman *et al.*, 1975). Comparisons of subunit reassociation rates, constants for cAMP-dependent activation, thermolability, and sodium thiocyanate-mediated dissociation of kinases from wild-type and two $K_a$ mutant sublines suggested that $K_a$ muta-

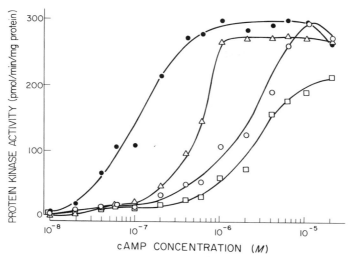

FIG. 3. Activation of cAMP-dependent protein kinase in extracts from wild-type and $K_a$ mutant sublines of S49 cells. Transfer of [$^{32}$P]phosphate from ATP to histone subfraction 2b was measured as described by Hochman *et al.* (1975) using enzymatic activities from extracts of wild-type (-●-●-) or $K_a$ mutant cells (-○-○-, -△-△-, -□-□-).

tions fell into two categories: those primarily affecting cAMP binding, and those primarily affecting the interaction of R with C subunit (Hochman *et al.*, 1977). More recent results discussed later (this section and Section VI) indicate that this dichotomy is overly simple.

Two-dimensional gel electrophoresis of [$^{35}$S]methionine-labeled R subunits from a variety of $K_a$ mutant sublines revealed altered forms of R shifted in charge from wild-type R by amounts consistent with single amino acid substitutions (Steinberg *et al.*, 1977; R. A. Steinberg, unpublished results). Figure 4 illustrates the variety of R subunit patterns that have been observed in cAMP affinity column-purified preparations from "charge-shift" $K_a$ mutant cells. Such patterns have always revealed coexpression of mutant and wild-type R in mutant cells suggesting that the mutants are heterozygous. Furthermore, relative labeling and phosphorylation of the mutant allele products has been invariably greater than labeling and phosphorylation of wild-type R in affinity-purified preparations from $K_a$ mutant cells. S49 subline U36 carries a phenotypically silent charge shift mutation in one R subunit allele (Steinberg *et al.*, 1978). Analysis of R subunit gel patterns from 130 Bt$_2$cAMP-resistant subclones of U36 (of which 120 had $K_a$ phenotypes) revealed total correlation between $K_a$ phenotypes and unequal phosphorylation of R subunit allele products (R. A. Steinberg, C. S. Murphy, and E. F. McHugh, unpublished results).

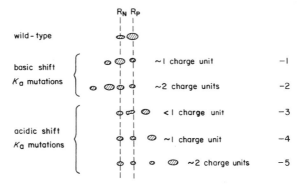

FIG. 4. Isoelectric focusing patterns of $R_I$ subunit from wild-type and $K_a$ mutant S49 cells. Patterns were traced from autoradiograms of two-dimensional gels of cAMP affinity-purified extracts from [$^{35}$S]methionine-labeled cells; more acidic species are at the right. $R_N$ and $R_P$ indicate positions of the two forms of wild-type R.

The experiment of Fig. 5 shows that unequal labeling of mutant and wild-type R in purified preparations from $K_a$ mutant cells reflects an artifact of affinity chromatography. In affinity-purified material (Fig. 5b), radioactivity in mutant forms of R (upward-pointing arrows) was about twice that in wild-type forms (downward-pointing arrows); in the extract from which this material was purified (Fig. 5a), radioactivity in mutant and wild-type R subunits was about equal. The missing wild-type R was found in flow-through fractions from the affinity column (Fig. 5c). (Resolution in the region of phosphorylated wild-type R is not good in these gel patterns, but, since very little wild-type R is phosphorylated, this does not pose a major obstacle to interpreting the experiment.) In another experiment with labeled extracts from the mutant strain used for Fig. 5, the flow-through fraction from an affinity column was applied to a second column; wild-type R subunit that passed through the first column did not bind to the second column (R. A. Steinberg, unpublished result). For this experiment and for the experiment of Fig. 5, extractions and purifications were performed in the cold; at room temperature, relative recovery of wild-type R from mutant extracts was somewhat higher (R. A. Steinberg, unpublished observations). These results imply that expression from wild-type and mutant R subunit alleles is equal in $K_a$ mutant cells but that a portion of wild-type R (wild-type R homodimer) is sequestered in a form incapable of binding to cAMP affinity resins in the cold. The very low proportion of wild-type kinase in $K_a$ mutant extracts (Fig. 3) and the slow dissociation of bound cAMP from R subunit in the cold (Gilman, 1970; Corbin and Rannels, 1981) suggest that wild-type R excluded from affinity purification represents a pool of "free" R subunit complexed

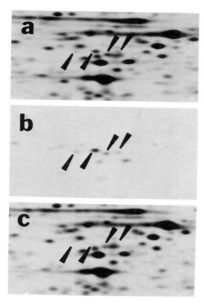

FIG. 5. Unequal recoveries of mutant and wild-type R in affinity-purification of extracts from $K_a$ mutant cells. Cells from $K_a$ mutant subline U200.65 (Steinberg *et al.*, 1977) were labeled for 2.5 hours with [35]methionine, extracted, and subjected to purification on N6-(2-aminoethyl)-cAMP Sepharose as described previously (Steinberg *et al.*, 1977). $10^6$ acid-precipitable cpm from the centrifuged extract (a) or the fraction excluded from column binding (c), or $10^5$ cpm from the affinity-bound fraction (b) were subjected to two-dimensional gel separation. Autoradiograms were exposed for 2 days. Wild-type and mutant forms of $R_I$ are indicated, respectively, with downward- and upward-pointing arrows.

with cAMP rather than with C subunit. Wild-type R that does bind to affinity columns from $K_a$ mutant extracts appears to be associated with holoenzyme, since the relative proportion of mutant and wild-type R in affinity-purified material is unaffected by prepurification steps that separate holoenzyme from free R subunit (R. A. Steinberg, unpublished results). Despite the fact that about one-third of total holoenzyme-associated R subunit is wild type in $K_a$ mutant cells (Fig. 5b), the proportion of kinase activity with wild-type activation parameters is insignificant (Fig. 3). These observations argue that holoenzyme-associated wild-type R subunits are in heterodimers with mutant R subunits and that dimer interactions in these complexes alter the activation properties of the wild-type subunits. The dominance (and, therefore, selectibility) of $K_a$ mutations is explained by both the modification of wild-type R subunit properties through heterodimer formation and the inability of wild-type R homodimers to compete effectively with dimers containing mutant R for binding to C subunit.

$K_a$ phenotypes have been reported in studies of cAMP-resistant variants of mouse neuroblastoma cells (Simantov and Sachs, 1975), J774.2 macrophage-like cells (Rosen *et al.*, 1979), Y1 adrenal carcinoma cells (Gutmann *et al.*, 1978; Rae *et al.*, 1979), and CHO cells (Evain *et al.*, 1979; Gottesman *et al.*, 1980). Kinases from several Y1-cell $K_a$ mutants and from one CHO-cell $K_a$ mutant have been analyzed in some detail. At least some of the Y1 mutants bear lesions in R subunit as determined by both reconstitution analysis and isoelectric focusing gel analysis of immunoprecipitated $R_I$ (Doherty *et al.*, 1982). R subunit lesions have not been described in CHO cells, which differ from S49 and Y1 cells in having about equal proportions of type I and type II kinases (Gottesman, 1980). A $K_a$ phenotype in the CHO cell line apparently results from a lesion in C subunit that affects both R–C interaction and protein substrate specificity (Evain *et al.*, 1979).

## D. Kinase-Negative Mutants

*Kin*⁻ mutations affect levels of both R and C subunits in S49 cells; C subunit activity is undetectable, and cAMP-binding activity is reduced by about 80–85% (Insel *et al.*, 1975; Steinberg *et al.*, 1978). The primary lesion is apparently one affecting C subunit expression; affects of C on R subunit metabolism can explain the reduced expression of R (Steinberg and Agard, 1981a,b; see Section V). Enzyme deficiency mutations resulting from loss of a gene function should be recessive in hybrids formed between mutant and wild-type cells, but *kin*⁻ mutations are either fully or partially dominant in such hybrids (Steinberg *et al.*, 1978). Figure 6 illustrates this dominance in terms of the effects of a *kin*⁻ mutation on expression of R and C subunit activities in diploid cells and tetraploid hybrids. Failure to identify recessive *kin*⁻ mutations and the very low frequency of *kin*⁻ mutants among $Bt_2$cAMP-resistant S49 subclones (Friedrich and Coffino, 1977; R. A. Steinberg and C. S. Murphy, unpublished results) suggest that S49 cells are diploid for C as well as for R subunit genes.

A variety of studies rule out explanations of the *kin*⁻ phenotype based on structural mutations in kinase subunits or overproduction of the heat-stable kinase inhibitor protein (Steinberg *et al.*, 1978). Reconstitution of apparently normal kinase holoenzyme from wild-type C subunit and R subunit from *kin*⁻ cells argues against a primary lesion in R subunit leading to formation of cryptic holoenzyme complexes incapable of being activated. Chromatographic properties of R from *kin*⁻ cells resemble those of "free" wild-type R; this argues that R subunit in *kin*⁻ cells is not prevented from associating with wild-type C subunit by irreversible binding to mutant C subunit. Mixing experiments rule out the presence in *kin*⁻ cells of excessive

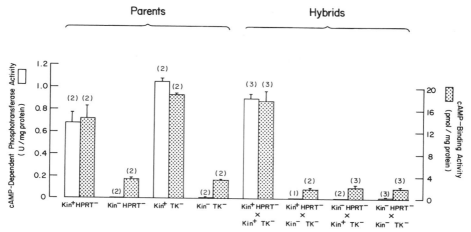

F*ig*. 6. Dominance of an S49 *kin⁻* mutation in hybrids between *kin⁻* and wild-type cells. Tetraploid hybrids were selected after polyethylene glycol-mediated fusion of *kin⁻* and wild-type (*kin⁺*) cells that were deficient in either hypoxanthine phosphoribosyltransferase (HPRT⁻) or thymidine kinase (TK⁻) by cloning in medium containing hypoxanthine, aminopterin, and thymidine. Several clones from parental sublines and from hybridization mixtures were grown into mass culture and assayed for cAMP-dependent protein kinase (phosphotransferase) activity and cAMP-binding activity; numbers of subclones assayed for each determination are shown in parentheses. [Reprinted with permission from Steinberg *et al.* (1978). Copyright 1978 by M.I.T. Press.]

levels of kinase inhibitor protein. In recent unpublished studies, T. van Daalen Wetters and M. Murtaugh have employed radioiodinated anti-C subunit antibodies in "Western blotting" experiments to search for C subunit protein in extracts of *kin⁻* cells. Although the protein is easily identified as a 39,000 MW species in extracts of wild-type cells, it has not been detected in extracts of *kin⁻* cells (T. van Daalen Wetters, personal communication). These results indicate that *kin⁻* cells lack immunoreactive C subunit. Comparisons of two-dimensional gel patterns of proteins from wild-type and *kin⁻* cells show that the mutation is fairly specific for kinase expression; no other significant differences can be detected in more than 1000 protein species resolved (Steinberg and Coffino, 1979; R. A. Steinberg, unpublished observations). Taken together, studies on *kin⁻* mutants of S49 cells suggest that the mutant phenotype results from structural mutations in a trans-acting regulatory element that normally facilitates C subunit expression but, when mutated in appropriate ways, inhibits expression. Dominance might result from competitive displacement of wild-type regulatory molecules from their sites of action by mutant molecules. Consistent with such a model for *kin⁻*

mutations, cAMP-sensitive revertants of *kin*⁻ mutants often express C subunit at levels intermediate between mutant and wild-type; in some revertants, expression of C activity is temperature dependent (T. van Daalen Wetters, personal communication).

## V. REGULATION OF KINASE SUBUNIT METABOLISM

Despite the importance of cAMP-dependent protein kinase in physiological regulation, very little is known about the regulation of its expression. Measurements of R and C subunit activities in a variety of rabbit tissues have revealed apparent coordination of R and C subunit levels over a range of kinase specific activities (Hofmann *et al.*, 1977). Ratios of type I to type II kinase isozymes vary among tissues and among the same tissues from different animal species (Sugden and Corbin, 1976; Weber *et al.*, 1981a). A number of studies have reported regulation of kinase levels and/or isozyme distribution by cell or tissue differentiation (Lee *et al.*, 1976; Knight and Skala, 1977; Malkinson and Butley, 1981; Setchenska *et al.*, 1981; Liu, 1982; Plet *et al.*, 1982), cell cycle progression (Haddox *et al.*, 1980), animal treatments with hormones or vitamin D (Fuller *et al.*, 1978; Richards and Rolfes, 1980; Rudack-Garcia and Henry, 1981), or tumorigenic transformation of mouse 3T3 cells (Gharret *et al.*, 1976; Wehner *et al.*, 1981). Altered kinase isozyme patterns have also been found in human leukemic cells (Elias *et al.*, 1981; Weber *et al.*, 1981b), but tumorigenic transformation does not invariably affect cAMP-dependent protein kinases (Kudlow *et al.*, 1981; Roth *et al.*, 1982). Unfortunately, many studies on kinase isozyme regulation require reevaluation, since, as discussed by Weber *et al.* (1981a), serious methodological problems are associated with attempts to assess kinase isozyme ratios by DEAE-cellulose chromatography or photoaffinity labeling.

Marked increases in levels of $R_I$ have been observed in neuroblastoma cells and neuroblastoma/glioma cell hybrids after prolonged incubation with $Bt_2cAMP$ (Prashad *et al.*, 1979; Walter *et al.*, 1979; Liu *et al.*, 1981). These increases are not accompanied by increases in C subunit (Prashad *et al.*, 1979; Liu *et al.*, 1981) and are attributable, in part, to increased synthesis of $R_I$ (Morrison *et al.*, 1980). Although changes in intracellular concentrations of protein kinase subunits must have effects on the intracellular activation of kinase and/or the rate and extent of phosphorylation of endogenous kinase substrates, the parameters for such effects remain unexplored. Whether the different kinase isozymes have distinct roles in mediating cAMP effects or merely allow enhanced flexibility in fine-tuning cAMP response sensitivity through differences in activation parameters for the different isozymes (Hofmann, 1980; Walter and Greengard, 1981) remains to be determined.

As discussed above (Section IV,C and D), $kin^-$ mutations cause reduced expression of both subunits of kinase in S49 cells, and $K_a$ mutations inhibit the phosphorylation of wild-type R subunits in mutant cells. $Kin^-$ mutations also cause marked reductions in the phosphorylation of wild-type R subunit (Steinberg *et al.*, 1978; Steinberg and Agard, 1981b). Studies of kinase subunit metabolism in S49 cells were initiated to investigate the mechanisms underlying these phenotypic changes. For technical reasons, studies of C subunit expression have lagged behind those of R subunit. Our approach for studying R subunit metabolism has been to incubate intact cells with [$^{35}$S]methionine using either pulse-labeling or label-chase protocols, extract total cellular proteins in a highly denaturing solvent, and subject the entire cell extract to high resolution two-dimensional gel electrophoresis (O'Farrell, 1975). Since resolution of R is not always complete in two-dimensional gel patterns of crude cell extracts, a computer-assisted densitometry and image enhancement procedure was developed to quantify radioactivity in R subunit species (Agard *et al.*, 1981). Although the two-dimensional gel analysis procedure is laborious, it provides information on both labeling of R relative to other cell proteins and distribution of R label between phosphorylated and nonphosphorylated forms. Furthermore, since intracellular proteins are extracted with a strong denaturant, the procedure avoids potential artifacts of differential extraction, purification, or proteolysis that might pose problems for alternative approaches using affinity purification or immunoprecipitation.

Studies on the mechanisms underlying the 80–85% reduction in R subunit expression in $kin^-$ cells yielded rather unexpected results. We had reasoned that reduced levels of R in $kin^-$ cells reflected either a primary effect of the putative $kin^-$ regulatory mutation or a secondary effect resulting from absence of functional C subunit. If interaction with C affected R subunit metabolism, $Bt_2cAMP$-mediated kinase activation was expected to mimic effects of $kin^-$ mutations. Relative rates of R synthesis in wild-type and $kin^-$ cells were compared by pulse-labeling experiments (Steinberg and Agard, 1981b). R synthesis in $kin^-$ cells was about half that in untreated wild-type cells. Consistent with results in neuroblastoma cells, R synthesis was induced by 50–100% in wild-type cells treated for several hours with $Bt_2cAMP$; the drug had no effect on R synthesis in $kin^-$ cells. Figure 7 shows results from a label-chase experiment comparing R degradation in wild-type and $kin^-$ cells (Steinberg and Agard, 1981a). R turnover was exponential with a half-life of about 8.5 hours in untreated wild-type cells; $Bt_2cAMP$ inhibited turnover. In $kin^-$ cells, on the other hand, R turnover was markedly stimulated with an estimated half-life of 50 minutes. The effects of the $kin^-$ mutation on synthesis and degradation of R provide a basis for reduced expression of R subunit activity in $kin^-$ cells, but they also pose a new problem: a 20-fold reduction in level of R should result from the 2-fold inhibition of R synthesis and 10-fold stimulation of R degradation, but only a 5- to 7-fold reduction is observed. Bt$_2$cAMP had effects on both synthesis and degradation of R, but, contrary to our expectations, the effects were opposite to those of the *kin*⁻ mutation.

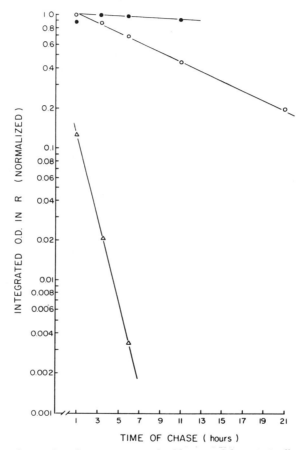

FIG. 7. Degradation of R subunit in untreated wild-type and *kin*⁻ S49 cells and in wild-type cells treated with Bt$_2$cAMP. Cells labeled for 1 hour with [³⁵S]methionine in the absence of drugs were chased in the absence or presence of 1 mM Bt$_2$cAMP. Whole cell extracts from samples harvested at various times of chase were subjected to two-dimensional gel analysis, and radioactivity in R$_I$ was determined by computer-assisted densitometry of the resulting autoradiograms. Values were normalized to the radioactivity in untreated wild-type cells at 1 hour of chase. -O-O-, Untreated wild-type cells; -●-●-, Bt$_2$cAMP-treated wild-type cells; -△-△-, *kin*⁻ cells. [From Steinberg and Agard (1981a).]

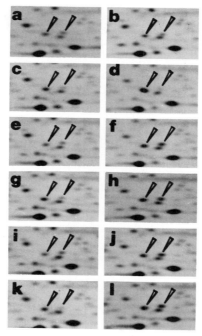

Fig. 8. Effects of several analogs and inducers of cAMP on phosphorylation and synthesis of R subunit in wild-type S49 cells. Cells were labeled for 30 minutes with [$^{35}$S]methionine after 6 hours of preincubation in low-methionine medium. Drugs were added at the start of the preincubation period or shortly before addition of the radioactive tracer as noted below. $10^6$ acid-precipitable cpm of whole cell extracts were subjected to two-dimensional gel electrophoresis; autoradiograms were exposed for 2 days. a and b, No drug controls; c and d, 1 mM Bt$_2$cAMP added 15 minutes or 6 hours before label; e and f, 2 mM BrcAMP added 15 minutes or 6 hours before label; g and h, 100 ng/ml cholera toxin added 90 minutes or 6 hours before label; i and j, 50 μM MIX added 5 minutes or 6 hours before label; k and l, 10 μM isoproterenol plus 50 μM MIX added 5 minutes or 6 hours before label. Arrows indicate positions of R$_N$ (left) and R$_P$ (right). [From Steinberg and Agard (1981b).]

Pulse-labeling experiments revealed not only a Bt$_2$cAMP-mediated induction of R synthesis but also a Bt$_2$cAMP-dependent inhibition of R phosphorylation in wild-type S49 cells (Steinberg and Coffino, 1979; Steinberg and Agard, 1981b). Further studies showed that Bt$_2$cAMP reduced both the rate and the final extent of R subunit phosphorylation (Steinberg and Agard, 1981b). Figure 8 shows R subunit patterns from a study with additional analogs and inducers of cAMP that demonstrates that inhibition of R subunit phosphorylation is not an inevitable consequence of intracellular kinase activation (Steinberg and Agard, 1981b). Wild-type cells were labeled for 30 minutes with [$^{35}$S]methionine after either short or long exposures to a variety of agents. R synthesis was induced in cells treated for 6 hours with any of the effectors that activate intracellular kinase (compare Fig. 8d,f,h,j, and l with Fig. 8a,b,c,e,g,i, and k). Bt$_2$cAMP inhibited phosphorylation of R with either short or long treatment (Fig. 8c and d), but neither 8-bromo cAMP (BrcAMP) nor methyl isobutylxanthine (MIX) had significant effects on phosphorylation (Fig. 8e,f,i, and j). Cholera toxin and isoproterenol plus MIX inhibited R phosphorylation after short treatment times (Fig. 8g and k), but their effects decayed after long treatment times (Fig. 8h and l). Short exposure to isoproterenol alone did not inhibit R phosphorylation (Steinberg and Coffino, 1979). Since phosphorylation of free wild-type R is inhibited in $kin^-$ cells (that lack C subunit) and in $K_a$ mutant cells (in which C subunit is bound up in mutant holoenzyme complexes) but not in wild-type cells activated with BrcAMP or elevated cAMP (in which C subunit is also free), it appears likely that the phosphorylation results from the catalytic activity of C subunit. Nevertheless, C subunit-dependent phosphorylation of R$_I$ has not been observed in purified kinase preparations (Hofmann et al., 1975; Walter et al., 1977).

Cholera toxin and isoproterenol plus MIX promote increases in intracellular cAMP to levels far in excess of those required for complete activation of kinase in S49 cells; isoproterenol alone produces a more moderate increase in cAMP level (Shear et al., 1976; Steinberg, 1981). After prolonged treatments with any of these agents, intracellular cAMP declines significantly (Shear et al., 1976; R. A. Steinberg, unpublished observations). These considerations suggest that cAMP effects on R subunit phosphorylation vary with cAMP concentrations: concentrations just sufficient to activate kinase are without effect on phosphorylation, but superphysiological concentrations inhibit phosphorylation. These differences in effects of low and high intracellular cAMP concentrations on R subunit phosphorylation can be reconciled with the differences in effects of Bt$_2$cAMP and BrcAMP by the different specificities of the two cAMP-binding sites in R (Section II,B). Site 1 has greater affinity for cAMP and BrcAMP, and site 2 has greater affinity for $N^6$-monobutyryl cAMP, the physiologically active form of Bt$_2$cAMP (Steinberg et al., 1979). The site of phosphorylation is near the aminoterminal end of R subunit in a region far from the cAMP-binding sites (Section VI), so it is likely that inhibition of phosphorylation results from a conformational change in R rather than from steric interference by nucleotide bound to site 2.

Effects of kinase activation on R turnover were reexamined in light of the differential effects of cAMP and cAMP analogs on R phosphorylation. Figure 9 shows gel patterns from an experiment in which wild-type cells were labeled with [$^{35}$S]methionine for an hour, washed, and chased for 1, 8, or 15

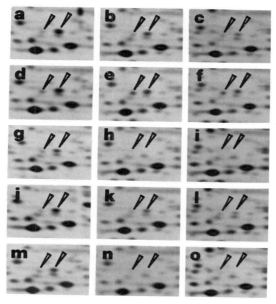

FIG. 9. Differential effects of Bt$_2$cAMP and other analogs and inducers of cAMP on R subunit degradation. Wild-type S49 cells were labeled for 1 hour with [$^{35}$S]methionine, then chased in the presence or absence of drugs as noted below. Samples were harvested after 1 hour (a,d,g,j, and m), 8 hours (b,e,h,k, and n), or 15 hours (c,f,i,l, and o) of chase, and 10$^6$ acid-precipitable cpm of cell extracts were subjected to two-dimensional gel electrophoresis; autoradiograms were exposed for 6 days. a–c, No drug addition; d–f, 1 mM Bt$_2$cAMP; g–i, 2 mM BrcAMP; j–l, 50 μM MIX; m–o, 10 μM isoproterenol plus 50 μM MIX. Arrows indicate positions of R$_N$ and R$_P$ as in Fig. 8. [From Steinberg and Agard (1981a).]

hours in media containing no drugs (Fig. 9a,b,c), Bt$_2$cAMP (Fig. 9d,e,f), BrcAMP (Fig. 9g,h,i), MIX alone (Fig. 9j,k,l), or isoproterenol plus MIX (Fig. 9m,n,o) (Steinberg and Agard, 1981a). Although Bt$_2$cAMP stabilized R as before (Fig. 7), both BrcAMP and isoproterenol plus MIX destabilized R to the extent that it was undetectable in labeled patterns after 8 or 15 hours of chase. In label-chase experiments using shorter time intervals, the half-life of R in wild-type cells stimulated with BrcAMP or isoproterenol was similar to that of R in *kin*$^-$ cells. Bt$_2$cAMP-mediated R stabilization is unrelated to kinase activation since it occurs in *kin*$^-$ as well as in wild-type cells (Steinberg and Agard, 1981a). Enhanced degradation of R in untreated *kin*$^-$ cells can be seen, therefore, as a simple consequence of its dissociation from C subunit. Like the inhibition of R subunit phosphorylation, R stabilization appears to result from analog binding to cAMP-binding site 2. The site 2-directed analogs $N^6$-monobutyryl cAMP, $N^6$-benzoyl cAMP, and $N^6$-

aminohexylcarbamoylmethyl cAMP all stabilize R, but the 5'AMP derivative, $N^6$-aminohexylcarbamoylmethyl AMP, and several site 1-directed
cAMP analogs do not stabilize R (R. A. Steinberg, unpublished results).

The effects of cAMP elevation on synthesis and degradation of R in wild-
type cells suggest that R should decrease to about 20% of basal level after
several hours of treatment with appropriate effectors. To test this prediction,
cAMP-binding activity was assayed in extracts of cells treated for various
times with isoproterenol or forskolin in the presence of MIX; extracts were
pretreated with charcoal to remove free and R subunit-bound cAMP (R. A.
Steinberg and E. F. McHugh, unpublished results). Cyclic AMP-binding
activity decreased with the expected half-time of about 50 minutes after
initiating treatment with either agent, but the maximum decrease was only
50–60%. This discrepancy between predicted and measured values of R
subunit activity is similar to that found in comparisons of *kin⁻* and wild-type
cells. A number of explanations for these discrepancies are possible, but we
have not yet been able to distinguish among them. They include possibilities
that our assay values are in error, that stable cAMP-binding fragments are
generated as products of turnover, and that decreases in levels of $R_I$ are
compensated in part by increases in levels of $R_{II}$. The last possibility is
supported by chromatographic studies showing that a large proportion of
cAMP-binding activity from *kin⁻* cell extracts has characteristics of $R_{II}$
(Steinberg *et al.*, 1978), but attempts to visualize $R_{II}$ in affinity column-
purified material from wild-type or *kin⁻* S49 cells have been unsuccessful
(R. A. Steinberg, unpublished results).

To fully understand the consequences of cAMP-mediated decreases in R
level, it is necessary both to resolve the discrepancies between results from
binding assays and labeling studies and to assess the effect of persistent
kinase activation on C subunit levels. Russell *et al.* (1981) have reported
decreases in type I and type II kinase activities in S49 cells treated for 2 or
more hours with $Bt_2cAMP$; for these studies, cytosolic extracts were prepared in buffer of low ionic strength and fractionated on DEAE-cellulose. I
am skeptical of these results because they depend on complete reassociation
of dissociated kinase subunits in chilled extracts: both dissociation of bound
cAMP and subunit reassociation of type I kinase are known to be inefficient
in the cold (Corbin and Keely, 1977; Corbin and Rannels, 1981). Absence of
a free C subunit peak is taken as evidence against incomplete kinase reassociation in these experiments (Russell *et al.*, 1981), but this absence might
also reflect binding of C to particulate cell fractions under the low ionic
strength extraction conditions used (Keely *et al.*, 1975; Rousseau *et al.*, 1976;
Zick *et al.*, 1979). Our own results suggest that there may be a decrease in C
subunit activity following activation, but that it is considerably slower than
the decrease in R subunit activity (R. A. Steinberg, unpublished results).

Studies on $R_I$ metabolism in *kin*⁻ and wild-type S49 cells provide a plausible mechanism for coordination of R and C subunit expression. C subunit synthesis is assumed to be constitutive at a level that depends, perhaps, on tissue-specific regulatory factors such as those thought to be altered by *kin*⁻ mutations. Under basal conditions, inhibition of C subunit function requires that R subunit be maintained at levels slightly higher than those of C. There appears to be a basal level of R synthesis that is regulated upward by the activity of C subunit. The higher basal synthesis of R in wild-type than in *kin*⁻ cells suggests that C has an effect even when it is confined mostly to holoenzyme; kinase activation leads to greater stimulation of R synthesis. Significant accumulation of free C is prevented in basal cells by this positive feedback of C activity on R synthesis and by the stabilization of R in holoenzyme. The half-life for R measured in untreated wild-type cells may underestimate the true half-life for holoenzyme-associated R, since the observed value will be affected by equilibration of R between free and holoenzyme-bound pools. Enhanced degradation of free R prevents a significant disproportion between R and C subunit levels. Recent experiments of van Daalen Wetters and Coffino (1983) have demonstrated that many cAMP-sensitive revertants of a $K_a$ mutant S49 subline are functionally hemizygous for R subunit yet express wild-type levels of both R and C subunit activities. This dosage compensation probably reflects full induction of synthesis from the one functional R allele and further illustrates the capacity of C subunit to regulate expression of R.

## VI. MAPPING MUTATIONS IN R SUBUNIT: AN APPROACH TO STRUCTURE–FUNCTION RELATIONSHIPS

A variety of structural mutations in R subunit of S49 cell protein kinase cause charge alterations in the mutant proteins. These mutations include $K_a$ mutations (Section IV,C), a phenotypically silent mutation in one R allele in S49 subline U36 (Steinberg *et al.*, 1978), and second-site mutations in cAMP-sensitive revertants of a $K_a$ mutant subline (van Daalen Wetters and Coffino, 1983). Correlation of functional consequences of these lesions with the regions of R in which they occur should provide a unique perspective on the functional organization of R subunit. To implement such an approach, we have developed procedures for rapid mapping of charge-shift mutations to locations within the R polypeptides. Figure 10 summarizes our results to date (Steinberg, 1983a; R. A. Steinberg, manuscripts submitted).

Initial studies took advantage of the domain structure of $R_I$ discussed above (Section II,C). Proteolysis of [35S]methionine-labeled S49 cell extracts

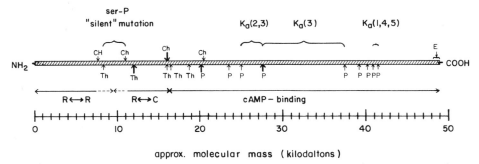

FIG. 10. Map of phosphate and charge-shift mutations in S49 R subunit. Sites are shown for chymotryptic (Ch), thermolytic (Th), and endogenous (E) proteolysis of native R and for papain (P) proteolysis of denatured R. Locations of endogenous phosphate (ser-P), the "silent" allele marker in subline U36, and $K_a$ mutations causing charge shifts of types 1–5 were determined as described in the text (Section VI). Regions involved in dimer interaction (R↔R), C subunit-binding (R↔C), and cAMP binding were inferred from published studies (Section II,C). Map scale is based on mobilities of R and its fragments in sodium dodecyl sulfate gel electrophoresis.

with thermolysin, trypsin, or chymotrypsin generated a collection of R sub-unit fragments that could be purified by cAMP-affinity chromatography and displayed by two-dimensional gel electrophoresis. Fragments containing mutations (or the endogenous phosphate) exhibited charge shifts similar to those in undigested R. Since chymotryptic and thermolytic cleavage sites were distributed throughout the hinge region of R (Fig. 10), features within this region could be mapped with high resolution. For mutations within the carboxyterminal cAMP-binding domain, however, proteolysis of native R was not very useful. To localize sites of mutation within the cAMP-binding region, we adopted an alternative strategy involving proteolysis of denatured R subunit. Limited papain digestion of affinity-purified R yielded a collec-tion of R peptides with endpoints distributed throughout the carboxytermi-nal portion of the molecule (Fig. 10). Two-dimensional gels were used again to identify fragments containing charge-shift mutations.

Proteolysis of native R was limited to the hinge region by structural con-straints, so virtually all cAMP-binding fragments contained the carboxyter-minus. Both terminal and internal fragments were obtained by papain diges-tion of denatured R, but cleavages could be limited to a single site per molecule by choosing appropriate concentrations of protease. Molecular weights of amino- or carboxyterminal fragments were used to localize sites of proteolytic cleavage within R; estimates of these molecular weights were based on peptide mobilities in second dimension sodium dodecyl sulfate gels. Aminoterminal fragments were distinguished from carboxyterminal fragments by a variety of end-specific markers, including the endogenous phosphate, specific charge-shift mutations, size heterogeneity caused by an endogenous protease (indicated by "E" in Fig. 10), and papain peptides released by further proteolysis. The map of proteolytic cleavage sites was oriented both by the known carboxyterminal location of cAMP-binding sites (Potter and Taylor, 1979a) and by preferential labeling of carboxyterminal peptides during runoff in the presence of the protein-initiation inhibitor, pactamycin.

Sites of endogenous phosphorylation and the U36 marker allele mutation were mapped to a 2.5-kd interval in the hinge region by chymotryptic and thermolytic proteolysis of native R. $K_a$ mutations, on the other hand, were clustered within the carboxyterminal half of the molecule. More than 30 independent $K_a$ mutations representing all five of the charge-shift patterns shown in Fig. 4 were mapped to intervals between papain cleavage sites. As shown in Fig. 10, the mutations fell into 3 discrete regions: mutations causing charge-shifts of types 2 and 3 were found in a 2.5-kd interval about 26 kd from the aminoterminus of R; type 1, 4, and 5 mutations were found in a very small interval about 8 kd from the carboxyterminus; and 3 (probably identical) type 3 mutations were found in a poorly defined interval between these two clusters. Two second-site mutations causing phenotypic reversion of a single type 2 mutant were mapped to either side of the original mutation (not shown).

Although the R subunit map is far from being saturated with mutations, a number of interesting conclusions can be drawn already from the mapping studies summarized above. Sites of endogenous phosphorylation and the "silent" mutation in subline U36 are near the region implicated in interaction between R and C subunits (Section II,C), yet neither phosphorylation nor mutation at these sites affects kinase activation significantly (Geahlen *et al.*, 1981; R. A. Steinberg, unpublished results). Furthermore, the U36 mutation has little or no effect on R subunit phosphorylation (Steinberg *et al.*, 1978). On the other hand, $K_a$ mutations (and their revertants), which do affect kinase activation properties, map to locations within the cAMP-binding domain. By proteolysis studies, this cAMP-binding region is structurally isolated from R-C interaction sites in the hinge region. As discussed previously (Section IV,C), $K_a$ mutations not only affect the properties of the R subunits in which they are found but also modify wild-type R subunits by heterodimer formation; this interaction causes reduced phosphorylation and altered parameters for cAMP and/or C subunit binding in the wild-type subunit. Since the region involved in dimer association is thought to be aminoterminal (Potter and Taylor, 1980), the ability of $K_a$ mutations in the carboxyterminal half of R to affect wild-type R properties through heterodimer interaction suggests that there are significant conformational interactions between aminoterminal and carboxyterminal domains of R and between individual subunits in R dimers. Allosteric linkage of R monomers might contribute to cooperative release of C subunits from wild-type holoenzyme.

Because of the complex properties suggested by intermolecular dominance of $K_a$ mutations, they cannot be regarded as specific lesions in cAMP- or C subunit-binding sites; mutations at all three loci identified in Fig. 10 promote resistance to both site 1- and site 2-directed analogs of cAMP and have comparable effects on kinase activation and R subunit phosphorylation (R. A. Steinberg and C. S. Murphy, unpublished results). Dominance of $K_a$ mutations appears to be a consequence of their selection in heterozygous diploid cells. Recent experiments, however, indicate that charge-shift $K_a$ mutations can also be isolated in cells that are functionally hemizygous for R subunit alleles (van Daalen Wetters and Coffino, 1983). Recessive $K_a$ mutations should be selectible in a hemizygous background, and such mutations are likely to affect discrete R subunit functions.


## VII. ANALYSIS OF cAMP ACTION IN INTACT CELLS

Investigation of the effects of metabolic and structural changes in protein kinase on cAMP action requires methods for analysis of kinase-mediated responses in intact cells. We have developed an approach using high resolution two-dimensional gel electrophoresis of proteins from cells labeled with [35S]methionine that has wide applicability for studying such responses (Steinberg and Coffino, 1979; Steinberg, 1980; Steinberg, 1981). Phosphorylation is monitored by the relative labeling of species corresponding to nonphosphorylated and phosphorylated forms of substrate proteins, and effects on protein synthesis are monitored by changes in relative rates of methionine incorporation into species of interest. In contrast to studies using well-characterized kinase substrates to monitor cAMP-dependent phosphorylation (e.g., Yeaman and Cohen, 1975; Sheorain et al., 1982) or enzyme-specific reagents to monitor changes in enzyme-specific mRNA (e.g., Iynedjian and Hanson, 1977; Lamers et al., 1982), the two-dimensional gel approach provides a global view of cAMP responses. Furthermore, since it does not depend on responsiveness of any particular protein, the gel approach can be used for studies in virtually any cell system that permits radiolabeling to high specific activities. Use of charge modification in [35S]methionine-labeled proteins also offers advantages over procedures using changes in [32P]phosphate labeling for monitoring phosphorylation of substrate proteins; these advantages include improved resolution and sensitivity, a capacity to study metabolic properties of substrate proteins, and, most importantly, the ability to determine extents of conversion of substrates from nonphosphorylated to phosphorylated forms.

Figure 11 compares response "domains" (Tomkins, 1975) of S49 mouse lymphoma cells treated with $Bt_2cAMP$ for short or long durations. Figure 11a shows a two-dimensional gel pattern from untreated S49 cells labeled for 15 minutes with [$^{35}$S]methionine; Fig. 11b shows a pattern from cells treated for 20 minutes with $Bt_2cAMP$ (including the 15-minute labeling period); and Fig. 11c shows a pattern from cells treated for 6 hours with $Bt_2cAMP$. All cells for this experiment were treated identically except for the time of drug addition, and incorporations were terminated by immediately extracting proteins with a strongly denaturing solvent to prevent postlysis modifications by the actions of proteases, kinases, or phosphatases. Proteins exhibiting acute responses to kinase activation are designated with arrows in the figure; inductions or repressions of specific protein synthesis are indicated, respectively, with circles and diamonds. The acute responses appear to reflect protein phosphorylation since enhanced labeling of the species indicated by arrows is generally accompanied by diminished labeling of species more basic by about a single charge unit; in several cases enhanced cAMP-dependent labeling of these putative phosphoproteins has also been seen with [$^{32}$P]phosphate labeling (Steinberg and Coffino, 1979; Steinberg, 1980; Steinberg, 1981). A number of phosphorylation substrates in S49 cells have been identified: protein I is the intermediate filament protein vimentin (Steinberg and Coffino, 1979); protein O includes β and γ forms of nonmuscle actin (Steinberg, 1980); proteins J and K are precursor and mature forms of β subunit of mitochondrial $F_1$ ATPase (R. A. Steinberg, manuscript in preparation); and protein A is either myosin light-chain kinase or an immunologically related protein (R. A. Steinberg, unpublished results). Cyclic AMP phosphodiesterase is inducible by cAMP treatment of S49 cells (Bourne *et al.*, 1973), and ornithine decarboxylase and S-adenosylmethionine decarboxylase are repressible (Insel and Fenno, 1978); these changes in enzyme activities have not been correlated with the inducible and repressible species indicated in Fig. 11. Activation of cAMP-dependent protein kinase is implicated in both rapid and slow responses to $Bt_2cAMP$: both types of responses are specifically elicited by a variety of agents that activate kinase; and they do not occur in *kin$^-$* mutant cells (Steinberg and Coffino, 1979).

The domain of cAMP-dependent phosphorylation substrates in S49 cells comprises about 1% of cellular proteins and includes two distinctly different classes of substrate. "Unorthodox" substrates, designated with open arrows in Fig. 11, are phosphorylated only as nascent polypeptide chains, and their relative extents of phosphorylation are low. Phosphorylated forms of unor-

*Robert A. Steinberg*

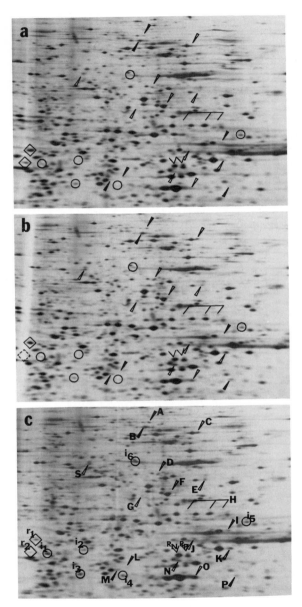

F<small>IG</small>. 11. Response domains of S49 cells to treatments with Bt₂cAMP. Wild-type cells were labeled for 15 minutes with [³⁵S]methionine after 5.75 hours preincubation in low methionine medium without drug (a) or with 1 m*M* Bt₂cAMP added 5 minutes before label (b) or at the start thodox substrates are generally stable to dephosphorylation (Steinberg and Coffino, 1979; Steinberg, 1980). "Orthodox" and "semi-orthodox" substrates, designated by filled arrows in Fig. 11, are phosphorylated posttranslationally; cAMP-mediated phosphorylation is essentially complete for orthodox substrates but relatively slight for semiorthodox substrates (Steinberg and Coffino, 1979). Phosphates on orthodox and semiorthodox substrates undergo rapid turnover both in the presence of elevated cAMP and after cAMP withdrawal (Steinberg, 1981).

Unorthodox phosphorylations probably result from exposure in protein nascent chains of phosphorylation sequences that are inaccessible in the fully folded mature proteins; stability of unorthodox phosphorylations might be another consequence of this inaccessibility. The existence of unorthodox substrates argues against the notion that primary sequence alone determines the substrate properties of proteins (Cohen, 1981). Since they constitute a form of memory response to cAMP elevation, unorthodox phosphorylations could serve a special regulatory function in cells. On the other hand, they may reflect physiological accidents that are tolerated because they involve relatively minor fractions of any substrate protein. In the case of the precursor to β subunit of mitochondrial $F_1$ ATPase, the phosphorylation appears to be a mistake, since, after proteolytic processing to mature β subunit, the phosphorylated form is specifically eliminated (Steinberg and Coffino, 1979; R. A. Steinberg, manuscript in preparation).

Consistent with their serving enzymatic functions, orthodox phosphorylation substrates in S49 cells are all species of very low abundance. The two semiorthodox substrates in S49 cells are proteins of relatively high cellular abundance and may constitute structural proteins; this is known to be the case for vimentin (protein I). In kinetic studies, phosphorylation and dephosphorylation of orthodox substrates closely follows intracellular activation and deactivation of cAMP-dependent protein kinase (Steinberg, 1981). The cAMP-dependent phosphorylations in S49 cells all appear to involve single phosphorylation sites, since labeling of only a single electrophoretic form of

---

of the preincubation period (c) as described elsewhere (Steinberg and Coffino, 1979) except that 5% dialyzed calf serum plus 5% dialyzed fetal calf serum replaced dialyzed horse serum in labeling media. $10^6$ acid-precipitable cpm of whole cell extracts were subjected to two-dimensional gel electrophoresis; autoradiograms were exposed for 10 days. Arrows indicate products of putative cAMP-dependent phosphorylations: closed arrows designate posttranslational modifications; open arrows designate modifications limited to nascent polypeptide chains. Circles enclose species whose synthesis is induced by long exposures to $Bt_2cAMP$, and diamonds enclose species whose synthesis is repressed. The two forms of R subunit are indicated by carets. Alphanumeric designations correspond to those used in previous reports (Steinberg and Coffino, 1979; Steinberg, 1981).

substrate proteins is enhanced by cAMP treatment.* Basal phosphorylation of orthodox substrates is observed in both wild-type and *kin⁻* cells (Steinberg and Coffino, 1979); preliminary experiments suggest that for some substrates basal phosphorylation may be at sites distinct from those for cAMP-dependent phosphorylation (R. A. Steinberg, unpublished results).

Figure 12 shows two-dimensional gel patterns from $GH_3$ rat pituitary tumor cells (Dannies and Tashjian, 1973) labeled with [$^{35}$S]methionine in the absence (Fig. 12a) or in the presence of $Bt_2cAMP$ after short (Fig. 12b) or long (Fig. 12c) treatment. Changes attributable to protein phosphorylation or changes in synthesis rates are indicated as in Fig. 11. Orthodox phosphorylations were distinguished from unorthodox phosphorylations by their appearance in an experiment in which cells were exposed to $Bt_2cAMP$ after labeling (not shown). Comparisons of acute $Bt_2cAMP$-mediated changes in S49 cells and $GH_3$ cells revealed extraordinary conservation of substrates for cAMP-dependent phosphorylation (Figs. 11 and 12). If species-specific alterations in protein charge are discounted (A′, B′, J′, and K′ are more acidic than their S49 cell counterparts by about one charge unit), about half the substrates from each cell type were identical. Shared substrates included species subject to orthodox, semiorthodox, and unorthodox phosphorylations. In no case was a protein detected in both cell types but phosphorylated in only one. Many of the cAMP-dependent phosphorylations were less pronounced in $GH_3$ than in S49 cells, but the basis of this difference is unknown. The conservation of substrates between S49 and $GH_3$ cells is consistent with other comparative studies; essentially, complete overlaps of substrate domains were found among S49 and three other murine cell lines of lymphoid origin and partial overlap was found between S49 cells and primary rat adrenocortical cells (Steinberg, 1981). Vimentin phosphorylation has been investigated in a number of additional cell systems and appears to be subject to cAMP-dependent regulation in C-6 glioma cells and chick myogenic cells (Groppi and Browning, 1980; Browning and Sanders, 1981; Gard and Lazarides, 1982); cAMP-independent, but not cAMP-dependent, phosphorylation of vimentin has been observed in CHO cells (Cabral and Gottesman, 1979).

In contrast to proteins subject to cAMP-dependent phosphorylation, proteins whose synthesis is regulated by cAMP are not well conserved between S49 and $GH_3$ cells (Figs. 11 and 12). Insufficient data are available, however, to define fully the domains of inducible and repressible species in the $GH_3$ system. Previous studies revealed only moderate conservation of inducible and repressible species among lymphoid cell lines; there was almost no

---

*Heterogeneity in phosphoprotein H reflects heterogeneity of the substrate rather than multiple sites for cAMP-dependent phosphorylation (R. A. Steinberg, unpublished results).

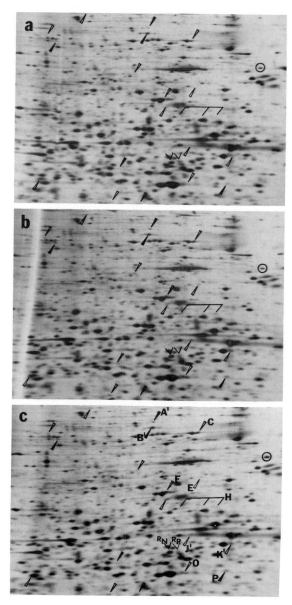

FIG. 12. Response domains of GH₃ rat pituitary tumor cells to treatments with Bt₂cAMP. Subconfluent monolayer cultures of GH₃ cells from clonal subline D6 (Ivarie *et al.*, 1981) were labeled for 15 minutes with [³⁵S]methionine in the absence (a) or presence of 1 m$M$ Bt₂cAMP after 5 minutes (b) or 5.75 hours (c) prior exposure as for Fig. 11 but with slight modifications appropriate for monolayer cultures (Steinberg, 1983b). Electrophoresis and autoradiography were as for Fig. 11; arrows, circles, and carets are used as before (Fig. 11). Letters designate cAMP-dependent changes observed in both GH₃ and S49 cells as discussed in the text (Section VII).

conservation of such species between primary rat adrenal cells and mouse lymphoid cells (Steinberg, 1981; R. A. Steinberg, unpublished observations). On the other hand, cAMP phosphodiesterase induction has been reported in a large number of cell types (D'Armiento *et al.*, 1972; Schwartz and Passonneau, 1974; Ross *et al.*, 1977). $R_I$ synthesis has been induced by cAMP treatment in S49 cells (Section V; note also $R_N$ and $R_P$ species in Fig. 11b and c), neuroblastoma cells (Morrison *et al.*, 1980), other mouse lymphoid cells, mouse embryo fibroblasts, and rat adrenal cells (Steinberg and Agard, 1981b). $R_I$ was not induced in $GH_3$ cells, although its basal synthesis in these cells was equivalent to that in S49 cells (Fig. 12b and c). It is not known whether this noninduction of $R_I$ in $GH_3$ cells represents a genetic defect or reflects physiologically important plasticity in cAMP-dependent regulation. In a similar vein, it should be noted that, although ornithine decarboxylase is repressed by cAMP treatment of S49 cells, the enzyme is induced by cAMP in a variety of other cell types (reviewed in Kudlow *et al.*, 1980).

Cyclic AMP-mediated inductions and repressions of specific protein synthesis have been correlated with changes in levels of protein-specific mRNA in several systems (Iynedjian and Hanson, 1977; Noguchi *et al.*, 1978; Brown and Papaconstantinou, 1979; Kellems *et al.*, 1979; Derda *et al.*, 1980; Morrison *et al.*, 1980). Recent studies on the $Bt_2cAMP$-mediated induction of rat liver phosphoenolpyruvate carboxykinase suggest that induction results from enhanced transcription of enzyme-specific mRNA (Beale *et al.*, 1981; Lamers *et al.*, 1982). The mediator for cAMP-specific effects on gene expression is not known, but the absence of such effects in $kin^-$ mutants of S49 cells implicates C subunit in the induction and repression processes. Models for C-dependent effects on mRNA transcription include the following: nuclear translocation of dissociated C subunit followed by C-dependent phosphorylation of chromosome-associated regulatory proteins (Jungmann and Russell, 1977; Johnson, 1977); cytoplasmic activation of a regulatory protein by C-dependent phosphorylation followed by nuclear migration of the regulator (Jost and Avener, 1975); and transcriptional regulation by a ternary complex of R subunit, C subunit, and cAMP (Cho-Chung, 1980). Basal synthesis of $R_I$ and other inducible proteins appears to be lower in $kin^-$ than in wild-type S49 cells (Section V; Bourne *et al.*, 1973; R. A. Steinberg, unpublished observations); this is consistent with a role for holoenzyme-associated C subunit in expression of cAMP-inducible genes. Involvement of R subunit in cAMP-mediated induction is suggested by recent experiments using $K_a$ mutants of Y1 adrenocortical cells (Kudlow *et al.*, 1980). In these studies, marked dissociation was observed between mutational effects on cAMP-dependent protein kinase and on corticotropin-mediated induction of ornithine decarboxylase. One structural lesion in $R_I$ (Doherty *et al.*, 1982) appeared to cause only a moderate shift in the cAMP dependence of kinase activation but complete inhibition of ornithine decarboxylase induction.

## VIII. PROSPECTS

The molecular genetic approaches reviewed in this chapter present a fresh outlook on cAMP action: they offer new methods of attacking long-standing problems and also pose intriguing new questions. C subunit-dependent regulation of R subunit synthesis and turnover in S49 cells (Section V) provides a mechanism for intracellular coordination of kinase subunit levels. This regulation of R expression also raises questions about the effects of long-term kinase activation on cellular responsiveness to cAMP elevation. It is not yet clear whether or not regulation of kinase metabolism in S49 cells will serve as a paradigm for regulation in other cell types. Mutational mapping studies of R subunit (Section VI) complement enzymological studies on functional organization of R and offer new insights into the interactions of structural domains of R. Additional structural mutations should help to define binding sites for cAMP and C subunit and regions affecting R turnover. Two-dimensional gel analysis of cAMP response domains (Section VII) has revealed both unexpected complexity in cellular responses to cAMP and remarkable conservation of proteins responsive to cAMP-dependent phosphorylation in unrelated cell types. The two-dimensional gel approach also provides a powerful technique for monitoring intracellular phosphorylation kinetics and for comparing the actions of different effector-mediated phosphorylation systems alone or in combination.

Studies in the kinase system also have relevance to a number of peripheral areas of biological interest. $R_I$ subunit has unique attributes for studying mechanisms of intracellular protein degradation: it is a constituent of nearly all cell types; its turnover is rapid in the free state but slow in holoenzyme complexes; its degradation can be inhibited with specific analogs of cAMP; and there is potential for identifying structural mutations affecting its turnover. We have already identified mutations affecting the proteolytic susceptibility of R (R. A. Steinberg, unpublished observations), so we are in a position to test the hypothesis that protein turnover *in vivo* reflects susceptibility to proteolysis.

Another area for which studies in the kinase system have relevance is mammalian cell mutagenesis. Mapping studies on S49 $K_a$ mutations represent the first extensive effort to localize and distinguish different induced structural mutations in a mammalian gene. We are accumulating data on hot spots for spontaneous and chemically-induced mutagenesis, and preliminary results suggest that N-methyl-N'-nitro-N-nitrosoguanidine and ethyl methanesulfonate, two DNA alkylating agents, induce distinct classes of $K_a$ mutations. Using the allelically marked strain U36, we are also finding differences in frequencies for $K_a$ mutations at the two R subunit alleles.

Although studies discussed in this chapter have not exhausted the potentially fruitful applications of available methodologies, they have raised questions whose elucidation requires technical innovations. Some of these questions include the following: What is the nature of the putative regulator of C subunit expression that is altered in $kin^-$ mutants of S49 cells? How is kinase expression phenotypically suppressed in unstable $V_{max}$ variants of S49 cells? What are the mechanisms underlying functional inactivation of one R subunit allele in hemizygous revertants of $K_a$ mutants? How many genes encode subunits for kinase? What is the basis for cell-specific regulation of kinase isozyme expression? Many of these questions could be approached using cloned DNA probes specific for kinase subunit genes.

The low abundance of kinase subunits and their mRNA's has retarded progress in isolating kinase genes, but several recent developments make such gene isolations feasible. Elucidation of complete amino acid sequences for kinase subunits (Shoji *et al.*, 1981; Takio *et al.*, 1982) offers the possibility of synthesizing oligonucleotide probes complementary to kinase gene sequences. Such probes could be used as primers for synthesizing large cDNA copies of kinase-specific mRNA's, or they could be used to screen libraries of cloned mammalian DNA for clones containing kinase genes. Dominant $K_a$ and $kin^-$ mutations in S49 cells offer possibilities for isolation of genes for $R_I$ subunit and the $kin^-$ regulator using DNA-mediated transformation of mammalian cells (Wigler *et al.*, 1978; Perucho *et al.*, 1980). We are presently involved in collaborative studies exploring the feasibility of such transformation using CHO cells as recipients. A scheme for isolation of functional genes for C subunit might employ DNA-mediated transformation of yeast cells deficient in adenylate cyclase. These cells require cAMP for growth, and their cAMP requirement can be overcome by mutations inactivating kinase R subunit (Matsumoto *et al.*, 1982); overproduction of C subunit by expression of newly introduced genes should also overcome the cAMP growth requirement.

Combinations of biochemical, physiological, pharmacological, and genetic investigations have contributed to make the cAMP system one of the most thoroughly elucidated pathways for regulation in mammalian cells. Nevertheless, questions about the mechanisms underlying cAMP action continue to mount. Gene-specific probes will provide new approaches for analyzing regulation of components of the cAMP response system, but it appears certain that such studies will also raise additional, more sophisticated questions. All in all, the study of cAMP action offers the prospect of continued challenge for many years to come.

## ACKNOWLEDGMENTS

I thank Theodoor van Daalen Wetters and Philip Coffino for generously and openly discussing their unpublished studies, David Borst for suggesting improvements in the manuscript, and Robert Ivarie and Julie Morris for providing $GH_3D_6$ cells for the experiment of Fig. 12. I also acknowledge the generous support provided me by grants CA 14733 and AM 27916 from the National Institutes of Health.

## REFERENCES

Adhya, S., and Garges, S. (1982). *Cell* **29**, 287–289.
Agard, D. A., Steinberg, R. A., and Stroud, R. M. (1981). *Anal. Biochem.* **111**, 257–268.
Armstrong, R. N., and Kaiser, E. T. (1978). *Biochemistry* **17**, 2840–2845.
Beale, E. G., Katzen, C. S., and Granner, D. K. (1981). *Biochemistry* **20**, 4878–4883.
Bourne, H. R., Tomkins, G. M., and Dion, S. (1973). *Science* **181**, 952–954.
Bourne, H. R., Beiderman, B., Steinberg, F., and Brothers, V. M. (1982). *Mol. Pharmacol.* **22**, 204–210.
Brothers, V. M., Walker, N., and Bourne, H. R. (1982). *J. Biol. Chem.* **257**, 9349–9355.
Brown, P. C., and Papaconstantinou, J. (1979). *J. Biol. Chem.* **254**, 9379–9384.
Browning, E. T., and Sanders, M. M. (1981). *J. Cell Biol.* **90**, 803–808.
Builder, S. E., Beavo, J. A., and Krebs, E. G. (1980a). *J. Biol. Chem.* **255**, 2350–2354.
Builder, S. E., Beavo, J. A., and Krebs, E. G. (1980b). *J. Biol. Chem.* **255**, 3514–3519.
Cabral, F., and Gottesman, M. M. (1979). *J. Biol. Chem.* **254**, 6203–6206.
Carmichael, D. F., Geahlen, R. L., Allen, S. M., and Krebs, E. G. (1982). *J. Biol. Chem.* **257**, 10440–10445.
Carr, S. A., Biemann, K., Shoji, S., Parmelee, D. C., and Titani, K. (1982). *Proc. Natl. Acad. Sci. U.S.A.* **79**, 6128–6131.
Cho-Chung, Y. S. (1980). *J. Cyclic Nucl. Res.* **6**, 163–177.
Coffino, P. (1981). *In* "Cellular Controls in Differentiation" (C. W. Lloyd and D. A. Rees, eds.), pp. 107–121. Academic Press, New York.
Coffino, P., Bourne, H. R., and Tomkins, G. M. (1975). *J. Cell. Physiol.* **85**, 603–610.
Coffino, P., Bourne, H. R., Friedrich, U., Hochman, J., Insel, P. A., Lemaire, I., Melmon, K. L., and Tomkins, G. M. (1976). *Recent Prog. Hormone Res.* **32**, 669–684.
Cohen, P., ed. (1980). "Recently Discovered Systems of Enzyme Regulation by Reversible Phosphorylation, Molecular Aspects of Cellular Regulation," Vol. I. Elsevier, New York.
Cohen, P. (1981). *In* "Cellular Controls in Differentiation" (C. W. Lloyd and D. A. Rees, eds.), pp. 81–103. Academic Press, New York.
Cooper, D. M. F. (1982). *FEBS Lett.* **138**, 157–163.
Corbin, J. D., and Keely, S. L. (1977). *J. Biol. Chem.* **252**, 910–918.
Corbin, J. D., and Rannels, S. R. (1981). *J. Biol. Chem.* **256**, 11671–11676.
Corbin, J. D., Sugden, P. H., West, L., Flockhart, D. A., Lincoln, T. M., and McCarthy, D. (1978). *J. Biol. Chem.* **253**, 3997–4003.
Corbin, J. D., Rannels, S. R., Flockhart, D. A., Robinson-Steiner, A. M., Tigani, M. C., Døskeland, S. O., Suva, R. H., Suva, R., and Miller, J. P. (1982). *Eur. J. Biochem.* **125**, 259–266.
Daniel, V., Litwack, G., and Tomkins, G. M. (1973). *Proc. Natl. Acad. Sci. U.S.A.* **70**, 76–79.
Dannies, P. S., and Tashjian, A. H., Jr. (1973). *In* "Tissue Culture: Methods and Applications" (P. P. Kruse, Jr., and M. K. Patterson, Jr., eds.), pp. 561–569. Academic Press, New York.

D'Armiento, M., Johnson, G. S., and Pastan, I. (1972). *Proc. Natl. Acad. Sci. U.S.A.* **69**, 459–462.

Derda, D. F., Miles, M. F., Schweppe, J. S., and Jungmann, R. A. (1980). *J. Biol. Chem.* **255**, 11112–11121.

Doherty, P. J., Tsao, J., Schimmer, B. P., Mumby, M. C., and Beavo, J. A. (1982). *J. Biol. Chem.* **257**, 5877–5883.

Elias, L., Li, A. P., and Longmire, J. (1981). *Cancer Res.* **41**, 2182–2188.

Erlichman, J., Rosenfeld, R., and Rosen, O. M. (1974). *J. Biol. Chem.* **249**, 5000–5003.

Erlichman, J., Sarkar, D., Fleischer, N., and Rubin, C. S. (1980). *J. Biol. Chem.* **255**, 8179–8184.

Evain, D., Gottesman, M., Pastan, I., and Anderson, W. B. (1979). *J. Biol. Chem.* **254**, 6931–6937.

Fischer, E. H., and Krebs, E. G. (1955). *J. Biol. Chem.* **216**, 121–132.

Francke, U., and Gehring, U. G. (1980). *Cell* **22**, 657–664.

Friedman, D. L., and Chambers, D. A. (1978). *Proc. Natl. Acad. Sci. U.S.A.* **75**, 5286–5290.

Friedrich, U., and Coffino, P. (1977). *Proc. Natl. Acad. Sci. U.S.A.* **74**, 679–683.

Fuller, D. J. M., Byus, C. V., and Russell, D. H. (1978). *Proc. Natl. Acad. Sci. U.S.A.* **75**, 223–227.

Gard, D. L., and Lazarides, E. (1982). *Mol. Cell. Biol.* **2**, 1104–1114.

Geahlen, R. L., and Krebs, E. G. (1980a). *J. Biol. Chem.* **255**, 1164–1169.

Geahlen, R. L., and Krebs, E. G. (1980b). *J. Biol. Chem.* **255**, 9375–9379.

Geahlen, R. L., Allen, S. M., and Krebs, E. G. (1981). *J. Biol. Chem.* **256**, 4536–4540.

Gharret, A. J., Malkinson, A. M., and Sheppard, J. R. (1976). *Nature (London)* **264**, 673–675.

Gilman, A. G. (1970). *Proc. Natl. Acad. Sci. U.S.A.* **67**, 305–312.

Gottesman, M. M. (1980). *Cell* **22**, 329–330.

Gottesman, M. M., LeCam, A., Bukowski, M., and Pastan, I. (1980). *Somat. Cell Genet.* **6**, 45–61.

Granot, J., Mildvan, A. S., Hiyama, K., Kondo, H., and Kaiser, E. T. (1980a). *J. Biol. Chem.* **255**, 4569–4573.

Granot, J., Mildvan, A. S., and Kaiser, E. T. (1980b). *Arch. Biochem. Biophys.* **205**, 1–17.

Groppi, V. E., Jr., and Browning, E. T. (1980). *Mol. Pharmacol.* **18**, 427–437.

Gutmann, N. S., Rae, P. A., and Schimmer, B. P. (1978). *J. Cell. Physiol.* **97**, 451–460.

Haddox, M. K., Magun, B. E., and Russell, D. H. (1980). *Proc. Natl. Acad. Sci. U.S.A.* **77**, 3445–3449.

Hashimoto, E., Takio, K., and Krebs, E. G. (1981). *J. Biol. Chem.* **256**, 5604–5607.

Hayes, J. S., and Brunton, L. L. (1982). *J. Cyclic Nucl. Res.* **8**, 1–16.

Hayes, J. S., Brunton, L. L., Brown, J. H., Reese, J. B., and Mayer, S. E. (1979). *Proc. Natl. Acad. Sci. U.S.A.* **76**, 1570–1574.

Hochman, J., Insel, P. A., Bourne, H. R., Coffino, P., and Tomkins, G. M. (1975). *Proc. Natl. Acad. Sci. U.S.A.* **72**, 5051–5055.

Hochman, J., Bourne, H. R., Coffino, P., Insel, P. A., Krasny, L., and Melmon, K. L. (1977). *Proc. Natl. Acad. Sci. U.S.A.* **74**, 1167–1171.

Hofmann, F. (1980). *J. Biol. Chem.* **255**, 1559–1564.

Hofmann, F., Beavo, J. A., Bechtel, P. J., and Krebs, E. G. (1975). *J. Biol. Chem.* **250**, 7795–7801.

Hofmann, F., Bechtel, P. J., and Krebs, E. G. (1977). *J. Biol. Chem.* **252**, 1441–1447.

Insel, P. A., and Fenno, J. (1978). *Proc. Natl. Acad. Sci. U.S.A.* **75**, 862–865.

Insel, P. A., Bourne, H. R., Coffino, P., and Tomkins, G. M. (1975). *Science* **190**, 896–898.

Ivarie, R. D., Baxter, J. D., and Morris, J. A. (1981). *J. Biol. Chem.* **256**, 4520–4528.

Iynedjian, P. B., and Hanson, R. W. (1977). *J. Biol. Chem.* **252**, 655–662.

Jastorff, B., Hoppe, J., and Morr, M. (1979). *Eur. J. Biochem.* **101,** 555–561.

Johnson, E. M. (1977). *Adv. Cyclic Nucleotide Res.* **8,** 267–309.

Johnson, G. L., Bourne, H. R., Gleason, M. K., Coffino, P., Insel, P. A., and Melmon, K. L. (1979). *Mol. Pharmacol.* **15,** 16–27.

Jost, J.-P., and Averner, M. (1975). *J. Theoret. Biol.* **49,** 337–344.

Jungmann, R. A., and Russell, D. H. (1977). *Life Sci.* **20,** 1787–1798.

Keely, S. L., Corbin, J. D., and Park, C. R. (1975). *Proc. Natl. Acad. Sci. U.S.A.* **72,** 1501–1504.

Kellems, R. E., Morhenn, V. B., Pfendt, E. A., Alt, F. W., and Schimke, R. T. (1979). *J. Biol. Chem.* **254,** 309–318.

Kerlavage, A. R., and Taylor, S. S. (1980). *J. Biol. Chem.* **255,** 8483–8488.

Kerlavage, A. R., and Taylor, S. S. (1982). *J. Biol. Chem.* **257,** 1749–1754.

Knight, B. L., and Skala, J. P. (1977). *J. Biol. Chem.* **252,** 5356–5362.

Krebs, E. G. (1972). *Curr. Top. Cell. Regul.* **5,** 99–133.

Krebs, E. G., and Beavo, J. A. (1979). *Annu. Rev. Biochem.* **48,** 923–959.

Kudlow, J. E., Rae, P. A., Gutmann, N. S., Schimmer, B. P., and Burrow, G. N. (1980). *Proc. Natl. Acad. Sci. U.S.A.* **77,** 2767–2771.

Kudlow, J. E., Watson, R. K., and Gill, G. N. (1981). *J. Cyclic Nucleotide Res.* **7,** 151–159.

Kuo, J. F., and Greengard, P. (1969). *Proc. Natl. Acad. Sci. U.S.A.* **64,** 1349–1355.

Lai, E., Rosen, O. M., and Rubin, C. S. (1982). *J. Biol. Chem.* **257,** 6691–6696.

Lamers, W. H., Hanson, R. W., and Meisner, H. M. (1982). *Proc. Natl. Acad. Sci. U.S.A.* **79,** 5137–5141.

Langan, T. A. (1973). *Adv. Cyclic Nucleotide Res.* **3,** 99–153.

Lee, P. D., Radloff, D., Schweppe, J. S., and Jungmann, R. A. (1976). *J. Biol. Chem.* **251,** 914–921.

Lemaire, I., and Coffino, P. (1977a). *J. Cell. Physiol.* **92,** 437–446.

Lemaire, I., and Coffino, P. (1977b). *Cell* **11,** 149–155.

Liu, A. Y.-C. (1982). *J. Biol. Chem.* **257,** 298–306.

Liu, A. Y.-C., Chan, T., and Chen, K. Y. (1981). *Cancer Res.* **41,** 4579–4587.

Malkinson, A. M., and Butley, M. S. (1981). *Cancer Res.* **41,** 1334–1341.

Martin, T. F. J., and Kowalchyk, J. A. (1981). *Science* **213,** 1120–1122.

Martin, T. F. J., and Ronning, S. A. (1981). *J. Cell. Physiol.* **190,** 289–297.

Matsumoto, K., Uno, I., Oshima, Y., and Ishikawa, T. (1982). *Proc. Natl. Acad. Sci. U.S.A.* **79,** 2355–2359.

Moreno, S., and Passeron, S. (1980). *Arch. Biochem. Biophys.* **199,** 321–330.

Morrison, M. R., Pardue, S., Prashad, N., Croall, D. E., and Brodeur, R. (1980). *Eur. J. Biochem.* **106,** 463–472.

Moyle, W. R., Kong, Y. C., and Ramachandran, J. (1973). *J. Biol. Chem.* **248,** 2409–2417.

Nimmo, H. G., and Cohen, P. (1977). *Adv. Cyclic Nucleotide Res.* **8,** 145–266.

Noguchi, T., Diesterhaft, M., and Granner, D. (1978). *J. Biol. Chem.* **253,** 1332–1335.

O'Farrell, P. H. (1975). *J. Biol. Chem.* **250,** 4007–4021.

Øgreid, D., Døskeland, S. O., and Miller, J. (1983). *J. Biol. Chem.* **258,** 1041–1049.

Pall, M. L. (1981). *Microbiol. Rev.* **45,** 462–480.

Perucho, M., Hanahan, D., Lipsich, L., and Wigler, M. (1980). *Nature (London)* **285,** 207–210.

Plet, A., Evain, D., and Anderson, W. B. (1982). *J. Biol. Chem.* **257,** 889–893.

Pollack, R., ed. (1981). "Readings in Mammalian Cell Culture, Second Edition," pp. 95–166. Cold Spring Harbor Laboratory, New York.

Potter, R. L., and Taylor, S. S. (1979a). *J. Biol. Chem.* **254,** 2413–2418.

Potter, R. L., and Taylor, S. S. (1979b). *J. Biol. Chem.* **254,** 9000–9005.

Potter, R. L., and Taylor, S. S. (1980). *J. Biol. Chem.* **255**, 9706–9712.

Prashad, N., Rosenberg, R. N., Wischmeyer, B., Ulrich, C., and Sparkman, D. (1979). *Biochemistry* **18**, 2717–2725.

Rae, P. A., Gutmann, N. S., Tsao, J., and Schimmer, B. P. (1979). *Proc. Natl. Acad. Sci. U.S.A.* **76**, 1896–1900.

Rangel-Aldao, R., and Rosen, O. M. (1976). *J. Biol. Chem.* **251**, 3375–3380.

Rangel-Aldao, R., Kupiec, J. W., and Rosen, O. M. (1979). *J. Biol. Chem.* **254**, 2499–2508.

Rannels, S. R., and Corbin, J. D. (1980). *J. Biol. Chem.* **255**, 7085–7088.

Rannels, S. R., and Corbin, J. D. (1981). *J. Biol. Chem.* **256**, 7871–7876.

Richards, J. S., and Rolfes, A. I. (1980). *J. Biol. Chem.* **255**, 5481–5489.

Rickenberg, H. V. (1974). *Annu. Rev. Microbiol.* **28**, 353–369.

Robinson-Steiner, A. M., and Corbin, J. D. (1983). *J. Biol. Chem.* **258**, 1032–1040.

Robison, G. A., Butcher, R. W., and Sutherland, E. W. (1971). "Cyclic AMP." Academic Press, New York.

Rosen, N., Piscitello, J., Schneck, J., Muschel, R. J., Bloom, B. R., and Rosen, O. M. (1979). *J. Cell. Physiol.* **98**, 125–136.

Rosen, O. M., and Krebs, E. G., eds. (1981). "Protein Phosphorylation, Cold Spring Harbor Conferences on Cell Proliferation," Vol. 8. Cold Spring Harbor Laboratory, New York.

Rosen, O. M., Rangel-Aldao, R., and Erlichman, J. (1977). *Curr. Top. Cell. Regul.* **12**, 39–74.

Ross, E. M., and Gilman, A. G. (1980). *Annu. Rev. Biochem.* **49**, 533–564.

Ross, P. S., Manganiello, V. C., and Vaughan, M. (1977). *J. Biol. Chem.* **252**, 1448–1452.

Roth, C. W., Singh, T., Pastan, I., and Gottesman, M. M. (1982). *J. Cell. Physiol.* **111**, 42–48.

Rousseau, G. G., Martial, J., and De Visscher, M. (1976). *Eur. J. Biochem.* **66**, 499–506.

Rubin, C. S. (1979). *J. Biol. Chem.* **254**, 12439–12449.

Rubin, C. S., and Rosen, O. M. (1975). *Annu. Rev. Biochem.* **44**, 831–887.

Rudack-Garcia, D., and Henry, H. L. (1981). *J. Biol. Chem.* **256**, 10781–10785.

Russell, D. H., Haddox, M. K., and Gehring, U. (1981). *J. Cell. Physiol.* **106**, 375–384.

Sampson, J. (1977). *Cell* **11**, 173–180.

Schwartz, J. P., and Passonneau, J. V. (1974). *Proc. Natl. Acad. Sci. U.S.A.* **71**, 3844–3848.

Schwechheimer, K., and Hofmann, F. (1977). *J. Biol. Chem.* **252**, 7690–7696.

Schwoch, G., Hamann, A., and Hilz, H. (1980). *Biochem. J.* **192**, 223–230.

Setchenska, M. S., Vassileva-Popova, J. G., and Arnstein, H. R. V. (1981). *Biochem. J.* **196**, 893–897.

Shear, M., Insel, P. A., Melmon, K. L., and Coffino, P. (1976). *J. Biol. Chem.* **251**, 7572–7576.

Sheorain, V. S., Khatra, B. S., and Soderling, T. R. (1982). *J. Biol. Chem.* **257**, 3462–3470.

Shoji, S., Parmelee, D. C., Wade, R. D., Kumar, S., Ericsson, L. H., Walsh, K. A., Neurath, H., Long, G. L., Demaille, J. G., Fischer, E. H., and Titani, K. (1981). *Proc. Natl. Acad. Sci. U.S.A.* **78**, 848–851.

Simantov, R., and Sachs, L. (1975). *Eur. J. Biochem.* **59**, 89–95.

Singh, T. J., Roth, C., Gottesmann, M. M., and Pastan, I. H. (1981). *J. Biol. Chem.* **256**, 926–932.

Smith, S. B., White, H. D., Siegel, J. B., and Krebs, E. G. (1981). *Proc. Natl. Acad. Sci. U.S.A.* **78**, 1591–1595.

Steinberg, R. A. (1980). *Proc. Natl. Acad. Sci. U.S.A.* **77**, 910–914.

Steinberg, R. A. (1981). *In* "Protein Phosphorylation, Cold Spring Harbor Conferences on Cell Proliferation" (O. M. Rosen and E. G. Krebs, eds.), Vol. 8, pp. 179–193. Cold Spring Harbor Laboratory, New York.

Steinberg, R. A. (1983a). *J. Cell Biol.* **97**, 1072–1080.

Steinberg, R. A. (1983b). *In* "Methods in Enzymology, Vol. 99: Hormone Action, Part F" (J. D. Corbin and J. G. Hardman, eds.), pp. 233–243. Academic Press, New York.

Steinberg, R. A., and Agard, D. A. (1981a). *J. Biol. Chem.* **256**, 10731–10734.

Steinberg, R. A., and Agard, D. A. (1981b). *J. Biol. Chem.* **256**, 11356–11364.

Steinberg, R. A., and Coffino, P. (1979). *Cell* **18**, 719–733.

Steinberg, R. A., O'Farrell, P. H., Friedrich, U., and Coffino, P. (1977). *Cell* **10**, 381–391.

Steinberg, R. A., van Daalen Wetters, T., and Coffino, P. (1978). *Cell* **15**, 1351–1361.

Steinberg, R. A., Steinberg, M. G., and van Daalen Wetters, T. (1979). *J. Cell. Physiol.* **100**, 579–588.

Sugden, P. H., and Corbin, J. D. (1976). *Biochem. J.* **159**, 423–437.

Sutherland, E. W., Jr., and Wosilait, W. D. (1955). *Nature (London)* **175**, 169–171.

Takio, K., Smith, S. B., Krebs, E. G., Walsh, K. A., and Titani, K. (1982). *Proc. Natl. Acad. Sci. U.S.A.* **79**, 2544–2548.

Thorner, J. (1982). *Cell* **30**, 5–6.

Tomkins, G. M. (1975). *Science* **189**, 760–763.

Trevillyan, J. M., and Pall, M. L. (1982). *J. Biol. Chem.* **257**, 3978–3986.

van Daalen Wetters, T., and Coffino, P. (1982). *Mol. Cell. Biol.* **2**, 1229–1237.

van Daalen Wetters, T., and Coffino, P. (1983). *Mol. Cell. Biol.* **3**, 250–256.

Walter, U., and Greengard, P. (1981). *Curr. Top. Cell. Regul.* **19**, 219–256.

Walter, U., Uno, I., Liu, A. Y.-C., and Greengard, P. (1977). *J. Biol. Chem.* **252**, 6588–6590.

Walter, U., Costa, M. R. C., Breakefield, X. O., and Greengard, P. (1979). *Proc. Natl. Acad. Sci. U.S.A.* **76**, 3251–3255.

Weber, W., and Hilz, H. (1979). *Biochem. Biophys. Res. Commun.* **90**, 1073–1081.

Weber, W., Schröder, H., and Hilz, H. (1981a). *Biochem. Biophys. Res. Commun.* **99**, 475–483.

Weber, W., Schwoch, G., Wielckens, K., Gartemann, A., and Hilz, H. (1981b). *Eur. J. Biochem.* **120**, 585–592.

Wehner, J. M., Malkinson, A. M., Wiser, M. F., and Sheppard, J. R. (1981). *J. Cell. Physiol.* **108**, 175–184.

Wigler, M., Pellicer, A., Silverstein, S., and Axel, R. (1978). *Cell* **14**, 725–731.

Witters, L. A., Kowaloff, E. M., and Avruch, J. (1979). *J. Biol. Chem.* **254**, 245–248.

Yeaman, S. J., and Cohen, P. (1975). *Eur. J. Biochem.* **51**, 93–104.

Zick, Y., Cesla, R., and Shaltiel, S. (1979). *J. Biol. Chem.* **254**, 879–887.

Zoller, M. J., Kerlavage, A. R., and Taylor, S. S. (1979). *J. Biol. Chem.* **254**, 2408–2412.

# CHAPTER 3

# Molecular Mechanism of Gonadotropin Releasing Hormone Action

## P. Michael Conn

Department of Pharmacology
Duke University Medical Center
Durham, North Carolina

67

BIOCHEMICAL ACTIONS OF HORMONES, VOL. XI

## I. INTRODUCTION

Gonadotropin releasing hormone (GnRH)* is a hypothalamic decapeptide ($pGlu^1$-$His^2$-$Trp^3$-$Ser^4$-$Tyr^5$-$Gly^6$-$Leu^7$-$Arg^8$-$Pro^9$-$Gly^{10}NH_2$) that stimulates pituitary gonadotropin [luteinizing hormone (LH) and follicle stimulating hormone (FSH)] release. These protein hormones regulate steroidogenesis and gamete maturation in gonadal tissue. For simplicity, we proposed (Conn *et al.*, 1981b) a "Three-Step" model for the mechanism by which GnRH stimulates gonadotropin release from the pituitary. In this model, GnRH-stimulated gonadotropin release action is viewed as being divided into three sequential and interrelated steps: (1) Interaction of GnRH with a specific plasma membrane receptor: (2) mobilization of ionic calcium ($Ca^{2+}$); and (3) expulsion of the contents of the gonadotropin secretory granule to the extracellular space. Since proposal of this model, a major goal of our laboratory has been to determine the means by which these steps are interrelated. How, for example, does receptor occupancy activate the effector system? What is the means by which $Ca^{2+}$ mobilization stimulates gonadotropin release? Are other actions of the releasing hormone mediated by a similar mechanism? We have recently obtained evidence about the means by which receptor occupancy appears to result in activation of the effector system. These findings and evidence to indicate the involvement of calmodulin in mediating the response mechanism are described in the present chapter in terms of the Three-Step Mechanism (Table I).

*GnRH is variously referred to as luteinizing hormone releasing hormone (LHRH) and luteinizing hormone releasing factor (LRF). Since its status as a hormone is unquestionable and it functionally stimulates release of both LH and FSH, the abbreviation GnRH is used in the present review. The nomenclature system for naming GnRH analogs specifies the alterations from the native sequence. For example, D-$Lys^6$-GnRH is the molecule $pGlu^1$-$His^2$-$Trp^3$-$Ser^4$-$Tyr^5$-D-$Lys^6$-$Leu^7$-$Arg^8$-$Pro^9$-$Gly^{10}NH_2$.

TABLE I

"Three-Step" Mechanism for GnRH-Stimulated LH Release[a]

1. GnRH binding to its plasma membrane receptor (Marian and Conn, 1983)
   a. Receptor regulation by endocrine status of the animal (Marian *et al.*, 1981)
   b. Likely receptor microaggregation (Conn *et al.*, 1982a; Conn *et al.*, 1982b; Blum and Conn, 1982)
   c. Patching, capping, and internalization of the GnRH-receptor complex (Hazum *et al.*, 1980)
   d. Step "b" does not appear to be required for gonadotropin release (Conn *et al.*, 1981d; Conn and Hazum, 1981)
   e. Receptor-mediated desensitization (Smith and Conn, 1983b; Conn *et al.*, 1984; Smith and Conn, 1984)
2. Calcium mobilization
   a. Increased calcium flux (Conn *et al.*, 1981b)
      Requirement for extracellular calcium (Marian and Conn, 1979, 1980; Stern and Conn, 1981)
      Reversibility of depletion (Conn and Rogers, 1979)
      Gonadotropin release by ionophores, liposomes, and activators of endogenous ion channels (Conn *et al.*, 1979; Conn *et al.*, 1980a; Conn and Rogers, 1980)
   b. Calcium action is postreceptor (Marian and Conn, 1980)
   c. Occupancy and redistribution of calmodulin (Conn *et al.*, 1981a)
      Block of stimulated release by anticalmodulin drugs (Conn *et al.*, 1981c; Hart *et al.*, 1983; Conn, 1982)
   d. Altered cellular function
3. Release of gonadotropin via granule exocytosis

[a]Representative references from the author's laboratory.

## II. DISTRIBUTION, CHARACTERIZATION, AND MOLECULAR BIOLOGY OF THE GnRH RECEPTOR

### A. Binding Characteristics

A reliable radioligand assay for the GnRH receptor took many years to develop. It was obvious that a good probe should have high specific activity yet retain a high percentage of specific binding to the GnRH receptor. It was possible to label authentic GnRH either by tritiation or by iodination (since a $Tyr^5$ is present). Both labeled compounds were highly susceptible to proteolytic degradation by enzymes in the pituitary (Kochman *et al.*, 1975), serum (Benuck and Marks, 1976), and hypothalamus (Griffiths and Kelly, 1979). Thus, the concentration of intact GnRH present in binding assays might be expected to change with time and complicate the reaction kinetics. The tritiated derivatives were of lesser specific activity (16–25 Ci/mMol, Perrin *et al.*, 1980) compared to the iodinated ones (1000 Ci/mMol, Clayton *et al.* 1979; Marian and Conn, 1980), although tritiation had the advantage of not introducing atoms not present in the native molecule. Problems in development of assays were further complicated because GnRH was found to dissociate rapidly from its receptor.

A major step in development of the radioligand assay came from the observation that insertion of D-amino acids at the principal degradation site in the GnRH molecule provided a relatively stable radioligand (Clayton *et al.*, 1979; a recent review of GnRH analogs has been presented, Bex and Corbin, 1982). In native GnRH, the bond adjacent to the sixth amino acid appears to be preferentially cleaved by endopeptidases (Koch *et al.*, 1974). A carboxyamide peptidase has also been characterized which cleaves the $Pro^9$-$Gly^{10}$-$NH_2$ bond (Marks, 1970). Thus, substitution of six-position D-amino acids (often $D$-$Leu^6$, $D$-$Trp^6$, $D$-$Ala^6$, $D$-(*tert*-butyl) $Ser^6$, or $D$-$Lys^6$) offers considerable protection against degradation during the assay. In addition, removal of the C-terminal amino acid (which is a blocked Gly-amide in native GnRH) and termination by $Pro^9$-ethylamide (the so-called "Fujino modification," Fujino *et al.*, 1974) has been found to result in superagonist activity. Because agonists that contain these modifications can be conveniently radioiodinated (Clayton *et al.*, 1979; Marian and Conn, 1980; Marian *et al.*, 1981; Conn and Hazum, 1981; Conn *et al.*, 1981d), these have served as useful probes of the GnRH receptor.

Accordingly, for the reasons of superagonist activity and enhanced metabolic stability, we have selected to use Buserelin (a trade name of Hoechst Pharmaceuticals for $D$-ser(*tert*-butyl)$^6$-des$^{10}$-$Pro^9$-ethylamide-GnRH, see Fig. 1) to prepare a radioligand for use in studies of the GnRH receptor. Iodination with $^{125}I$ of this GnRH analog was done (Marian and Conn, 1980) in a reaction mixture that contained 5 μg analog in 10 μl 0.1 $M$ phosphate buffer, pH 7.5, 1–2 mCi $^{125}$-iodide, and 250 ng chloramine T in 0.1 $M$ phosphate. After 2 minutes at room temperature, the reaction mixture was stopped by dilution with 2 m$M$ ammonium acetate, pH 4.5, and the mixture was applied to a 3.0 ml carboxymethyl cellulose column (0.7 mEq/g, fine mesh) previously equilibrated in the same buffer. The column was washed first with the equilibration buffer to remove unbound iodide then with 60 m$M$ ammonium acetate, pH 4.5, to elute the labeled analog. Typical specific activity was 850–1250 μCi/μg (assessed by selfdisplacement) and maximum binding ranged from 30–50% in different batches. This procedure has been useful for labeling a large number of GnRH analogs. Readers who attempt to use this method should note that elevation of the concentration of the elution buffer to 200 m$M$ acetate is needed to elute other GnRH analogs containing $D$-$Lys^6$ substitutions (Conn *et al.*, 1981d; Conn and Hazum, 1981). We have also found that equimolar HEPES or phosphate (buffers) may be substituted

GnRH Analogs (All May Be Radiolabeled By Iodination Of Tyr$^5$)

GnRH (Natural Sequence):

pyroGlu$^1$-His$^2$-Trp$^3$-Ser$^4$-Tyr$^5$-Gly$^6$-Leu$^7$-Arg$^8$-Pro$^9$-Gly$^{10}$NH$_2$

D-Lys$^6$-GnRH (Lysyl$^6$ Allows Derivatizations; D-amino acid$^6$ Leads to Metabolic Stability)

pyroGly$^1$-His$^2$-Trp$^3$-Ser$^4$-Tyr$^5$-D-Lys$^6$-Leu$^7$-Arg$^8$-Pro$^9$-Gly$^{10}$NH$_2$

D-Lys$^6$-Fuj-GnRH (D-amino acid$^6$ and C Terminal Alteration Leads to 10X Higher Ka)

pyroGlu$^1$-His$^2$-Trp$^3$-Ser$^4$-Tyr$^5$-D-Lys$^6$-Leu$^7$-Arg$^8$-Pro$^9$-ethylamide

Buserelin (Radioligand, Stable, High Affinity)

pyroGlu$^1$-His$^2$-Trp$^3$-Ser$^4$-Tyr$^5$-D(tBu)Ser$^6$-Leu$^7$-Arg$^8$-Pro$^9$-ethylamide

D-GPT-GnRH (Antagonist With D-Lys$^6$)

D-pyro-Glu$^1$-D-Phe$^2$-D-Trp$^3$-Ser$^4$-Tyr$^5$-D-Lys$^6$-Leu$^7$-Arg$^8$-Pro$^9$-Gly$^{10}$NH$_2$

Des-His$^2$-GnRH (Antagonist)

D-pyroGlu$^1$-D-Trp$^3$-Ser$^4$-Tyr$^5$-Gly$^6$-Leu$^7$-Arg$^8$-Pro-Gly$^{10}$NH$_2$

FIG. 1. Analogs of gonadotropin releasing hormone (GnRH). The availability of analogs has greatly expedited work in this area. Specific substitutions are known that allow preparation of GnRH antagonists and superagonists as well as compounds that are blocked against degradation. All shown GnRH analogs may be iodinated at the Tyr$^5$ position.

without loss of yield when acetate cannot be tolerated for a particular experiment.

Agonist binding occurs with high affinity and high specificity to pituitary and ovarian membranes. No specific binding was found in heart, lung, spleen, adrenal, kidney, or cerebral cortex. Gonadal receptor has been characterized and reviewed (Hsueh and Jones, 1981). Evidence is also available to support binding sites in the brain (Liscovitch and Koch, 1982).

## B. CHEMICAL NATURE OF THE RECEPTOR

Photoaffinity labeling (Hazum, 1981) of pituitary plasma membrane fractions using D-Lys$^6$-N$^e$-azidobenzoyl-GnRH followed by polyacrylamide gel electrophoresis in sodium dodecyl sulfate indicated specific photolabeling of two protein classes. These were of estimated molecular weight 60,000 (major band) and 48,000 (minor band). Dalton components of 60,000 and 54,000 were also observed when a similar technique was applied to rat ovarian granulosa cell membranes (Hazum and Nimrod, 1982). The ability of wheat germ agglutinin to inhibit agonist and antagonist binding by rat pituitary membranes indicates that sugar moieties may be located near the binding site. Binding inhibition was reversed by N-acetyl glucosamine and not observed for Concanavalin A or soybean agglutinin (Hazum, 1982).

## C. SUBCELLULAR LOCALIZATION OF THE GnRH RECEPTOR

The first step in the mechanism of GnRH action is binding of the releasing hormone to its receptor (Conn *et al.*, 1981b). Radioligand assays have been used to characterize binding in membrane fractions (Spona, 1973; Marshall *et al.*, 1976; Wagner *et al.*, 1979; Clayton *et al.*, 1979; Conne *et al.*, 1979; Perrin *et al.*, 1980; Marian *et al.*, 1981), homogenates (Pedroza *et al.*, 1977; Clayton *et al.*, 1980), and cultured cells (Grant *et al.*, 1973; Naor *et al.*, 1980; Meidan and Koch, 1981). When expressed on a "per cell" basis and allowing for reasonable yields, the number of GnRH receptors in plasma membrane fractions is reasonably close to that found in homogenates. Thus, it seems likely that binding to the plasma membrane receptor is the primary action of the releasing hormone. This belief appears to be supported by morphological studies.

Even so, some reports have questioned whether the plasma membrane is the sole, or even predominant, locus of GnRH receptors. Sternberger and Petrali (1975) and Sternberger (1978) were able to demonstrate immunocytochemical staining for GnRH in the large secretory granules of gonadotropes. The enhancement of granule staining following GnRH was attributed to specific binding of exogenous GnRH to granule receptors. Bauer *et al.* (1981), also using GnRH antibodies, reported localization of endogenous immunoreactive GnRH itself in the secretory granules. Following injection of rats with a GnRH agonist, EM autoradiography showed grains in the plasma membrane, lysosomes, and secretory vesicles (Duello *et al.*, 1981). These later observations, however, were likely due to internalized plasma membrane patches containing receptor enroute to degradation (see Section II,H). Specific binding sites for GnRH have also been proposed in the nuclear membrane (Millar *et al.*, 1982) and lysosomes (Jayatilak, 1982).

In order to clarify the sites of specific GnRH receptors, we examined (Marian and Conn, 1983) subcellular fractions of the pituitary that had been characterized by enzymatic and chemical markers. The major portion of specific GnRH-receptor binding, in both pituitary and ovarian tissue, was indeed associated with a membranous fraction sedimenting at 11,000 $g$. The distribution of ligand binding in more purified membrane subfractions, obtained from sucrose gradient centrifugation, paralleled the distribution of 5'-nucleotidase activity (a marker of the plasma membrane). Electron micrographs of the membrane subfraction most enriched with GnRH binding sites were distinguished by smooth, irregular vesicular structures characteristic of plasma membrane fragments. The specific ligand binding associated with the 600 g (plasma membrane and nuclear fraction) pellet may be due to plasma membrane contamination of this fraction by trapping of large cell debris or by the presence of some intact cells. Because of their size heterogeneity (Maunsbach, 1974), we were unable to obtain a single fraction enriched in lysosomes (assessed by acid phosphatase activity). Since at least some acid phosphatase activity was associated with all of our fractions, it was not possible to completely eliminate lysosomes as a minor compartment for GnRH receptors. However, since some fractions that were enriched with acid phosphatase were not also enriched with radioligand binding, it seems likely that any contribution is minimal. The migration of LH in the sucrose gradients of pituitary tissue also differed significantly from the distribution of GnRH binding sites measured by our assay. This suggests that if receptors were present in the granules, they were either undetectable by conventional radioligand methods or represent only a very minor component of the whole receptor population. These results are consistent with the report of Clayton *et al.* (1978) that specific binding of [$^{125}$I]GnRH in bovine pituitary is enriched in fractions, shown by electron microscopy and the presence of adenylate cyclase activity, to contain a plasma membranes. These authors also found no displaceable binding of [$^{125}$I]GnRH in the bovine pituitary fraction (density >1.20 g/cm$^3$) containing secretory vesicles. Thus, it appears that the plasma membrane is the predominant, possibly exclusive, site of functional GnRH receptors in unstimulated cells. The plasma membrane fraction is an appropriate site to examine for quantitation of this receptor.

## D. ONTOGENY OF THE GnRH RECEPTOR

A comprehensive developmental study of pituitary and gonadal GnRH receptors in the rat has been presented (Dalkin *et al.*, 1981). This study used the metabolically stable agonist D-Ala$^6$-des-Gly$^{10}$-ethylamide-GnRH and found that receptor binding affinities did not change throughout maturation and were similar in the pituitary, testes, and ovaries. Pituitary GnRH-receptor concentration (fmol/mg protein) increased twofold in both sexes. In females, the peak values (720 ± 52 fmol/mg protein) occurred at 20 days of age, and in males the peak value (594 ± 54) occurred at 30 days. The changes in receptor correlated well with plasma follicle stimulating hormone (FSH). Age-dependent changes in gonadal receptors were also noted and were maximal (271 ± 25) on day 20 in females and in males (256 ± 13) on day 40, despite the undetectable levels at day 30. These studies further substantiate the key role of the receptor in regulating tissue responsiveness and suggest that substances that cross-react with the GnRH receptor may be important in regulating steroidogenesis at puberty. The gonadal GnRH receptor is one of the extrapituitary GnRH receptors, which are discussed more fully later.

### E. Changes in Receptor Number through the Estrous Cycle

The labeled superactive analogs have been used by us (Marian *et al.*, 1981) and others (Savoy-Moore *et al.*, 1980; Clayton *et al.*, 1980) to characterize GnRH levels in the pituitary during the rat estrous cycle. The results of these studies from three different laboratories are nearly identical; they indicate a low concentration of GnRH receptors on the morning of estrus and a gradual increase to a plateau on the afternoon of diestrus II through proestrus (time of the LH surge). There is no marked change in receptor affinity for the radioligand (in our own study the range was $K_a = 1.6$–$2.7 \times 10^{10}$ $M^{-1}$). These observations suggest that GnRH receptors may be important in regulation of LH release. A recent study suggests that the apparent loss of receptor binding activity beginning on the afternoon of proestrous may result from occupancy (White and Ojeda, 1982).

### F. Receptor Changes following Ovariectomy and Steroid Replacement

We additionally assessed the contribution of estrogen *in vivo* to the regulation of the GnRH receptor in ovariectomized rats (Marian *et al.*, 1981). At 24 days of age, rats that had been ovariectomized at 14 days of age had twice the number of pituitary GnRH receptors compared with sham-operated rats of the same age. Receptor affinity did not vary significantly ($K_a = 1.1$–$1.9 \times 10^{10} M^{-1}$). Within 3 hours of administration of 10 μg estradiol benzoate (in oil, s.c.), receptor number returned to sham levels, and LH serum concentration dropped 86% from nontreated ovariectomized rats. Twelve hours after the initial estradiol injection, both receptor number and LH serum concentration were again above sham levels, although not as high as for nontreated ovariectomized rats. Marshall's group (Frager *et al.*, 1981) has provided convincing evidence that administration of antiserum to GnRH concomitant with castration inhibits the rise in both GnRH receptor number and LH release, which follow castration. They have shown that changes in pituitary GnRH receptors parallel previously demonstrated changes in hypothalamic secretion of GnRH. The authors have suggested that GnRH probably regulates its own receptor *in vivo* and gonadal steroids may influence pituitary GnRH receptors by changing hypothalamic GnRH secretion.

## G. Receptor Changes during Normal Aging

Because of the marked reproductive changes associated with aging (for review, Smith and Conn, 1983a), we also examined receptor number and binding affinity in pituitaries from pseudopregnant (PP) and constant estrus (CE) rats (20–24 months) in comparison to 30-day-old pups (Marian *et al.*, 1981). Since these old animals differ from weanlings both in age and in endocrine status, 6 and 12 month spontaneously CE rats (controls for endocrine status) were also examined. For all ages of CE rats, receptor binding was dramatically decreased compared to weanling females. A similar decrease was observed for old PP rats. Receptor affinity was not different between the groups, while receptor concentration in the CE and the old animals was 18–24% of that in the young. It was observed that the number of GnRH receptors in lactating rats (when LH levels are low) are also diminished compared with nonlactating animals. Accordingly, it appeared that alterations in GnRH receptor, but not binding affinity, occur during different endocrine states. Because functional receptor levels can effectively alter target cell sensitivity and because relatively elevated receptor levels appear necessary for elevated serum LH, the possibility remains that gonadotrope sensitivity is regulated in part by altered receptor levels.

## H. Occupancy of the GnRH Receptor Leads to Patching, Capping, and Internalization

We have found chemical properties in a number of GnRH agonists, which make them particularly useful for determining some of the biological characteristics of the GnRH receptor. Because of the free $\epsilon$ amino group in D-Lys[6]-GnRH, it was possible to prepare a rhodamine derivative of this compound (Hazum *et al.*, 1980). The presence of the D-amino acid has the advantage of adding stability against proteolytic degradation. The rhodamine-D-Lys[6]-GnRH derivative retained high affinity (3 n$M$) binding to the GnRH receptor. This derivative, then, was suitable for visualization and localization of GnRH receptors in cultured cells using the technique of image intensification. The fluorescently labeled receptors were initially distributed on the cell surface and formed patches that subsequently internalized (at 37° C) into endocytic vesicles. These processes were dependent on specific binding sites for the peptide and conceivably could be the vesicular, intracellular binding sites of GnRH reported previously (Sternberger and Petrali, 1975). An independent report (Naor *et al.*, 1981) subsequently confirmed the sequence of events described above using the identical technique. Duello and Nett (1980) and Hazum (1982) have used autoradiography to show internalization of GnRH and its analogs. They indicated that uptake and length of retention correlate well with biological potency. Studies (Jennes *et al.*, 1983) using ferritin and colloidal gold derivatives of GnRH have produced high-resolution microscopic views, suggesting movement of the GnRH-receptor complex to the Golgi and lysosomal compartments is consistent with observations made in other systems.

### I. GnRH INTERNALIZATION IS NOT REQUIRED FOR STIMULATION OF GONADOTROPIN RELEASE

Our interest in internalization of the GnRH-receptor complex was that this phenomena might be involved in the mechanism by which GnRH stimulates gonadotropin release. In order to determine whether patching, capping, and internalization were involved, we examined gonadotropin release under circumstances in which internalization was blocked (either by GnRH-analog immobilization or by incubation in the presence of vinblastine) or when the cells were stimulated under conditions in which only internalized GnRH was available. In one approach (Conn *et al.*, 1981d) a GnRH analog, D-Lys$^6$-GnRH (Fig. 1), was coupled by its $\epsilon$ amino group with an *N*-hydroxy succinimide ester, then, through a 10 Å spacer arm, to a cross-linked agarose matrix. Exposure of the product to proteases, soaps, detergents, solvents, chaotropic agents, or cell cultures resulted in dissociation of at most $< 0.28\%$ of biologically active releasing hormone. Although the apparent potency of the immobilized analog was one-fourth that of the free form, it was still capable of evoking a full LH secretory response. In other covalent immobilization studies, a more potent agonist, D-Lys$^6$-des$^{10}$-Pro$^9$ethylamide GnRH, was prepared with a high ratio of agonist to bead. This resulted in a derivative that stimulated LH release with full efficacy. Because of the increased potency of this compound and the increased molar coupling ratio, the quantity of LH release was restricted, however, by the number of beads added at concentrations of releasing hormone sufficient to evoke release. This finding was interpreted as added evidence that the immobilization of the agonist was stable during the bioassay and indicated that LH release could be stimulated with full efficacy without the requirement for GnRH internalization.

In order to confirm these findings by an independent means, a comparative study (Conn and Hazum, 1981) was undertaken using image-intensified microscopy and the cell-culture bioassay. With these techniques, it was possible to show that vinblastine markedly inhibited large-scale patching and capping of the GnRH receptor (viewed by image intensification) but did not alter the $EC_{50}$ or efficacy of LH release stimulated by GnRH or by the agonist described above. Another approach demonstrated that exposure of cells to GnRH evoked LH release, which underwent prompt extinction following removal of GnRH from the incubation medium. Accordingly, a continuous supply of externally applied GnRH appeared to be required for stimulation of LH release. These observations indicated that internalization as well as large-scale patching and capping of the GnRH receptor are not required for LH release. They did not exclude the possibility discussed below that microaggregation (small numbers of receptors, too small to be seen by image intensification) is involved in the mechanism of action of GnRH.

## J. Microaggregation of the GnRH Receptor Leads to Stimulation of LH release

While large-scale patching, capping, and internalization of the GnRH receptor do not appear to be needed for the release process, we have been interested in the possibility that microaggregation of the receptor plays a role in receptor-response coupling. Small receptor microaggregates would provide too small a signal to measure by image intensification (which has a sensitivity of about 40–50 molecules of hormone, Conn and Hazum, 1981; Hazum *et al.*, 1980).

In these studies (Conn *et al.*, 1982a), we have taken advantage of a GnRH *antagonist* [D-pyroGlu$^1$-D-Phe$^2$-D-Trp$^3$-D-Lys$^6$-GnRH ("GnRH-Ant")], which binds to the pituitary GnRH receptor. This antagonist inhibits GnRH-stimulated LH release and alone had no measurable agonist activity up to $10^{-6}$ $M$. The presence of the D-Lys$^6$ both afforded protection against proteolysis (see Section II,A) and introduced a single amino group into this molecule, which could be used for derivatization without loss of receptor-binding activity. Formation of the GnRH-Ant dimer by cross-linking of the (lysyl) amino groups of two molecules with ethylene glycol bis(succinimidyl succinate) (EGS) resulted in a GnRH-Ant dimer joined through a 12–15 Å chain. Since there was only a single reactive group, the reaction of EGS with GnRH-Ant does not lead to larger polymers. The dimer could be purified by gel filtration. Like the parent compound, this dimer was purely an antagonist. When antibody (AB) prepared against D-Lys$^6$-GnRH (which cross-reacts with GnRH-Ant) was incubated with excess dimer, a product was formed that consists of a divalent antibody with a GnRH-Ant dimer attached to each arm {AB-[(GnRH-Ant)EGS-(GnRH-Ant)]2} (Fig. 2). One molecule of

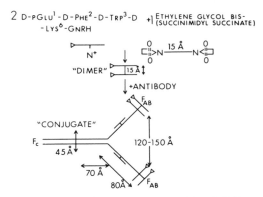

FIG. 2. Formation of the GnRH antagonist conjugate. The GnRH antagonist (D-pGlu[1]-D-Phe[2]-D-Trp[3]-D-Lys[6]-GnRH) is first dimerized through the $\epsilon$ amino group with the bridge ethylene glycol bis(succinimidyl succinate). This dimer of GnRH antagonist is then combined with antibody as shown. The resulting compound consists of two GnRH antagonists, which are available to the receptor (the remaining two being bound to the antibody) and separated by approximately 120–150 Å.

each GnRH-Ant dimer was attached to each antigenic binding site and therefore unavailable to the receptor. The other molecule of each dimer was available to the receptor although bound to the antibody via the 15 Å chain and the other molecule of GnRH-Ant. Thus, the product consisted of two molecules of GnRH-Ant available to the receptor although separated from each other by about 150 Å. In contrast to the parent compounds, this conjugate showed *agonist* action, stimulating LH release from pituitary cultures. Release was calcium dependent and blocked by the anticalmodulin drug, Pimozide, as was stimulation in response to GnRH itself. Conjugate prepared from monovalent AB fragment did not stimulate release; neither the GnRH-Ant dimer nor AB alone stimulate release. Thus, a pure antagonist became an agonist when it was capable of bringing two receptor molecules within a critical distance, $d$ (15 Å $< d <$ 150 Å). The data indicate that formation of the receptor microaggregate itself is sufficient to stimulate a transmembrane response system.

The behavior of the antibody conjugate (A) was modeled on the assumption that it could react with a plasma membrane receptor (R) to form a complex (A·R). The complex could interact with a second receptor to form A·R$_2$. This dimeric receptor could react with a quiescent effector, E (for example, a closed Ca$^{2+}$ ion channel) to form A·R$_2$·E which, now activated, leads to LH release (Fig. 3). An alternate suggestion that the receptors each contain a portion of the ion channel seems unlikely since agents exist which open the Ca$^{2+}$ channel in the absence of GnRH (see Section III,C). The equilibrium equations governing the behavior of the former model were derived, solved, and found to yield a good fit to the experimental data (Blum and Conn, 1982).

In other studies (Conn *et al.*, 1982b), it was possible to show potency enhancement of a GnRH agonist under conditions that favored receptor microaggregation. The EGS dimer of D-Lys⁶-GnRH was prepared and the dose–response curve obtained. The $ED_{50}$ values of D-Lys⁶-GnRH and D-Lys⁶-GnRH dimer (molar in terms of D-Lys⁶-GnRH) were $5 \times 10^{-10}$ $M$ and $8 \times 10^{-10}$ $M$. The $ED_{10}$ value for the dimer was approximately $3 \times 10^{-11}$ $M$ in terms of D-Lys⁶-GnRH concentration or $1.5 \times 10^{-11}$ $M$ in terms of dimer. This concentration was selected for further study.

Figure 4 shows (solid symbol) the effect of adding the indicated titer of antibody after addition of $1.5 \times 10^{-11}$ $M$ dimer followed by cross-reactive antisera. Optimum potentiation is seen at antibody titer $1:10^5–1:10^6$. For comparison, $10^{-7}$ $M$ D-Lys⁶-GnRH-stimulated LH release was $58 \pm 6$ ng (100 ng DNA in this study). The antibody cross-linked dimer thus stimulated response at about the $ED_{40}$ level. Monovalent antibody (i.e., reduced pep-

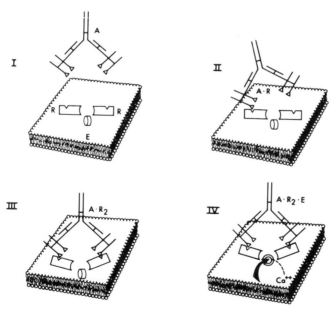

Fig. 3. The ligand receptor effector model (LREM). In this model the GnRH antagonist conjugate is seen as binding to two separate receptor molecules. The complex of this conjugate and the two receptors are then able to activate the effector (in this system, a calcium ion channel). The mathematics of fit for this model has been presented in Blum and Conn (1982). [From Blum and Conn (1982).]

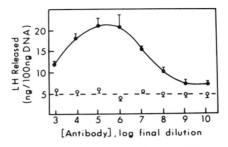

FIG. 4. Potentiation of the action of $1.5 \times 10^{-11}$ $M$ GnRH agonist dimer by indicated addition of antisera to D-Lys6-GnRH. GnRH agonist (D-Lys6-GnRH) was dimerized by using ethylene glycol bis(succinimidyl succinate) as described for GnRH antagonist in Fig. 2. An $ED_{10}$ dose of the dimer was allowed to incubate with gonadotrope cell cultures; then antibody was added at the indicated final dilution (solid symbol). The open symbol shows lack of activity of antisera alone. Maximal LH release was $58 \pm 6$ ng LH per 100 ng DNA in response to $10^{-7}$ $M$ D-Lys6-GnRH. Unstimulated release was $5 \pm 0.5$ ng per 100 ng DNA in this experiment. [Reprinted with permission from Conn *et al.* (1982b). © 1982 by the Endocrine Society, the Williams and Wilkins Company, agent.]

sin fragments) was ineffective in stimulating release in the presence of $1.5 \times 10^{-11}$ $M$ dimer (mean release $= 5.1 \pm 0.5$ ng/100 ng DNA at all titers). Likewise, addition of 5 μ$M$ Pimozide or 2 m$M$ EGTA diminished LH release ($\geq$ 90%, at all titers in the presence of $1.5 \times 10^{-11}$ $M$ dimer). Addition of antibody alone did not stimulate LH release over basal levels ($5.0 \pm 0.5$ ng/100 ng DNA). Thus, addition of antibody prepared against D-Lys6-GnRH to (D-Lys6)$_2$-EGS dimer enhances the potency of the dimer; that is, the dimer was able to stimulate gonadotropin release at concentrations which, in the absence of antibody, were minimally effective. These observations support the view that formation of a microaggregate of the GnRH receptor is sufficient to transduce the signal across the plasma membrane and elicit cell responses if the separation distance between ligands is increased to a critical point. The dimer alone, with only a 15 Å bridge length, is unable to do this, while the conjugate [i.e., (dimer)$_2$-antibody complex about 150 Å bridge length] is apparently of sufficient length.

While it is clear that microaggregation of the receptor is a sufficient criteria to stimulate release, it is of interest to consider whether GnRH itself acts via this mechanism. It is unlikely that the releasing hormone itself bridges two receptors since it is neither multivalent nor sufficiently long to do so. A more likely possibility is that receptor occupancy by an agonist alters the receptor structure in such a way as to increase the probability of microaggregation. For example, occupancy (by an agonist) might increase freedom of lateral mobility of the receptor in the plasma membrane by releasing it from an anchoring attachment; alternatively, a conformational change might occur such that complementary binding sites are exposed. It is also possible that occupancy activates enzymes that catalyze the formation of disulfide, or peptide, or tyrosyl bonds and thereby link receptors (Davies *et al.*, 1980; King and Cuatrecases, 1981; Hazum *et al.*, 1981). An antagonist would be viewed as occupying the binding site without affecting these changes.

It is interesting to note that Concanavalin A inhibits GnRH-stimulated LH release (Ponsin *et al.*, 1980). Since this lectin does not interfere with GnRH binding by the receptor (Hazum, 1982), it is tempting to speculate that it may interfere with receptor mobility in the lateral plane of the plasma membrane.

Several lines of evidence indicate that microaggregation of plasma membrane receptors is required for activation of some other plasma-membrane regulated systems. In the case of epidermal growth factor (EGF)-stimulated mitogenesis in 3T3 fibroblasts (Shechter *et al.*, 1979), it has been shown that cyanogen bromide treatment of EGF results in a molecule (CN-EGF) that binds to the EGF receptor but does not elicit mitogenesis. Addition of bivalent EGF antibody, which presumably brings together the occupied receptors, results in activation of mitogenesis. For insulin receptors, the importance of microaggregation has been suggested by the observation that anti-insulin receptor antibodies stimulate insulin-like functions in target tissues (Jacobs *et al.*, 1978). Bivalent antibodies are required for such stimulation (Kahn *et al.*, 1978), indicating the importance of a receptor microaggregation in this process. While intellectually attractive, it can not yet be stated with certainty that the microaggregate is the precursor of large-scale patching, capping, and internalization. Alternatively, both processes may compete for receptors.

## III. CALCIUM AS A SECOND MESSENGER FOR GnRH

It was apparent from early studies with hemipituitaries and pituitary slices (Samli and Geschwind, 1968) that the ionic makeup of the incubation medium, especially with regard to $Ca^{2+}$, influenced the release of pituitary hormones. While these studies were not conclusive since they relied on crude hypothalamic extracts (synthetic releasing hormones had not yet been prepared), they indicated the importance of calcium (Geschwind, 1969; McCann, 1971; Vale *et al.*, 1967). It was shown (Samli and Geschwind, 1968) that while $Ca^{2+}$ was required for optimal release of LH, changes in extracellular $Ca^{2+}$ levels did not alter the pattern of incorporation of [$^{14}C$]leucine into pituitary LH. In addition, metabolic inhibitors (dinitrophenol and oligomycin) at concentrations sufficient to inhibit 75% of the leucine incorporation into LH did not alter gonadotropin release. These observations suggested that LH biosynthesis and LH release are distinct processes and that $Ca^{2+}$ was involved in pituitary LH release but not in its biosynthesis. Wakabayashi *et al.* (1969) showed that optimal stimulation of pituitary LH release in response to hypothalamic extract required extracellular $Ca^{2+}$ and that ethylenediaminetetraacetic acid (EDTA) inhibited release. Although these studies demonstrated that $Ca^{2+}$ was needed for the release process, its status as a "second messenger" was not established. We proposed (Marian and Conn, 1979) criteria that would have to be fulfilled to establish $Ca^{2+}$ as a second messenger of GnRH action. First, removal of $Ca^{2+}$ from its site of action must block LH release in response to GnRH. Second, as a direct consequence of stimulation with GnRH, it should be possible to demonstrate the movement of $Ca^{2+}$ (either from internal stores or from the extracellular spaces) into a site that can be linked directly to LH release. Third, any manipulation that results in movement of $Ca^{2+}$ to this site should evoke LH release independent of stimulation by GnRH.

## A. The Locus of Calcium Action Is Subsequent to GnRH Recognition

The first criterion that was fulfilled in order to implicate $Ca^{2+}$ in the mechanism of GnRH action was the demonstration that GnRH did not stimulate gonadotropin release in the absence of extracellular $Ca^{2+}$ or in the presence of drugs that blocked $Ca^{2+}$ entry from the extracellular medium (Marian and Conn, 1979; Conn *et al.*, 1980b; Stern and Conn, 1981). This requirement has been fulfilled in rat (Marian and Conn, 1979; Stern and Conn, 1981), pig (Hopkins and Walker, 1978), and sheep (Adams and Nett, 1979). The structure–function relationships for $Ca^{2+}$ ion-channel antagonists suggest that the channel is not identical to that described in contractile tissue (Conn *et al.*, 1983).

In the rat-cell culture system we have demonstrated that return of $Ca^{2+}$ to the medium of cells preincubated without $Ca^{2+}$ serves to restore responsiveness to GnRH (Conn and Rogers, 1979). Because the $Ca^{2+}$ requirement for responsiveness could reflect a permissive action for the binding of GnRH to its plasma membrane receptor, we examined (Marian and Conn, 1980) the ionic requirements for binding. In these studies, we employed a superactive, degradation-resistant GnRH analog, D-ser-(t-Bu)[6]-des gly[10]EA-GnRH (Buserelin, Hoechst Pharmaceutical Company). This molecule (fully described in Section II,A) can be derivatized with [125]I to high specific activity with retention of about 30–50% binding (Marian *et al.*, 1981). $Ca^{2+}$ did not exert a permissive effect for binding of the analog to this site; in fact, at high concentrations (>10 m$M$) it actually inhibited specific binding due to an effect on affinity, which dropped from $4 \times 10^9 \ M^{-1}$ at $<10^{-6} \ M$ $Ca^{2+}$ to $9 \times 10^8 \ M^{-1}$ at $10 \ mM \ Ca^{2+}$. Accordingly, the $Ca^{2+}$ requirement for GnRH-stimulated release cannot be explained simply by a permissive effect at the receptor as clearly demonstrated by the inverse correlation between the $Ca^{2+}$ requirement for GnRH-stimulated LH release and the effect at the receptor. The inhibitory effects observed with $Ca^{2+}$ are not specific for this ion since inhibition of receptor binding is also seen with $Ba^{2+}$, $Mn^{2+}$, $Co^{2+}$, $Mg^{2+}$, $Na^+$, and $La^{3+}$. While all of the ions listed decrease specific binding to the GnRH receptor, their effects on GnRH-stimulated LH release are markedly different. At the concentration used, $Ba^{2+}$ acts as a secretogogue; $Mg^{2+}$ has no effect; and $La^{3+}$, $Mn^{2+}$, and $Co^{2+}$ are inhibitory. Thus, these studies suggest that the specific action of $Ca^{2+}$ occurs at a locus after the initial recognition of GnRH by its receptor.

## B. EVIDENCE FOR CALCIUM FLUX AS THE FIRST MEASURABLE EVENT AFTER GnRH BINDING

The second criterion for $Ca^{2+}$ as an intracellular mediator for GnRH action required demonstration of movement of $Ca^{2+}$ into an active site prior to release of LH. Technical problems make direct demonstration of $^{45}Ca^{2+}$ uptake difficult (Putney, 1979), although it has been possible to do so in some cases (Hopkins and Walker, 1978) by relying on special manipulations. By preloading cells with $^{45}Ca^{2+}$ and using the efflux of this isotope to measure channel activity, Williams (1976) first used a perifusion system of hemipituitaries to demonstrate that opening of a $Ca^{2+}$ channel could be seen at an early time following administration of GnRH. Ovariectomy appears to enhance the magnitude of the $Ca^{2+}$ flux relative to the background. The samples were not collected at small enough intervals, however, to determine the precise temporal relation between LH release and $Ca^{2+}$ flux. Although there was a dose–response relation between GnRH and $Ca^{2+}$ flux, the flux was not shown to be a specific action of GnRH. We have confirmed (Conn et al., 1981b) Williams' observations and extended them by demonstrating that $Ca^{2+}$ mobilization actually *precedes* LH release and is a specific function of GnRH. Release of $^{45}Ca^{2+}$ from preloaded cells was measured at short intervals following addition of either GnRH or an inactive analog [des[1] GnRH (2–10)] to the pituitary slices (Conn et al., 1981b). LH was determined in aliquots taken at the same times. Our results extend Williams' findings and suggest that (1) GnRH specifically stimulates efflux of $^{45}Ca^{2+}$ from preloaded gonadotropes; (2) flux occurs rapidly ($<1.5$ minutes) after GnRH administration, preceding measurable LH release, and (3) $^{45}Ca^{2+}$ flux and LH release cannot be uncoupled.

## C. Increases in Intracellular Calcium Also Evoke LH Release

The third requirement that implicated $Ca^{2+}$ as a mediator of GnRH action was the observation that compounds which themselves stimulated increased $Ca^{2+}$ levels in the cytosol also stimulated LH release. We showed that this occurs even in the absence of GnRH. Thus, the connection may be made between $Ca^{2+}$ mobilization itself and LH release even in the absence of GnRH receptor occupancy. Three approaches to assessing $Ca^{2+}$ mobilization have been useful. Cytosolic $Ca^{2+}$ can be increased by the following: (1) Addition of bacterial ionophores; (2) insertion by liposome fusion; or (3) activation of endogenous ion channels by membrane depolarizing agents.

We have used the three calcium ionophores that are currently available; are all bacterial products that bind $Ca^{2+}$ and, due to their hydrophobic nature, insert themselves into the plasma membrane to provide a specific conduit for $Ca^{2+}$. When ionophore A23187 (Lilly) was added to the pituitary cultures in the presence of 1 m$M$ $Ca^{2+}$, the cells responded with release of LH (Conn *et al.*, 1979). This response was dose and time dependent and required extracellular $Ca^{2+}$. Ionomycin (Squibb; Conn *et al.*, 1980a) and X537A (Roche; Conn *et al.*, 1979) also stimulated LH release; but in contrast to A23187 and Ionomycin, however, X537A did not require extracellular $Ca^{2+}$. A series of experiments suggested that X537A may have released $Ca^{2+}$ from intracellular pools (such as those in the mitochondria, Conn *et al.*, 1979).

Liposomes (lipid vesicles) have the interesting characteristics of inserting their contents into living cells and, accordingly, have been used for insertion of drugs, messenger RNA, and ions. We showed that $Ca^{2+}$-bearing liposomes, but neither $Mg^{2+}$-bearing nor monovalent ion-containing liposomes, successfully evoked LH release from pituitary cells (Conn *et al.*, 1979). Thus, it appeared that in addition to a $Ca^{2+}$ requirement for GnRH-stimulated LH release, insertion of $Ca^{2+}$ even in the absence of GnRH was sufficient to stimulate LH release.

In order to explore possible routes of ion entry into the gonadotrope, we used drugs that exert direct effects on ion channels and determined their effects on the release of LH. Veratridine, which activates the $Na^+$ channel of electrically excitable cells and on depolarization allows extracellular $Ca^{2+}$ to enter, stimulated LH release from the cultures (Conn and Rogers, 1980). The response was measurable 15 minutes after the addition of veratridine and was maximal at 180 minutes, displaying an efficacy similar to that for GnRH. The time course for veratridine-stimulated LH release was similar to that seen in response to GnRH or ionophoretic $Ca^{2+}$ mobilization and was consistent with the view that the rate-limiting step in stimulated LH release from these cells occurs after $Ca^{2+}$ mobilization. Veratridine-stimulated LH release was blocked by tetrodotoxin (TTX, $10^{-5} M$), by chelation of $Ca^{2+}$ with EGTA, by low $Na^+$-containing medium, or by D600. Both GnRH-stimulated and veratridine-stimulated LH release required extracellular $Ca^{2+}$; however, GnRH was not blocked by TTX or by low $Na^+$.

In addition to veratridine, aconitine and batrachotoxin produced TTX-sensitive LH release which additionally required $Ca^{2+}$ and $Na^+$. This suggests that the site of action for all these agents is similar to that reported in nervous tissue. Veratridine appears to stimulate LH release via $Ca^{2+}$ mobilization resulting from activation of the $Na^+$ channel, while GnRH-stimulated $Ca^{2+}$ mobilization is not mediated via the $Na^+$ channel. Indeed, the ability of D600 (which blocks the $Ca^{2+}$ channels) to block GnRH action suggests that the GnRH receptor may be functionally coupled, perhaps as a result of microaggregation, to a distinct $Ca^{2+}$ channel. In addition to providing a method for $Ca^{2+}$ mobilization by stimulation of endogenous ion channels, these results suggest considerable functional homology between the pituitary gonadotrope and neural tissue, which also contain these channels.

## D. Calmodulin Appears to Be the Site of Calcium Action in the Pituitary

One likely intracellular target for $Ca^{2+}$ action is calmodulin (CaM), a ubiquitous intracellular $Ca^{2+}$ receptor that has been shown to modulate many cellular processes, including cyclic nucleotide and glycogen metabolism, protein phosphorylation, microtubule assembly and disassembly, and $Ca^{2+}$ flux, as well as the activity of NAD kinase, tryptophan 5' monoxidase, and phospholipase $A_2$. In order to explore this possibility, a specific and sensitive radioimmunoassay for calmodulin was to used to determine its quantity and distribution in the gonadotrope before and during GnRH-stimulated LH release (Conn *et al.*, 1981a).

GnRH was administered by subcutaneous injection to ovariectomized rats 5–7 weeks old, which had been ovariectomized at 24 days of age. After 35 minutes (or as indicated in the time-course study), the rats were killed by decapitation. Trunk blood was collected and serum LH determined by RIA. The pituitary was removed, homogenized, and filtered through organza cloth. Nuclear, plasma membrane, mitochondrial/granule, microsomal, and cytosolic fractions were identified by marker enzymes (aldolase, glucose 6-phosphatase, malic dehydrogenase, NADH cytochrome C reductase, and 5' nucleotidase) and chemical analysis for DNA, protein, and LH using standard methods. These analyses indicated less than 10% cross-contamination between fractions. Aliquots of these fractions were stored at $-70°$ C, then heat treated and assayed for CaM by RIA.

The distribution of CaM in the fractions was expressed as a percentage of the total immunoassayable activity in the homogenate. There was an initial rise in the percentage of CaM associated with the plasma membrane, which appears concomitantly with the depletion of the cytosolic CaM. The increase occurs with a time course similar to secretion of LH into the blood. As the CaM begins to be cleared from the plasma membrane fraction, its level increases first in the mitochondrial/granule and microsomal fractions and finally in the cytosol. There is also a dose–response relation between plasma membrane accumulation of CaM and its cytosolic depletion. A chemically similar analog [des¹GnRH(2–10)], which has no efficacy in stimulating LH release and does not bind to the GnRH receptor (Marian *et al.*, 1981), also did not stimulate CaM redistribution.

Since CaM synthesis is constitutive in all systems examined (including the GnRH-stimulated pituitary, Chafouleas *et al.*, 1980), the possibility remains that the redistribution was caused by translocation between cellular compartments. The apparent initial accumulation at the plasma membrane may allow CaM to exert regulatory functions at that locus.

While translocation of CaM as such has not been reported previously, there are observations in other systems which indicate that such an event occurs. In the red blood cell, islet cell, and adipocyte (Larsen and Vincenzi, 1979; Pershadsingh and McDonald, 1980) CaM-activated ATPases are located at the plasma membrane. In the case of the adipocyte, $Ca^{2+}$ ATPases appear to be hormonally regulated and activated in response to insulin. Although CaM redistribution may be either a cause or a consequence of the secretory process, a role for CaM seems to be emerging. Steinhardt and Alderton (1982) have provided evidence to suggest that CaM confers calcium sensitivity on secretory exocytosis. CaM has been found at the postsynaptic membrane and appears to mediate the $Ca^{2+}$ effects on synaptic transmission (Grab *et al.*, 1979; Ilundain and Naftalin, 1979) and may, accordingly, have a role in the release of neurotransmitters.

### E.  Calmodulin Antagonists Inhibit GnRH-Stimulated LH Release at a Postreceptor and Postcalcium Mobilization Locus

Additional support for the involvement of CaM in the mechanism of action of GnRH comes from the observation that Pimozide is a noncompetitive antagonist of GnRH-stimulated LH release from pituitary cell cultures. For this and several other neurotropic agents (penfluridol, chlordiazepoxide, chlorpromazine), the concentration needed to inhibit 50% of LH release in response to GnRH correlated well with the ability to inhibit enzyme activation by CaM *in vitro* (Conn *et al.*, 1981c). Pimozide does not alter the $K_a$ or $N_o$ of releasing hormone binding by the GnRH receptor. The additional observation that Pimozide inhibits $Ca^{2+}$ ionophore (A23187 and Ionomycin)-stimulated LH release suggests that the locus of Pimozide action is after $Ca^{2+}$ mobilization. Because Pimozide is known to bind and inactivate the $Ca^{2+}$-CaM complex and because $Ca^{2+}$ is a second messenger for GnRH, it is likely that CaM is the target of action of these drugs. These observations may be useful to indicate the basis for the clinical reports of inhibition of LH release in humans receiving Pimozide (Ojeda *et al.*, 1974; Leppaluoto *et al.*, 1976) or other antipsychotics (DeWied, 1967). Recent studies (Conn, 1982) have indicated that naphthalenesulfonamide CaM antagonists (Hidaka and Tanaka, 1983; Hart *et al.*, 1983) also inhibit GnRH-stimulated LH release.

## IV. PITUITARY ACTIONS OF GnRH OTHER THAN STIMULATION OF GONADOTROPIN RELEASE

Occupancy of the GnRH receptor by an agonist results in gonadotropin release, homologous receptor regulation, gonadotropin biosynthesis, and possibly other unidentified actions. In order to develop a detailed model of GnRH action, it is significant to determine if these are proximal results of occupancy or due to other events, themselves stimulated by occupancy. For example, are biosynthesis and tissue desensitization proximally caused by receptor occupancy or, for example, are they caused by gonadotropin depletion due to release?

We recently (Smith and Conn, 1983b) examined a model for GnRH-stimulated homologous desensitization using immobilized perifused cells. It was possible to evoke desensitization within 1 hour following a 20-minute pulse of as little as $10^{-9} M$ GnRH. It quickly became apparent that desensitization: (1) Required receptor occupancy by an agonist (an antagonist was ineffective); (2) did not require extracellular $Ca^{2+}$, unlike LH release; and (3) was not evoked by $Ca^{2+}$ ionophore A23187 (unlike LH release). Thus, conditions could be established in which desensitization occurred without LH release and in which LH release occurred without desensitization. The data are summarized in Table II.

Accordingly, LH release and desensitization are both proximal actions of receptor occupancy by an agonist but appear to be mediated by different mechanisms.

TABLE II

COMPARISON OF REQUIREMENTS OF GONADOTROPE
DESENSITIZATION AND LH RELEASE IN RESPONSE TO GnRH[a]

|  | Desensitization | LH release |
|---|---|---|
| Stimulated by receptor oc-<br>cupancy by an agonist | Yes | Yes |
| Stimulation by receptor oc-<br>cupancy by an antagonist | No | No |
| Extracellular $Ca^{2+}$ |  |  |
| Inhibited by EGTA | No | Yes |
| Inhibited by $Ca^{2+}$ ion<br>channel antagonist | No | Yes |
| Stimulated by $Ca^{2+}$<br>ionophore | No | Yes |

[a] Evidence that gonadotrope desensitization to GnRH is not due to
gonadotropin depletion and may be uncoupled from LH release.

## V. EXTRAPITUITARY SITES OF ACTION OF GnRH AND CROSS-REACTIVE SUBSTANCES

While most of the work on the mechanism of action of GnRH and on its receptor have been done in the pituitary, it is apparent that GnRH (or substances that cross-react at its pituitary receptor) are present in gonadal, neural, and other tissues. Little information is available to indicate whether these compounds have similar mechanisms of action to GnRH in the pituitary; however, it is clear that nonpituitary tissues contain receptors which bind GnRH analogs with high affinity and specificity. Specific and direct biological effects can be attributed to occupancy of GnRH binding sites in several systems. Hypothalamic GnRH origin does not enter the circulation at concentrations that allow substantial occupancy of these receptors. Accordingly, it has been necessary to look for extrapituitary sites of synthesis of these compounds. A discussion of these has been presented previously (see Section V in Conn *et al.*, 1981b; Hsueh and Jones, 1981).

## VI. CONCLUSIONS

A large body of evidence from ours and other laboratories suggests that occupancy of the GnRH receptor (1) leads to mobilization of calcium (2) and release of gonadotropin from preexisting storage granules (3). While experimental evidence indicates that these steps are integrated, it is only very recently that progress has been made to indicate the molecular basis of this integration. It appears that while patching, capping, and internalization occur as early steps in the mechanism of GnRH action, these are not requisite for stimulation of release (although they have not been excluded as having a role in biosynthesis or other processes). Microaggregation of receptors (too small to see by image intensification) may form the basis for activation of receptors. Indeed, such findings indicate that the information needed for activating the response system (secretion) resides within the receptor, not the stimulating ligand. The observation that pituitary CaM redistribution follows pituitary stimulation with GnRH and that CaM-antagonistic drugs inhibit GnRH-stimulated release at a site of action after calcium mobilization indicates a possible role of CaM in this system.

NOTE ADDED IN PROOF

It has been possible to show that microaggregation of the GnRH receptor stimulates biphasic receptor regulation and desensitization much like the releasing hormone itself (Conn *et al.*, 1984; Smith and Conn, 1984). The role of $Ca^{2+}$ in receptor regulation has also been identified (Conn *et al.*, 1984).

## ACKNOWLEDGMENTS

Work described from the author's laboratory was supported by NIH grants HD13220, RCDA HD00337, and the Mellon Foundation. Aging studies were supported by NIH grant AG1204. The author is a senior fellow of the Center for the Study of Aging and Human Development.

## REFERENCES

Adams, T. E., and Nett, T. M. (1979). *Biol. Reprod.* **21**, 1073–1086.
Bauer, T. W., Moriarty, C. M., and Childs, G. V. (1981). *J. Histochem. Cytochem.* **29**, 1171–1178.
Benuck, M., and Marks, N. (1976). *Life Sci.* **19**, 1271–1276.
Bex, F., and Corbin, A. (1982). *In* "Hormone Antagonists" (M. K. Agarwal, ed.), pp. 609–622. de Gruyter, Berlin.
Blum, J. J., and Conn, P. M. (1982). *Proc. Natl. Acad. Sci. U.S.A.*, **79**, 7307–7311.
Chafouleas, J. A., Conn, P. M., Dedman, J. R., and Means, A. R. (1980). *Endocrinology (Baltimore)* **106A**, p. 289 (Abstract).
Clayton, R. N., Shakespear, R. A., and Marshall, J. C. (1978). *Mol. Cell. Endocrinol.* **11**, 63–78.
Clayton, R. N., Shakespear, R. A., Duncan, J. A., and Marshall, J. C. (1979). *Endocrinology (Baltimore)* **105**, 1369–1376.
Clayton, R. N., Solano, A. R., Garcia-Vela, A., Dufau, M. L., Catt, K. J. (1980). *Endocrinology (Baltimore)* **107**, 699–706.
Conn, P. M., (1982). *In* "Role of Drugs and Electrolytes in Hormonogenesis" (S. B. Pal, ed.). de Gruyter, Berlin, in press.

Conn, P. M., and Hazum, E. (1981). *Endocrinology (Baltimore)* **109**, 2040–2045.
Conn, P. M., and Rogers, D. C. (1979). *Life Sci.* **24**, 2461–2466.
Conn, P. M., and Rogers, D. C. (1980). *Endocrinology (Baltimore)* **107**, 2133–2134.
Conn, P. M., Rogers, D. C., and Sandhu, F. S. (1979). *Endocrinology (Baltimore)* **105**, 1122–1127.
Conn, P. M., Kilpatrick, D., and Kirshner, N. (1980a). *Cell Calcium* **1**, 129–133.
Conn, P. M., Marian, J., McMillian, M., and Rogers, D. (1980b). *Cell Calcium* **1**, 7–20.
Conn, P. M., Chafouleas, J., Rogers, D., and Means, A. R. (1981a). *Nature (London)* **292**, 264–265.
Conn, P. M., Marian, J., McMillian, M., Stern, J. E., Rogers, D. R., Hamby, M., Penna, A., and Grant, E. (1981b). *Endocr. Rev.* **2**, 174–185.
Conn, P. M., Rogers, D. R., and Sheffield, T. (1981c). *Endocrinology (Baltimore)* **109**, 1122–1126.
Conn, P. M., Smith, R. G., and Rogers, D. C. (1981d). *J. Biol. Chem.* **256**, 1098–1100.
Conn, P. M., Rogers, D. C., Stewart, J. M., Neidel, J., and Sheffield, T. (1982a). *Nature (London)* **296**, 653–655.
Conn, P. M., Rogers, D. C., and McNeil, R. (1982b). *Endocrinology (Baltimore)* **111**, 335–337.
Conn, P. M., Rogers, D. C., and Seay, S. G. (1983). *Endocrinology (Baltimore)*, in press.
Conn, P. M., Rogers, D. C., and Seay, S. G. (1984). *Mol. Pharmacol.*, in press.
Conne, B. S., Aubert, M. L., Sizonenko, P. C. (1979). *Biochem. Biophys. Res. Commun.* **90**, 1249–1256.
Dalkin, A. C., Bourne, G. A., Pieper, D. R., Regiani, S., and Marshall, J. C. (1981). *Endocrinology (Baltimore)* **108**, 1658–1663.
Davies, P. J. A., Davies, D. R., Levitzki, A., Maxfield, F. R., Milhaud, P., Willingham, M. C., and Pasten, I. H. (1980). *Nature (London)* **283**, 162–167.
DeWied, D. (1967). *Pharmacol. Rev.* **19**, 251–275.
Duello, T. M., and Nett, T. M. (1980). *Mol. Cell. Endocrinol.* **19**, 101–112.
Duello, T. M., Nett, T. M., Farquhar, M. G. (1981). *J. Cell Biol.* **91**, 220a (Abstract).
Frager, M. S., Pieper, D. R., Tonetta, J. A., and Marshall, J. C. (1981). *J. Clin. Invest.* **67**, 615–621.
Fujino, M., Fukuda, T., Shinagawa, S., Kobayashi, S., Yamazaki, I., and Nakayama, R. (1974). *Biochem. Biophys. Res. Commun.* **60**, 406–413.
Geschwind, I. I. (1969). *In* "Frontiers in Neuroendocrinology" (L. Martini and W. F. Ganong, eds.), pp. 389–431. Oxford Univ. Press, New York.
Grab, D. J., Berzins, K., Cohen, R. S., and Siekevitz, P. (1979). *J. Biol. Chem.* **254**, 8690–8696.
Grant, G., Vale, W. W., Rivier, J. (1973). *Biochem. Biophys. Res. Commun.* **50**, 771–778.
Griffiths, E. C., and Kelly, J. A. (1979). *Mol. Cell. Endocrinol.* **14**, 3–17.
Hart, R., Bates, M. D., Cormier, M. J., Rosen, G. M., and Conn, P. M. (1983). *In* "Methods in Enzymology, Vol. 102: Hormone Action, Part G" (A. R. Means and B. W. O'Malley, eds.), pp. 195–204. Academic Press, New York.
Hazum, E. (1981). *Endocrinology (Baltimore)* **109**, 1281–1283.
Hazum, E. (1982). *Mol. Cell. Endocrinol.* **26**, 217–222.
Hazum, E., and Nimrod, A. (1982). *Proc. Natl. Acad. Sci. U.S.A.* **79**, 1747–1750.
Hazum, E., Cuatrecasas, P., Marian, J., and Conn, P. M. (1980). *Proc. Natl. Acad. Sci. U.S.A.* **77**, 6692–6695.
Hazum, E., Chang, K.-J., and Cuatrecasas, P. (1981). *Nature (London)* **282**, 626–628.
Hidaka, H., and Tanaka, T. (1983). *In* Methods in Enzymology, Vol. 102: Hormone Action, Part G" (A. R. Means and B. W. O'Malley, eds.). pp. 185–194. Academic Press, New York.
Hopkins, C. R., and Walker, A. M. (1978). *Mol. Cell. Endocrinol.* **12**, 189–208.

Hsueh, A. J. W., and Jones, P. B. C. (1981). *Endocr. Rev.* **2**, 437–461.
Ilundain, A., and Naftalin, R. J. (1979). *Nature (London)* **279**, 446–448.
Jacobs, S., Chang, K.-J., and Cuatrecasas, P. (1978). *Science* **200**, 1283–1284.
Jayatilak, P. G. (1982). *Prog. 64th Annu. Meet. Endo. Soc.*, San Francisco, California, *1982*, p. 146 (abstract).
Jennes, L., Stumpf, W. E., and Conn, P. M. (1983). *Endocrinology (Baltimore)*, in press.
Kahn, C. R., Baird, K. L., Jarrett, D. B., and Flier, J. S. (1978). *Proc. Natl. Acad. Sci. U.S.A.* **75**, 4209–4213.
King, A. C., and Cuatrecasas, P. (1981). *N. Engl. J. Med.* **305**, 77–88.
Koch, Y., Baram, T., Chobsieng, P., and Fridkin, M. (1974). *Biochem. Biophys. Res. Commun.* **61**, 95–103.
Kochman, K., Kerdelhue, B., Zor, U., and Jutisz, M. (1975). *FEBS Lett.* **50**, 190–194.
Larsen, F. L., and Vincenzi, F. F. (1979). *Science* **204**, 306–308.
Leppaluoto, J., Mannisto, P., Ranta, T., and Linnoila, M. (1976). *Acta. Endocrinol.* **81**, 455–460.
Liscovitch, M., and Koch, Y. (1982). *Peptides* **3**, 55–60.
McCann, S. M., (1971). *In* "Frontiers in Neuroendocrinology" (L. Martini, and W. F. Ganong, eds.), pp. 209–235. Oxford Univ. Press, New York.
Marian, J. M., and Conn, P. M. (1979). *Mol. Pharmacol.* **16**, 196–201.
Marian, J. M., and Conn, P. M. (1980). *Life Sci.* **27**, 87–92.
Marian, J. M., and Conn, P. M. (1983). *Endocrinology (Baltimore)* **112**, 104–112.
Marian, J. M., Cooper, R., and Conn, P. M. (1981). *Mol. Pharmacol.* **19**, 399–405.
Marks, N. (1970). *In* "Subcellular Mechanisms in Reproductive Neuroendocrinology" (F. Naftolin, R. J. Ryan, and J. Davis, eds.), pp. 129–147. Elsevier, Amsterdam.
Marshall, J. C., Shakespear, R. A., Odell, W. D. (1976). *Clin. Endocrinol.* **5**, 671–677.
Maunsbach, A. B. (1974). *In* "Methods in Enzymology, Vol. 31: Biomembranes, Part A" (S. Fleisher and L. Packer, eds.), p. 330. Academic Press, New York.
Meidan, R., and Koch, Y. (1981). *Life Sci.* **28**, 1961–1967.
Millar, R., Rosen, H., Pasqualini, C., and Kerdelhue, B., (1982). *Prog. 64th Annu. Meet Endo. Soc., San Francisco, California*, p. 91 *(abstract)*.
*Naor, Z, Clayton, R. N., Catt, K. J. (1980). Endocrinology (Baltimore)* **107**, 1144–1152.
Naor, Z., Atlas, A., Clayton, R. N., Forman, D. S., Amsterdam, A., and Catt, K. J. (1981). *J. Biol. Chem.* **256**, 3049–3052.
Ojeda, S. R., Harms, P. G., and McCann, S. M. (1974). *Endocrinology (Baltimore)* **94**, 1650–1660.
Pedroza, E., Vilchez-Martinez, J. A., Fishback, J., Arimura, A., Schally, A. V. (1977). *Biochem. Biophys. Res. Commun.* **79**, 234–246.
Perrin, M. H., Rivier, J., and Vale, W. W. (1980). *Endocrinology (Baltimore)* **106**, 1289–1296.
Pershadsingh, H. A., and McDonald, J. M. (1980). *Nature (London)* **281**, 495–497.
Ponsin, G., Khar, A., Kunert-Radek, J., Bennardo, T., and Jutisz, M. (1980). *FEBS Lett.* **113**, 331–334.
Putney, J. W. (1979). *Pharmacol. Rev.* **30**, 209–245.
Samli, M. H., and Geschwind, I. I. (1968). *Endocrinology (Baltimore)* **82**, 225–231.
Savoy-Moore, R. T., Schwartz, N. B., Duncan, J. A., and Marshall, J. C. (1980). *Science* **209**, 942–944.
Shechter, Y., Hernaez, L., Schlessinger, J., and Cuatrecasas, P. (1979). *Nature (London)* **278**, 835–838.
Smith, W. A., and Conn, P. M. (1983a). *In* "Clinical and Experimental Intervention in the Pituitary during Aging" (R. Walker and R. L. Cooper, eds.). Dekker, New York, in press.
Smith, W. A., and Conn, P. M. (1983b). *Endocrinology (Baltimore)* **112**, 408–410.

Smith, W. A., and Conn, P. M. (1984). *Endocrinology (Baltimore)*, in press.

Spona, J. (1973). *FEBS Lett* **34**, 24–26.

Steinhart, R. A., and Alderton, J. M. (1982). *Nature (London)* **295**, 154–155.

Stern, J. E., and Conn, P. M. (1981). *Am. J. Physiol.* **240**, (Endocrinology Section), 504–509.

Sternberger, L. A. (1978). *Histochem. Cytochem.* **26**, 542–544.

Sternberger, L. A., and Petrali, J. P. (1975). *Cell. Tissue Res.* **162**, 141–176.

Vale, W., Burgus, R., and Guillemin, R. (1967). *Experientia* **23**, 853–859.

Wagner, T. O. F., Adams, T. E., Nett, T. M. (1979). *Biol. Reprod.* **20**, 140–149.

Wakabayashi, K., Kamberi, I. A., and McCann, S. M. (1969). *Endocrinology (Baltimore)* **85**, 1046–1056.

White, S. S., and Ojeda, S. R. (1982). *Endocrinology (Baltimore)* **111**, 353–355.

Williams, J. A. (1976). *J. Physiol. (London)* **260**, 105–115.

# CHAPTER 4

# Mechanisms of Biological Signaling by the Insulin Receptor

*Michael P. Czech, Joan Massagué, Jonathan R. Seals, and Kin-Tak Yu*

Department of Biochemistry
University of Massachusetts Medical School
Worcester, Massachusetts

BIOCHEMICAL ACTIONS OF HORMONES, VOL. XI

The sequence of molecular events, which comprises the mechanism of insulin action on the metabolism and growth of its target cells, has proven to be one of the more elusive mysteries in modern endocrinology. Extensive investigation of an impressive variety of hypotheses about this phenomenon has failed to reveal the unifying molecular feature that links the hormone's numerous, diverse actions into a coordinated scheme. Most of these investigations have been guided by the same assumption: the identification of a cellular regulatory molecule, which can act as a mediator or second messenger for insulin action, will provide the key to resolving this question. However, these studies have thus far been inconclusive. Recently, advances in the understanding of two other aspects of the insulin effector system have opened new perspectives on the problem. Studies of insulin receptor structure and function and of the covalent modification of cellular enzymes in response to insulin have become important elements in the investigation of insulin action. Ultimately, it will be necessary to integrate the findings from all three of these approaches to obtain a complete understanding of the mechanism of insulin action. This chapter will briefly review the status of each of these three lines of investigation and assess the possibilities for viewing them in terms of a coordinated mechanism. The role of enzyme phosphorylation–dephosphorylation as a unifying covalent modification observed in response to the insulin effector system will be considered first. Then, the role of the insulin receptor structure as the initiator of these responses will be considered. And finally, the linkage of these two elements by cellular signaling phenomena, such as the generation of insulin mediators, will be discussed.

## I. ENZYME PHOSPHORYLATION AND DEPHOSPHORYLATION AS THE COMMON TERMINAL MECHANISM IN METABOLIC REGULATION BY INSULIN

### A. Insulin Effects of Enzyme Phosphorylation

The concept that insulin action is expressed as a change in the phosphorylation of target proteins has developed in parallel with an increased awareness of the importance of protein phosphorylation as a cellular regulatory mechanism. The earliest investigations of phosphorylation as a modification that altered enzyme activity were carried out using enzymes of glycogen metabolism, which are regulated by insulin. These early studies also demonstrated that changes in enzyme phosphorylation could be associated with enzyme regulation by epinephrine and linked to the hormone–receptor interaction via the "second messenger" function of cAMP and the activation of cAMP-dependent protein kinase. In light of the antagonistic effects of insulin and epinephrine on most metabolic processes, it was hypothesized that these agents acted by respectively decreasing and increasing enzyme phosphorylation via the coordinate modulation of cellular cAMP levels. Subsequently, this simple model has not been borne out, but the concept that protein phosphorylation–dephosphorylation is the terminal covalent enzyme modification in insulin action has been strengthened and expanded by studies of this hypothesis. The corollary to this concept is that it should be possible to identify protein kinases and/or phosphatases whose activity is regulated by insulin in a manner that accounts for the observed phosphorylation changes. It should then be possible to establish a cause-effect linkage between the mechanism by which these enzymes are regulated and an insulin receptor-mediated function. Thus, the importance of specifying emzyme phosphorylation–dephosphorylation as the common link in insulin action is that it allows the hormone effector system to be experimentally and analytically approached from a specific terminal phenomenon. Studies of this type have not yet drawn a complete picture of the mechanism of insulin action but have begun to reveal regulatory components and processes, which may ultimately prove to be pieces of this puzzle.

Development of a scheme that integrates protein phosphorylation changes in insulin action has been complicated by the complex hormone-phosphorylation relationships that have been revealed by numerous studies (Fig. 1). All insulin-regulated enzymes that have been characterized have been

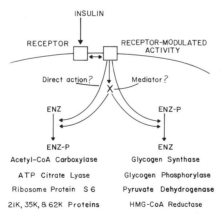

FIG. 1. Role of enzyme phosphorylation and dephosphorylation in insulin action. Insulin increases and decreases the phosphorylation of two separate groups of proteins, implying that the insulin-effector system, the details of which remain unknown, possesses at least two divergent branches.

found to undergo concomitant changes in phosphorylation. As predicted, regulation of the major enzymes of carbohydrate and lipid metabolism, including glycogen synthase (Sheorain *et al.*, 1982) and phosphorylase (Sobrino and Hers, 1980), pyruvate dehydrogenase (Hughes *et al.*, 1980), and HMG-CoA reductase (Ingebritsen *et al.*, 1979), appears to be associated with decreases in the phosphorylation of each enzyme. However, when $^{32}P$ incorporation into total cellular proteins has been studied, insulin has been found to even more dramatically *increase* the labeling of a set of components from various cellular loci (Avruch *et al.*, 1976; Belsham *et al.*, 1980; Benjamin and Singer, 1975; Forn and Greengard, 1976; Smith *et al.*, 1979). These effects did not correlate with any anticipated enzyme alterations; in fact, increases in phosphorylation were observed in some of the same proteins as with cAMP-mediated hormones, and the increases were additive when these hormones were used together with insulin (Avruch *et al.*, 1976; Forn and Greengard, 1976). However, the insulin-stimulated phosphorylations displayed characteristics consistent with biologically relevant actions of insulin (Avruch *et al.*, 1982a). Some of these proteins have since been identified as the enzymes ATP-citrate lyase (Alexander *et al.*, 1979) and acetyl-CoA carboxylase (Witters, 1981; Brownsey and Denton, 1982) and the ribosomal protein S6 (Smith *et al.*, 1979), but no functional change could initially be associated with the phosphorylation change in any of these proteins. The lack of an effect raised the question of whether the observed change in labeling actually represents a stoichiometric change in phosphate incorporation or simply an enrichment of label due to accelerated turnover. Although this issue has not been addressed in all cases, evidence for increased phosphorylation has been presented for ribosomal protein S6 (Nilsen-Hamilton *et al.*, 1981), ATP-citrate lyase (Alexander *et al.*, 1982), and acetyl-CoA carboxylase, the only enzyme in which a change in activity has been ascribed to the change in phosphorylation (Brownsey and Denton, 1982). If increased phosphorylation does occur in all of these cases, then the possibility that it represents a largely silent or noneffective modification must be considered in some cases, although functional effects may yet be revealed where none has previously been found. Regardless of whether increased phosphorylation is ultimately shown to mediate part of insulin's effects or to be physiologically silent, its existence requires that the insulin effector system include at least two separate pathways for the regulation of protein kinase and/or phosphatase activities, with exclusive specificity to discriminate between two classes of proteins. This concept increases the complexity of any hypothetical model, but it is not clear whether this expanded version yet accounts for all of insulin's effects. Many of insulin's effects, including stimulation of glucose transport, macromolecular synthesis, and cell growth, remain to be associated with a change in the phosphorylation of any protein. The ubiquity of protein phosphorylation as a regulatory phenomenon suggests that ultimately these hormone responses will also fall into one of the two categories of phosphorylation-mediated effects and that phosphorylation–dephosphorylation mechanisms will be the single unifying effector in insulin action.

Further analysis of the role of phosphorylation in insulin action requires consideration of the biochemistry of phosphorylation-regulated enzymes. Most protein-bound phosphate is covalently attached to serine or threonine residues, although a small but possibly significant percentage of phosphorylation is found on tryosine residues. All changes in enzyme phosphorylation due to insulin have been found to occur at serine residues. In addition, most enzymes do not contain single phosphorylation sites but contain as many as seven separate phosphorylatable residues (Soderling, 1979). The individual phosphorylation sites appear, in many cases, to be independently regulated and to possess different functional significance for the enzyme. Consistent with this observation, an enzyme may be a substrate for more than one protein kinase and/or phosphatase, each of which may express specificity for only a portion of those sites. This concept of multiple phosphorylation makes measurement of total enzyme phosphorylation potentially misleading. It becomes necessary to consider the specific locus of any change in phosphorylation and to interpret it in terms of the functional properties of that site. This complicates any experimental analysis but also raises the possibility that a unique specificity between enzyme phosphorylation site and protein kinase or phosphatase will provide a link in determining components involved in the hormone effector system. All of these factors must therefore be considered in arriving at an understanding of insulin-dependent, phosphorylation-mediated enzyme regulation.

## B. REGULATION OF GLYCOGEN SYNTHASE BY PHOSPHORYLATION AND BY INSULIN

The insulin-sensitive enzyme whose biochemistry of phosphorylation is best understood is glycogen synthase. The details of this system appear to be unique rather than representative of a general pattern applicable to all enzymes, but its complexity illustrates a wide range of concepts, at least some of which may operate on other enzymes as well. Discussion of this system is complicated by the fact that its numerous components have been studied in different laboratories that use different techniques and nomenclatures. In many cases, the available data are not adequate to determine whether two components with different names actually represent different components or merely a difference in nomenclature or experimental approach. The most comprehensive system of classification of glycogen synthase kinases and phosphatases is that of Cohen (1982). This system will be used here but, where possible, reference to other nomenclatures will be made. The phosphorylation of glycogen synthase will be discussed in terms of the seven phosphorylation sites that have been reported in the enzyme from skeletal muscle (Picton *et al.*, 1982a). All sites are serine residues. Site 2 is located seven residues from the N-terminus of the enzyme. The remaining six sites are located in a large cyanogen bromide fragment at the C-terminus of the enzyme. Sites 3a, 3b, 3c, 5, 1a, and 1b are located, respectively, 30, 34, 38, 46, 87, and 100 residues from the N-terminus of this fragment.

As many as eight distinct protein kinases have been reported to possess some activity toward glycogen synthase. The cAMP-dependent protein kinase, GSk-1, phosphorylates two sites, 1a and 1b (Proud *et al.*, 1977). Site 1a is phosphorylated more rapidly and appears to correlate with decreased enzyme activity. Phosphorylase kinase, GSk-2, phosphorylates a single residue, site 2, which also correlates with decreased enzyme activity (Embi *et al.*, 1979). A glycogen synthase kinase, which like phosphorylase kinase is $Ca^{2+}$ dependent and phosphorylates site 2, has also been reported but appears to be distinct since it exhibits exclusive specificity for glycogen synthase (Woodgett *et al.*, 1982). Several cAMP- and $Ca^{2+}$-independent glycogen synthase kinases have been reported in different tissues by various laboratories. Comparison of these activities is difficult because none exhibit known regulatory properties, their physical properties have been only randomly addressed, and the most discriminating characteristic, their phosphorylation site specificity, remains largely unknown. The available data are consistent with the interpretation that most of these activities can be identified as one of three kinases or as a mixture of them. The first activity, GSk-3, is defined by its ability to phosphorylate sites 3a, 3b, and 3c (Rylatt *et al.*, 1980). Phosphorylation of these sites potently inhibits the enzyme (Embi *et al.*, 1980). A second activity, GSk-4, displays similar physical and enzymatic properties but phosphorylates site 2 specifically (Cohen *et al.*, 1982). These enzymes appear to account for several other reported glycogen synthase kinase activities; they occur as mixtures of GSK-3 and GSK-4, such as CISk-1 (Itarte and Huang, 1979) and others (Schlender *et al.*, 1980; Vila *et al.*, 1982), or as GSk-4 alone, such as $PC_{0.4}$ (DePaoli-Roach *et al.*, 1979) and others (Soderling *et al.*, 1977). A third independent glycogen synthase kinase, GSk-5, uniquely phosphorylates site 5 on the enzyme (Cohen *et al.*, 1982). Phosphorylation of this site does not appear to directly alter enzyme activity. This enzyme appears to be identical with enzymes identified as glycogen synthase kinases $PC_{0.7}$ (DePaoli-Roach *et al.*, 1979) and CISk-2 (Itarte *et al.*, 1977) or as casein kinase 2 (Hathaway and Traugh, 1979), casein kinase TS (Meggio *et al.*, 1977), and troponin-T kinase (Risnik *et al.*, 1980).

In addition to the enzymes described above, several other kinases have been reported to phosphorylate glycogen synthase, but their site specificity and significance are unknown. These include the cGMP-dependent protein kinase (Lincoln and Corbin, 1977) and the $Ca^{2+}$ and phospholipid-stimulated protein kinase C (Kishimoto *et al.*, 1978).

The confusion that characterizes the identification of glycogen synthase phosphatase activities is even greater than that which reigns in the area of protein kinases. This is partially attributable to technical reasons, in that phosphatases appear to possess physical and enzymatic properties that are extremely sensitive to the conditions and methods of isolation and analysis. Thus, a great deal of the available data is conflicting or not comparable at all. In light of this problem, a single classification scheme for glycogen synthase phosphatase activities will be considered without reference to molecular characterization. Two types of phosphatase can be distinguished on the basis of their preference for catalyzing the dephosphorylation of the α or β subunit of phosphorylase kinase. Type 1 phosphatase activity preferentially dephosphorylates the β subunit and accounts for 70–80% of glycogen synthase phosphatase activity in skeletal muscle extracts (Ingebritsen *et al.*, 1980). Type 2 phosphatases preferentially dephosphorylate the α subunit of phosphorylase kinase (Cohen, 1978). Three forms of this activity, 2A, 2B, and 2C, that differ in their substrate specificity or regulatory properties have been identified (Cohen, 1982). Types 1 and 2 phosphatase activity can also be distinguished on the basis of their sensitivity to two protein inhibitors, inhibitor 1 and inhibitor 2 (Cohen, 1981). Type 1 activity is blocked by both inhibitors, while type 2 activity is not (Cohen, 1982). These two types of activity have now been distinguished in several tissues. Unlike protein kinases, these protein phosphatases have not been shown to exhibit any phosphorylation site specificity within glycogen synthase. In fact, phosphatases 1, 2A, and 2C show little substrate specificity and are active on a broad range of enzymes (Cohen, 1982). Phosphatase 2B shows a greater preference for phosphorylase kinase (Stewart *et al.*, 1982). In light of their overlapping activities, it is difficult to distinguish these enzymes with respect to their importance in the regulation of specific processes. The enzymes differ in their regulation. Phosphatase 2B is completely dependent on $Ca^{2+}$ for activity, while phosphatase 2C is completely dependent on $Mg^{2+}$ (Cohen, 1982). Phosphatase 1 is regulated by inhibitors 1 and 2 and also appears to exist in an inactive form, $F_c$, which can be activated in a $Mg^{2+}$ ATP-dependent process (Goris *et al.*, 1980a). Surprisingly, this activation requires GSk-3 activity (Hemmings *et al.*, 1981) and is modulated by inhibitor 2 (Yang *et al.*, 1981). It has been reported that the activation involves phosphorylation of inhibitor 2 with a consequent reduction of its ability to bind and inhibit phosphatase 1 (Hemmings *et al.*, 1982b).

The large number of phosphorylation effectors that act on glycogen synthase presents many opportunities for the regulation of enzyme phosphorylation. The regulatory mechanisms involve interactions among the phosphorylation effectors as well as with other cellular components. Any of these mechanisms may be considered a potential site of hormone action. The first level of regulation is the direct control of protein kinase and phosphatase activity by cellular regulatory components. GSk-1 is stimulated by cAMP in a well-characterized manner (Walsh *et al.*, 1968). GSk-2 (Roach *et al.*, 1978) and the $Ca^{2+}$-dependent glycogen synthase kinase (Woodgett *et al.*, 1982) are stimulated by $Ca^{2+}$, as is phosphatase 2B (Stewart *et al.*, 1982). These enzymes provide a mechanism by which hormones that modulate cAMP and $Ca^{2+}$ are able to directly alter enzyme phosphorylation. Other regulatory mechanisms for the control of enzyme phosphorylation involve interactions among the protein components of the phosphorylation–dephosphorylation system. These include kinase–kinase interactions, kinase–phosphatase interactions, and phosphatase–phosphatase interactions.

The regulation of kinase activity by other protein kinases is a phenomenon that has long been recognized. GSk-1 is known to phosphorylate and activate GSk-2 (Cohen, 1980). Thus, GSk-1 directly phosphorylates glycogen synthase and also indirectly effects its phosphorylation through GSK-2. Other examples of kinase phosphorylation have been reported, but in most cases the effect of this modification on enzyme activity remains unknown. For example, GSk-1 is phosphorylated by GSk-3, GSk-5 (Hemmings *et al.*, 1982a), and by an autophosphorylation reaction (Takio *et al.*, 1982).

The regulation of phosphatase activity by protein kinases does not appear to be direct but is mediated by the activity of inhibitors 1 and 2. Inhibitor 1 is active only when it is phosphorylated by GSk-1 on a threonine residue (Cohen *et al.*, 1977b). Thus, GSk-1 acts in two complementary ways to increase enzyme phosphorylation, either directly, or indirectly by activating an inhibitor of dephosphorylation. In contrast, a system has been described by which protein kinase activity can have the paradoxical effect of activating phosphatase activity. This system involves the activation of the inactive form of phosphatase 1 in a $Mg^{2+}$ ATP-dependent process catalyzed by GSk-3 and modulated by inhibitor 2. It has recently been reported that the inactive form of the enzyme, Fc, consists of a 1:1 complex of phosphatase 1 and inhibitor 2 (Hemmings *et al.*, 1982b). Interaction with $Mg^{2+}$ ATP and GSk-3 results in the phosphorylation of inhibitor 2 on a threonine residue with the resultant dissociation of the complex and activation of the enzyme.

The same processes that allow protein kinases to regulate other kinases and phosphatases should allow protein phosphatases to regulate these enzymes in the opposite direction by dephosphorylating them. Although little data are available concerning this phenomenon, one example has been characterized. The dephosphorylation of inhibitor 1 is catalyzed by phosphatases 1, 2A, and 2B, which is relatively specific for this process (Stewart *et al.*, 1982), as well as by a "deinhibitor protein" (Goris *et al.*, 1980b). In this way, phosphatases may alter the activity of another phosphatase.

A final type of interaction between phosphorylation effectors is an indirect interaction mediated by site–site interactions within the substrate. An example of this has recently been reported in the observation that GSk-3 phosphorylates sites 3a, 3b, and 3c only if site 5 has been phosphorylated by GSk-5 (Picton *et al.*, 1982b). This type of mechanism provides a means by which one kinase can affect the phosphorylation of other sites by altering their suitability as substrates for other kinases. All of the regulatory interactions cited above have the potential to play a role in the propagation of a hormone-induced signal and must be considered in the analysis of a hormone effector system.

The effects of insulin on glycogen synthase have not been conclusively attributed to any of the phosphorylation–dephosphorylation mechanisms described above. Arguments have been made in favor of several possible models, but no change in the activity of any protein kinase of phosphatase that acts on enzyme substrates has been convincingly demonstrated in response to insulin. The general concensus is that insulin does not act by altering cAMP or $Ca^{2+}$ levels (Fain, 1975), thus regulating GSk-1 or GSk-2 activity. An alternative hypothesis has been proposed that insulin acts by decreasing the sensitivity of GSk-1 to cAMP, thus decreasing its activity in the absence of altered cAMP levels (Larner, 1971). This hypothesis is attractive because GSk-1 regulates several cellular enzymes that are altered by insulin. Further, a decrease in GSk-1 activity would be expected to decrease. the phosphorylation and activity of inhibitor 1, leading to increased phosphatase-1 activity. The broad specificity of this enzyme also includes several insulin-sensitive enzymes. Together, these mechanisms could account for most, if not all, of the decreased phosphorylation due to insulin. Experimental support for this hypothesis includes the report that phosphorylation of inhibitor 1 is decreased by insulin (Foulkes *et al.*, 1980), although other reports have not found this to be true (Khatra *et al.*, 1980). In addition, there have been reports that GSk-1 from insulin-treated tissue displays a decreased sensitivity to cAMP (Walkenbach *et al.*, 1980). A report has also been made that an insulin-dependent chemical regulator extracted from muscle desensitizes GSk-1 to cAMP (Larner *et al.*, 1979), but this has not been confirmed. The most discriminating test of this hypothesis is whether the decrease in enzyme phosphorylation due to insulin occurs at sites 1a or 2, indicating decreased activity of GSk-1 or GSk-2. One report has been made that suggests the decrease in phosphorylation due to insulin occurs in the trypsin-insensitive, $NH_2$-terminal domain of the protein, suggesting that it may be at site 2, although no sequence data are provided (Sheorain *et al.*, 1981, 1982). In contrast, a recent report indicates that the effect of insulin is exclusively observed at sites 3a, 3b, and 3c, with no effect on other sites (Parker *et al.*, 1983). This report implies that insulin action involves a specific effect on GSk-3. No data are currently available that suggest a mechanism for the regulation of GSk-3. However, one corollary of an effect on GSk-3 might be an effect on the activity of phosphatase 1 by a modulation of its activation from the inactive precursor, $F_c$. To account for the decreased phosphorylation of sites 3a, 3b, and 3c, as well as a predicted activation of phosphatase 1, it is necessary to hypothesize that a modification occurs that decreases the activity of GSk-3 toward glycogen synthase and increases it toward the inhibitor-2 portion of the Fc complex. Such a mechanism would allow for a reciprocal relationship between GSk-3 and phosphatase 1, which could account for many of insulin's effects.

It is likely that neither of these models provides a full picture of the mechanisms involved in the regulation of glycogen synthase. In addition, it is likely that insulin regulation of the phosphorylation of other enzymes involves additional mechanisms. The question to be addressed in analyzing the overall effector system is the extent to which pathways leading to the regulation of different enzymes diverge from a common starting point, the hormone–receptor interaction. The effector system may consist of a single major pathway with branching only at the terminal effectors or it may include multiple, substantially different pathways initiated by the common stimulus. Comparison of other insulin-sensitive, phosphorylation-regulated enzymes with glycogen synthase should allow some conclusions to be drawn about the diversity of mechanisms that may be involved in insulin action.

## C. Regulation of Pyruvate Dehydrogenase by Phosphorylation and by Insulin

Another insulin-sensitive enzyme, which has been well-characterized but which presents a picture very different from glycogen synthase, is pyruvate dehydrogenase. Like glycogen synthase, pyruvate dehydrogenase is stimulated by insulin by a mechanism that involves decreased enzyme phosphorylation (Wieland, 1983). However, the phosphorylation characteristics of the two enzymes are completely distinct. Pyruvate dehydrogenase is a complex of three enzymes: pyruvate decarboxylase (sometimes referred to individually as pyruvate dehydrogenase), lipoate acetyl transferase, and dihydrolipoyl dehydrogenase. Pyruvate decarboxylase is the site of all known regulatory control of the complex. This enzyme consists of two α subunits ($M_r = 41,000$) and two β subunits ($M_r = 36,000$). The α subunit is the substrate for phosphorylation catalyzed by a specific pyruvate de-hydrogenase kinase and a specific pyruvate dehydrogenase phosphatase, both of which are also associated with the complex (Denton and Hughes, 1978). Sequence analysis has revealed the existence of three phosphorylated sites in the $\alpha$ subunit of the enzyme, all serine residues. The phosphoryla-tion of site 1 occurs most rapidly and is correlated with inactivation of the enzyme (Yeaman *et al.*, 1978). The phosphorylation of sites 2 and 3 occurs mainly after inactivation is complete. However, phosphorylation of the addi-tional sites decreases the rate of reactivation of the enzyme by pyruvate dehydrogenase phosphatase, since these sites are more rapidly de-phosphorylated than site 1 (Kerbey *et al.*, 1981). Pyruvate dehydrogenase kinase is tightly associated with the complex (Linn *et al.*, 1972). It requires $Mg^{2+}$ for activity but is cAMP and $Ca^{2+}$ independent (Wieland, 1983). It is regulated by the concentration of pyruvate and by the ratios of NAD/NADH and CoA/acetyl-CoA (Denton and Hughes, 1978). Pyruvate dehydrogenase phosphatase is loosely associated with the enzyme complex (Teague *et al.*, 1982). It also requires $Mg^{2+}$ and is activated by $Ca^{2+}$ ($K_a = 0.1\mu M$), which may function by facilitating binding of the phosphatase to the complex (Pettit *et al.*, 1972).

The mechanism by which insulin regulates enzyme phosphorylation has not been clearly established. Regulation of kinase activity secondary to an increase in the CoA/acetyl-CoA ratio by insulin has been reported (Paetzke-Brunner *et al.*, 1978) but not confirmed (Stansbie *et al.*, 1976). One model of insulin action on pyruvate dehydrogenase involves activation of the phos-phatase by increased mitochondrial $Ca^{2+}$ (Denton and Hughes, 1978). This model has been supported by studies suggesting alterations of mito-chondrial $Ca^{2+}$ by insulin (McDonald *et al.*, 1976) and would explain the failure to obtain persistent enzyme activation in broken mitochondria. This hypothesis has not been confirmed by the demonstration of a direct causal linkage between these phenomena, however. One conclusion that appears certain from the available data is that regulation of glycogen synthase and pyruvate dehydrogenase by insulin proceeds by pathways that differ at the level of their terminal effectors. No relationship has been reported, nor does one seem likely, between the mitochondrial kinase and phosphatase and their cytosolic counterparts. Thus the insulin effector system must be con-ceived of as branching in leading to effects on these two enzymes, even though their phosphorylation is similarly affected. The level and number of such branch points in the effector system will be determined only after all insulin-sensitive enzymes have been studied. This issue will be particularly interesting in the case of enzymes whose phosphorylation is increased by insulin, since they might be expected to proceed via different mechanisms than those whose phosphorylation is decreased.

## D. Regulation of Acetyl-CoA Carboxylase by Phosphorylation and by Insulin

The only enzyme whose phosphorylation is increased by insulin, which has also been reported to undergo a concomitant change in activity, is acetyl-CoA carboxylase. This association was initially obscured since insulin, glucagon, and epinephrine all increased the incorporation of $^{32}$P into the enzyme, but insulin increased while the other two agents decreased enzyme activity (Halestrap and Denton, 1974; Witters, 1981). Subsequent studies have explained these observations by showing that insulin and the cAMP-mediated agents increased the phosphorylation of residues in different tryptic peptides (Brownsey and Denton, 1982). These studies have correlated the phosphorylation of a specific peptide in response to insulin with activation of the enzyme. Thus, acetyl-CoA carboxylase appears similar to other enzymes in that it possesses multiple phosphorylation sites and is regulated by multiple protein kinases and phosphatases but appears unique in that phosphorylation at different sites appears to have functionally opposite effects on the enzyme. Analysis of the phosphorylation sites and their kinases and phosphatases is far from complete. All phosphorylation sites appear to be serine residues, but their number and location have not been determined beyond separation into two types on the basis of differential hormonal sensitivity of tryptic peptides. Several protein kinases have been reported to phosphorylate the enzyme, including the cAMP-dependent protein kinase (Tipper and Witters, 1982), a cAMP-and Ca$^{2+}$-independent kinase that copurifies with the enzyme (Hardie and Cohen, 1979), and a membrane-associated, cAMP-independent protein kinase (Brownsey *et al.*, 1981). Phosphorylation by cAMP-dependent protein kinase has been reported to inactivate the enzyme, while phosphorylation by the membrane kinase has been reported to activate it (Brownsey *et al.*, 1981). Dephosphorylation of the enzyme by protein phosphatase 1 from skeletal muscle or a similar enzyme from mammary tissue activates enzyme that has previously been phosphorylated by cAMP-dependent protein kinase or the copurified kinase (Hardie and Cohen, 1979). The available data are not yet adequate to assign the effect of insulin to a specific mechanism. However, the possibility has been raised that insulin activates the plasma membrane-associated protein kinase, which directly effects phosphorylation of the enzyme (Brownsey *et al.*, 1981). Although there is no direct evidence to support this model, it represents a potential effector pathway, which may be very different from the others discussed previously, involving direct enzyme–enzyme contact between the cytosolic target protein and a membrane component that is possibly linked to the receptor. This would mean that insulin may increase phosphorylation by a mechanism that is totally separate or diverges very early from the mechanism which has been most commonly considered as leading to decreased phosphorylation, involving a regulatory mediator or second messenger.

## E. ROLE OF ENZYME PHOSPHORYLATION IN THE INSULIN EFFECTOR SYSTEM

It is apparent from the few enzymes described here that the insulin-effector system is potentially very complex. Adequate data are not yet available to rationalize the information from individual enzymes into a total scheme. It should be emphasized that connections, which are not yet apparent, may be revealed between seemingly unrelated effectors from individual enzyme studies. Other examples of kinase–kinase, kinase–phosphatase, or phosphatase–phosphatase interactions may be revealed as further characterization is carried out. These mechanisms provide a means by which propagation of the hormone's signal can be amplified and diversified, even to the extent of linking increased and decreased phosphorylation effects in a unified pathway, and it is likely that they will play an important role in the effector system. Ultimately it will be necessary to establish a link between a phosphorylation–dephosphorylation mechanism and the hormone–receptor complex, either by a direct interaction or by means of a regulatory mediator.

## II. THE INSULIN RECEPTOR

### A. RECEPTOR STRUCTURE

The event that initiates the cellular actions of insulin is its recognition and binding by specific receptors in the target cells. Binding of insulin to cell surface receptors is thought to initiate transmembrane signals that set off a diversity of cellular responses. The insulin receptor is also the vehicle for internalization and degradation of receptor-bound ligand. This section will discuss the structural properties of the insulin receptor and how particular domains of the receptor structures may be involved in various receptor functions.

Receptors for insulin are present in almost every cell type in chordates, and the general structure of these receptors has been preserved for at least 500 million years of evolution (Czech and Massagué, 1982). Relatively high amounts of these receptors are present in human placenta, rat liver and rat adipocytes, and in the cultured cell lines 3T3-L1 adipocytes and IM-9 human lymphoblasts; for this reason, these tissues and cell lines have been extensively used in biological and structural studies of the insulin receptor. Like many other types of hormone receptors, insulin receptors exhibit a $K_d$ for its ligand in the low nanomolar range. A complication of the binding of insulin to its receptor is that the kinetics of this process do not reflect a simple interaction with one single class of binding sites but rather a more complex type of interaction. This atypical behavior has been attributed to either "negative cooperativity" among insulin-binding sites (De Meyts *et al.*, 1976), interaction of insulin with a heterogenous population of receptors (Olefsky *et al.*, 1978), or conformational and kinetic changes that occur in the receptor on insulin binding (Corin and Donner, 1982); in many cases it probably reflects the summation of various of these and perhaps other factors.

The methodology initially employed to attack the problem of insulin receptor isolation and structural characterization was affinity chromatography of solubilized receptor extracts using agarose-linked insulin as the affinity matrix (Cuatrecasas, 1972; Jacobs *et al.*, 1977). Initial electrophoretic analysis of receptor preparations obtained by this method resolved polypeptides of 135 kd, 95 kd, and 45 kd, respectively (Jacobs *et al.*, 1980b). More recently, receptor methodologies like photoaffinity labeling (Yip *et al.*, 1978; Wisher *et al.*, 1980) and affinity crosslinking (Pilch and Czech, 1979, 1980b), based on the formation of stable [$^{125}$I]insulin–receptor complexes that can be detected by autoradiography, have circumvented the need to purify the receptor prior to its study. The advent of affinity-labeling methodologies has allowed a rapid progress in the understanding of the insulin receptor subunit composition and stoichiometry. It is now recognized that the insulin receptor is a disulfide-linked structure that consists of 125–135 kd subunits and 90–95 kd subunits termed, respectively, $\alpha$ and $\beta$ receptor subunits (Massagué *et al.*, 1980). Two laboratories (Czech *et al.*, 1981; Jacobs and Cuatrecasas, 1981) have independently proposed that the disulfide-linked receptor subunits are arranged in an heterotetrameric ($\beta$-S-S-$\alpha$)S-S($\alpha$-S-S-$\beta$) complex with a general design analogous to that of an immunoglobulin (Fig. 2). In addition, this complex might be noncovalently associated to other membrane components yet to be identified. This model is based on the molecular mass values estimated for receptor in the unreduced form and after partial or complete reduction. In the absence of direct protein chemistry analysis this model accommodates virtually all the structural data available at present. In addition to this predominant insulin receptor structure, free $\alpha$ and $\beta$ insulin receptor subunits, partially reduced ($\alpha\beta$)- and ($\alpha$)$_2$-receptor fragments, and receptor complexes containing biosynthetic precursors of the $\alpha$ and $\beta$ subunits have been identified in various cell types by

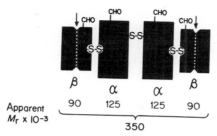

F<small>IG</small>. 2. Proposed minimum subunit structure of the insulin receptor. The basic features of this deduced structure are two copies of each of two glycoprotein subunit types, denoted α and β, disulfide bridges linking all subunits, and high susceptibility of the β subunit to cleavage near the center of its amino acid sequence by elastase-like enzymes (arrows). The disulfides linking one α subunit with one β subunit are protected from reduction in the native state. The presence of other subunits not covalently linked to this structure cannot be excluded. The apparent molecular weight values are estimates obtained on SDS gels in the nonreduced (intact complex, $M_r = 350,000$) and reduced (individual subunits), respectively.

receptor affinity labeling (Massagué and Czech, 1980) and immunoprecipitation with antiinsulin receptor antibodies (Kasuga *et al.*, 1982a).

The disulfide bonds that link the insulin receptor subunits have been classified according to their susceptibility to reductants (Massague and Czech, 1982b) (Fig. 2). The class I disulfides that link the two (α-S-S-β) receptor halves are very sensitive to low concentrations of dithiothreitol, even in the intact cell. The reduction of class I disulfides is in part reversible, and holoreceptor complexes can be obtained by incubation of partially reduced receptor halves in the presence of a redox buffer (Massagué and Czech, 1982b). Partially reduced receptor halves seem to occur naturally in rat liver and other tissues (Massagué and Czech, 1980; Kasuga *et al.*, 1982a), but their physiological significance is obscure. When the class I disulfides are eliminated by reduction *in vitro*, the resulting insulin receptor halves remain linked together by strong noncovalent interactions that resist cell disruption and solubilization with nonionic detergents. After reduction of class I disulfides, the insulin receptor in rat adipocytes is still capable of binding insulin and eliciting normal insulin effects (Massagué and Czech, 1982c). The disulfides linking one α receptor subunit to one β receptor subunit, or class II disulfides, are comparably well protected against reduction by dithiothreitol. Denaturation of the insulin receptor with ionic detergents is required to expose class II disulfides to the action of reductants.

The insulin receptor in intact cells or in isolated membranes is very susceptible to proteolytic attack. A short exposure of rat adipocytes to as low as 10 μg/ml trypsin will result in extensive insulin-receptor cleavage (Pilch *et al.*, 1981). A specific site in the β subunit of the insulin receptor is uniquely sensitive to cleavage by certain lysosomal enzyme(s), and this action can be mimicked *in vitro* by elastase but not other proteases (Massagué *et al.*, 1981b). The 45–49 kd fragment of the β subunit that remains attached by disulfide bonds to the receptor core after nicking by elastase-like enzymes (Fig. 2) has been referred to as the "$\beta_1$ receptor subunit." Partially pro-teolyzed $(\alpha\beta)(\alpha\beta_1)$ and $(\alpha\beta_1)_2$ receptor forms are commonly present in mem-brane preparations from virtually all tissues examined, even when these preparations are obtained in the presence of various protease inhibitors. The relative abundance of $(\alpha\beta)(\alpha\beta_1)$ and $(\alpha\beta_1)_2$ forms varies with each tissue, being typically low in human placental membranes and high in rat liver membranes. The varying amounts of 90–95 kd and 45–49 kd peptides pre-sent in purified insulin-receptor preparations normally reflect different ex-tents of β-receptor subunit proteolysis during the early steps of membrane isolation. The widespread occurrence of a lysosomal elastase-like protease(s) acting on the β insulin-receptor subunit suggests a possible role of this enzyme in the normal processing of the receptor. Another protease, an adipocyte membrane-associated thiol proteinase causes the rapid degrada-tion of the α insulin-receptor subunit into a free 80 kd fragment (Massagué and Czech, 1982b). Interestingly, after extensive cleavage by the proteolytic enzymes mentioned above, the insulin receptor is still capable of binding insulin and signaling for stimulation of glucose oxidation (Pilch *et al.*, 1981b), presumably due to coherence among the resulting peptide fragments pro-vided by hydrophobic and other noncovalent interactions.

## B. Receptor Biosynthesis and Turnover

The structural features of the insulin receptor suggest a relatively complex biosynthetic pathway for this membrane protein. Physical isolation and quantitation of *de novo* synthesized receptor has been obtained by incuba-tion of cultured cells in the presence of amino acids labeled with heavy ($^2$H, $^{13}$C, $^{15}$N) isotopes, followed by solubilization and isopycnic separation of cellular components (Reed and Lane, 1980). Results obtained using this strategy have indicated that translation of proreceptor polypeptide(s) in the rough endoplasmic reticulum of 3T3-L1 adipocytes is followed by $1\frac{1}{2}$ hours of processing that involves receptor glycosylation and gives rise to receptor forms capable of binding insulin (Ronnett *et al.*, 1983). Another 3 hours elapse before newly synthesized receptors reach the cell surface in the form of the $(\alpha\beta)_2$ complex discussed above. There is evidence indicating that the α- and β-receptor subunits may be products of cleavage of a 200–210 kd precursor(s) that can be immunoprecipitated in detergent extracts form various cell types (Kasuga *et al.*, 1982a; Deutsch *et al.*, 1983).

Another type of posttranslational modification that affects the insulin receptor is glycosylation. Glycosylation of the receptor was first inferred from its ability to bind to lectins (Cuatrecasas and Tell, 1973; Hedo *et al.*, 1981a) and to be partially digested by glycosidases (Jacobs *et al.*, 1980a). Biosynthetic labeling with radioactive sugar precursors (Hedo *et al.*, 1981b) has shown that both the α subunit and the β subunit are glycoproteins with extracellular domains. The binding capacity of *de novo* synthesized receptors in cultured cells can be blocked when cultures are maintained in the presence of tunicamycin, a drug that presumably prevents receptor glycosylation (Ronnett and Lane, 1981). Removal of this drug restores the cellular capacity to produce active insulin receptors (Ronnett and Lane, 1981). These findings indicated that glycosylation is required either as a structural component of the insulin receptor involved in ligand binding or as a step in the processing and full maturation of nascent receptors.

After insulin binding, the ligand–receptor complex is internalized (Kahn and Baird, 1978; Schlessinger *et al.*, 1978) through a pathway that involves some degree of receptor clustering (Schlessinger *et al.*, 1978). Internalized insulin is directed at least in part toward secondary lysosomes and degraded there (Marshall and Olefsky, 1979). This process presumably involves steps and subcellular structures similar to other ligand/receptor systems that also undergo internalization and ligand transformation inside the cell. However, the insulin receptor is not always degraded when it becomes internalized on ligand binding. Rather, the receptor can apparently escape the intracellular degradative route and be recycled back to the plasma membrane in a fully functional form. Quantitative measurements of ligand and receptor internalization rates (Ronnett *et al.*, 1983; Marshall *et al.*, 1981) as well as direct observation of [$^{125}$I]insulin-labeled receptor dynamics in intact cells (Fehlmann *et al.*, 1982) provide strong evidence for this receptor-recycling phenomenology.

The heavy-isotope labeling technique mentioned above has been also instrumental in showing that insulin and the insulin receptor are degraded through different pathways (Krupp and Lane, 1982). Receptor inactivation/degradation occurs in various cell types independently of the presence or absence of insulin in the medium (Ronnett *et al.*, 1983). This process has clear potential as a regulatory step for the number of insulin-receptor molecules present in the cell. For example, the decrease of cell-surface insulin receptor or "down regulation" that follows a prolonged exposure of 3T3-L1 adipocytes to insulin appears to result from a specific insulin-induced increase in the rate of receptor inactivation (Ronnett *et al.*, 1982). Similarly, glucocorticoids decrease the rate of insulin receptor degradation to cause receptor "up regulation" in 3T3-L1 cells (Knutson *et al.*, 1982). Regulation of insulin receptor levels by alteration of the receptor biosynthetic pathway also appears to take place in some systems (Fantus *et al.*, 1982).

## C. Functional Aspects of the Insulin Receptor

Information on what structural domains of the insulin structure may be involved in specific receptor functions has started to emerge from studies involving structural analysis following specific biochemical perturbations of the receptor. Tentative localization of the ligand binding site is based on results from receptor affinity-labeling studies. Linkage of several photoreactive [$^{125}$I]insulin derivatives to the receptor invariably resulted in the labeling of the α subunit (Yip *et al.* 1978, 1980; Jacobs *et al.*, 1979a) and, in some cases, the β subunit (Yip *et al.*, 1980). Similarly, crosslinking of [$^{125}$I]insulin with the insulin receptor by short-arm bifunctional succinimidyl esters effected the labeling of the α subunit and, to a lesser extent, the β subunit (Pilch and Czech, 1979; Massagué *et al.*, 1980, 1981a). Therefore, both receptors' subunits seem to contribute parts of their sequence to the insulin-binding site(s). It is not known whether interaction of insulin with both receptor subunits is simultaneous or sequential during the course of the receptor conformational change that accompanies ligand binding (Pilch and Czech, 1980a). It is interesting to note that the apparent structural symmetry of the insulin receptor suggests the presence of more than one insulin-binding site per holoreceptor complex, although some recent data are not consistent with this hypothesis (Pang and Shafer, 1983).

Insulin receptors immunoprecipitated or chromatographically isolated from a variety of tissues contain covalently bound phosphate attached mainly to the β receptor subunit (Kasuga *et al.*, 1982b). Importantly, the phosphorylation level of the receptor is increased on ligand binding. Insulin-stimulated phosphorylation of the insulin receptor was initially found in [$^{32}$P]ATP-labeled intact cells (Kasuga *et al.*, 1982b) and subsequently demonstrated in cell-free systems and in partially purified receptor preparations (Kasuga *et al.*, 1982d; Van Obberghen and Kowalski, 1982; Petruzzelli *et al.*, 1982; Avruch *et al.*, 1982b; Zick *et al.*, 1983; Machicao *et al.*, 1982). Insulin-induced receptor phosphorylation is generally rapid, occurs at physiological concentrations of insulin, and is mimicked with the corresponding relative potency by various insulin analogs but not by peptide hormones that do not interact with the insulin receptor (Zick *et al.*, 1983). Magnesium ions do not substitute for $Mn^{2+}$, which is required for the receptor phosphorylation reaction (Avruch *et al.*, 1982b; Zick *et al.*, 1983). Insulin-stimulated receptor phosphorylation occurs mainly at tyrosine residues. Phosphorylation on tyrosine residues is most remarkable since phosphotyrosine represents a very small fraction of the phosphoaminoacid content in normal cells. Ligand-induced receptor phosphorylation on tyrosine residues also occurs in receptors for epidermal growth factor (Cohen *et al.*, 1980) and platelet-derived growth factor (Ek *et al.*, 1982), being perhaps a trend common to several other peptide hormone receptors.

Recent evidence from various laboratories (Roth and Cassell, 1983; Van Obberghen *et al.*, 1983; Shia and Pilch, 1983) suggests that the insulin-sensitive tyrosine kinase activity that phosphorylates the β insulin receptor subunit resides in the receptor itself. Furthermore, receptor preparations partially purified by affinity chromatography, immunoprecipitation, or other methods can apparently act as a tyrosine kinase on several exogenous protein substrates added *in vitro* (Petruzzelli *et al.*, 1982). Localization of the receptor subunit that may contain this enzymatic activity has been attempted by affinity labeling of ATP-binding sites in receptor preparations with a radio-labeled photoreactive analog of ATP. In these experiments, only the β receptor subunit was labeled, substantiating the conclusion that this subunit is perhaps an insulin-sensitive tyrosine kinase with autophosphorylation capacity (Roth and Cassell, 1983; Van Obberghen *et al.*, 1983; Shia and Pilch, 1983). Unfortunately, this conclusion cannot yet be considered unequivocal because of the possibility that ATP binds to a site on the receptor subunit that is unrelated to a kinase catalytic site.

Proof of the hypothesis that the insulin receptor itself is the tyrosine kinase will depend on achieving purification of the homogeneous receptor and the assay of its putative kinase activity. Studies by one laboratory (Petruzzelli *et al.*, 1982) demonstrated that the insulin-sensitive kinase activity copurified with the insulin receptor until the final elution from the insulin–agarose affinity column. It is important to know whether the loss of the kinase activity is due to the inactivation of the receptor kinase by the denaturing conditions used to elute the receptor or due to the physical separation of the noncovalently bound kinase from the receptor. Studies in this laboratory (Yu and Czech, submitted for publication) have been directed toward this question and have suggested that highly purified insulin receptor, while immobilized on insulin–agarose, exhibits tyrosine kinase activity. Immobilized insulin receptor appears to contain kinase activity toward its own β subunit as well as added substrates such as histone and casein. The purification protocol involves sequential affinity chromatography of Triton X-100 extracts of placental membranes through wheat germ agglutinin–agarose to enrich the sugar-containing receptors, dithiothreitol and heat-inactivated insulin–agarose to absorb nonreceptor contaminants, and native insulin–agarose to absorb the insulin receptor. The specificity of absorption of the insulin receptor kinase to insulin–agarose was documented by the ability of free native insulin but not other proteins, such as cytochrome $c$, to displace the kinase activity.

The insulin-receptor-associated kinase immobilized on insulin–agarose exhibits an absolute dependence on $Mn^{2+}$ ion both for the phosphorylation of the β subunit of the receptor and added substrates and contains no endogenous phosphatase activity. Significantly, the kinase activity of this receptor preparation toward histone appeared to be enhanced four- to sixfold when the receptor was first incubated with ATP (Fig. 3). The magnitude of activation of this kinase activity is dependent on the concentration of ATP used for preincubation. A maximal 10-fold activation can be achieved at 400 μM ATP (K-T. Yu and M. P. Czech, unpublished data). The activation of the kinase activity is specific for ATP. A possible explanation for this phenomenon is that the receptor kinase is activated by prior phosphorylation. However, activation by other covalent or allosteric modifications cannot be excluded. Interestingly, prior incubation with unlabeled ATP increased the subsequent phosphorylation of the β subunit of the insulin receptor with ATP [γ-$^{32}$P] at the earlier time point (5 minutes). However, at later time points the level of phosphorylation in the untreated preparation became slightly higher compared to that of the ATP-treated preparations. The lack of marked inhibition on the subsequent incorporation of $^{32}$P into the β subunit of the insulin receptor after preincubation with unlabeled ATP for 40 minutes suggests that the phosphorylation of the β subunit may also be stimulated by pretreatment with ATP. Preliminary results (Yu and Czech, unpublished data) suggest that multiple sites on the β subunit may be exposed for phosphorylation after preincubation with ATP.

## D. Receptor Heterogeneity

Insulin receptors from various sources share many of the properties described above, but they frequently exhibit significant differences at both the structural and biochemical level indicative of some degree of insulin-receptor heterogeneity. An extreme example of this polymorphism is the receptor for insulin-like growth factor-I (IGF-I). IGF-I, like IGF-II, is a small polypeptide with extensive amino acid sequence homology to insulin (Rinderknecht and Humbel, 1978). The biological actions of IGF-I and IGF-II, like those of insulin, include activation of cellular metabolism and synthesis (Zapf *et al.*, 1978). IGF-I and IGF-II also exhibit a potent mitogenic activity in certain cell types (Zapf *et al.*, 1978). The multiple chemical and biological similarities between IGF-I, IGF-II, and insulin suggested that receptors for these peptides might have some trends in common. This possibility has been

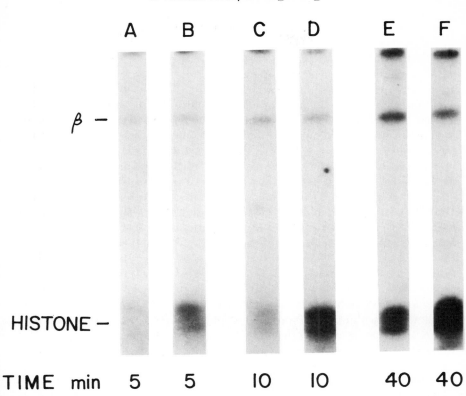

FIG. 3. Activation of insulin receptor kinase activity by ATP. Human placental membranes (5 mg/lane) were solubilized in 1% Triton X-100 and the insulin receptor was affinity purified through wheat germ agglutinin–agarose, dithiothreitol heat-inactivated insulin–agarose, and insulin–agarose. The receptor, while immobilized on insulin–agaorse (0.05 ml), was incubated with (lanes B, D, and F) or without (lanes A, C, and E) 20 μM of unlabeled ATP in 0.08 ml of 50 mM HEPES buffer containing 0.1% Triton X-100, 10 mM MgCl$_2$, 3 mM MnCl$_2$, 1 mM PMSF, and 10 μg/ml leupeptin, pH 7.4 for 40 minutes at 25°C. The preparation was then washed extensively to remove the unreacted ATP and suspended in 0.08 ml of the same buffer. [γ $^{32}$P]ATP was added to a final concentration of 5 μM (specific activity 50 μCi/nmol), and incubation was performed at 25°C for the indicated period of time. At the end of incubation, 0.1 ml of sample buffer containing 0.17 M Tris, 10% sodium dodecyl sulfate, 20 mM dithiothreitol, 30% glycerol pH 6.8 was added and the entire sample was boiled for 5 minutes to terminate the reaction. The samples were then electrophoresed on 8–16% SDS-polyacrylamide gradient gel. The gel was stained, destained, and autoradiographed.

recently confirmed by affinity labeling of IGF receptors using [125]I-labeled IGF-I or IGF-II and appropriate chemical crosslinking agents (Massagué *et al.*, 1981a; Massagué and Czech, 1982a; Bhaumick *et al.*, 1981; Chernausek *et al.*, 1981; Kasuga *et al.*, 1981; Kasuga *et al.*, 1982c). Two types of IGF receptor structures have been identified using this approach. One type is a 220–260 kd single-chain polypeptide with high affinity for IGF-II, lower affinity for IGF-I, and no affinity for insulin. This receptor type, with no obvious structural relationship to the insulin receptor, has been termed the IGF-II receptor (or "type II" IGF receptor). In contrast, a second type of receptor that exhibits the highest affinity for IGF-I is structurally very similar to typical high-affinity insulin receptors. Thus, the IGF-I receptor (or "type I" IGF receptor) is a disulfide-linked structure consisting of two 130–140 kd $\alpha$ subunits and two 95–97 kd $\beta$ subunits, all linked in a proposed $(\beta\text{-S-S-}\alpha)\text{-S-S}(\alpha\text{-S-S-}\beta)$ configuration (Massagué and Czech, 1982a). The relative susceptibility to reduction of the class I and class II disulfide bonds in the IGF-I receptor is similar to that of the corresponding disulfides in the insulin receptor (Massagué and Czech, 1983). The subunits in the IGF-I receptor contain a site approximately in the middle of their amino acid sequence highly susceptible to cleavage by elastase-like proteases, just like an homologous site in the $\beta$ insulin receptor subunit. However, the affinity of this receptor for insulin is generally very low (Massagué and Czech, 1982a; Kasuga *et al.*, 1982c). The results from recent studies using specific antiinsulin receptor and anti-IGF-I receptor antibodies indicate structural differences between the subunits of insulin receptors and IGF-I receptors and even between their respective precursor polypeptides (Jacobs *et al.*, 1983). These findings indicate that at least two, and possibly many, variations of the same basic $(\alpha\beta)_2$ structure serve as receptors for the insulin/IGF peptide hormone family. This conclusion is further supported by the finding that IGF-I receptors in different tissues can be distinguished by their relative affinity for insulin. Thus, the IGF-I receptor in chick embryo fibroblasts exhibits relatively high affinity for insulin, while a similar receptor form in an Ehrlich-Lettre mouse-ascites carcinoma cell lines has very low insulin-binding capacity (Massagué and Czech, unpublished observations). The polymorphism of receptors for insulin and IGF-I may be the result of multiple genes that code for a common polypeptide domain in these receptors but undergo rearrangements to determine a heterogeneity in other domains, including the ligand binding site. Alternatively, the heterogeneity of binding site in receptors for insulin and IGF-I may be the result of posttranslational modification of the same polypeptide(s). Whichever of these two explanations is correct, the close nature of the genetic expression of receptors for insulin and IGF-I is illustrated by several instances in which parallel modifications of receptor expression occur. For example, both the insulin and the IGF-I receptor types are induced simultaneously in differentiating 3T3-L1 cells (Massagué and Czech, 1982a). Parallel alterations of the expression of insulin receptors and IGF-I receptors have been observed in skin fibroblasts from patients with leprechaunism and insulin-resistance syndromes (Van Obberghen-Schilling *et al.*, 1981; Massagué *et al.*, 1983).

In view of the extensive homology that characterizes the insulin and IGF-I receptors at the structural and genetic levels, functional analogies may also be expected for these two receptors in terms of similar transmembrane signaling systems. This hypothesis is supported by the observation that the IGF-I receptor in rat muscle cells can mediate the rapid activation of glucose transport by IGF-I in a manner analogous to the mediation of this effect by the insulin receptor in rat adipocytes (Yu and Czech, 1983). Therefore, at least in rat muscle tissue the IGF-I receptor is coupled to an effector system similar to the one interacting with insulin receptors in rat adipocytes. Conversely, insulin acts as a potent mitogen in H-35 rat hepatoma cells because this cell line has insulin receptors that signal for stimulation of cell proliferation (Massagué *et al.*, 1982) in contrast to other cell lines in which the mitogenic action of insulin is induced through its relatively weak interaction with IGF-I receptors (King *et al.*, 1980). These examples illustrate the concept that the responsiveness of cells to insulin and the IGFs is regulated by the type and number of insulin/IGF-I cell-surface receptors and by the effector system to which these receptors are linked in every particular cell type.

## III. BIOLOGICAL SIGNALING BY THE RECEPTOR

The molecular basis of insulin's actions on cellular functions has been the focus of extensive investigations by large numbers of laboratories over the last several decades; yet we are still left without a satisfactory resolution to this problem. Many hypotheses have been put forward based on data provided by numerous experimental approaches, and several previous reviews are available that present comprehensive summaries of these efforts (Czech, 1977; Czech, 1981a,b). It is clear that several cellular systems involved in signaling, e.g., cyclic nucleotides and calcium, are indeed modulated by insulin action. However, our current thinking involves the hypothesis that a more primary signal or signals participate in mediating even these early effects of insulin. Two possible modes of primary signaling seem most attractive to us at present: (1) Insulin-receptor tyrosine kinase activity may directly or indirectly initiate the signaling process or (2) the release of one or more mediator substances into the cell from the plasma membrane may directly or indirectly regulate the insulin-sensitive cellular systems. It should be noted that these hypotheses are not mutually exclusive. Hypotheses related to the first of these possibilities will be treated in detail in this volume in the chapter by Kahn and colleagues and will thus not be further considered here. This section will review recent data and interpretations related to the hypothesis that soluble mediator or mediators are involved in cellular signaling by insulin.

## A. The Mediator Hypothesis

Several reviews are available that present the early framework for the mediator hypothesis (Seals and Czech, 1982; Jarett *et al.*, 1982; Larner *et al.*, 1982; Larner, 1982). Briefly, studies in Larner's laboratory using heat-treated acid extracts of control versus insulin-treated muscle suggested the presence of an insulin-dependent activity that could interfere with cAMP-dependent activation of protein kinase in vitro (Larner *et al.*, 1975). Subsequent results by Seals and Jarett (1980) and Seals *et al.*, (1978, 1979) indicated that biologically active material in isolated adipocyte membranes could be released from the membrane in response to the hormone *in vitro*. This material stimulated the insulin-dependent enzyme pyruvate dehydrogenase in isolated mitochondria. Further results by these laboratories (Larner *et al.*, 1979; Kiechle *et al.*, 1981; Saltiel *et al.*, 1981) and by Seals and Czech (1981) indicated the insulin-dependent activity in cell or membrane extracts was of low molecular weight in the range 1000–3000. We also reported that the release of pyruvate dehydrogenase-stimulating activity from isolated membranes in response to insulin could be blocked by antiproteases and esters of arginine and that the activity of putative mediator was destroyed by trypsin or chymotrypsin (Seals and Czech, 1980). Inhibited formation of the insulin-dependent enzyme regulator by the protease substrate TAME was also observed by Begum *et al.* (1982). Larner's group (Larner *et al.*, 1981) failed to observe protease sensitivity of the enzyme regulator from muscle extracts.

Several problems and issues related to the above work have been addressed in the past 2 years. A major concern has been the difficulty in reproducing the formation of putative mediator activity in response to insulin in several laboratories. Our group has also experienced this problem during certain periods, and there is no known explanation. Two possible characteristics of the insulin-dependent enzyme-modulating activity that may lead to confounding obstacles to its detection are as follows: (1) the biphasic nature of its action on enzyme activity and (2) a tendency to be more stable and identifiable following preliminary purification steps compared to its activity in crude extracts. This first point has been noted by several groups (Larner *et al.*, 1979; Saltiel *et al.*, 1982; Kiechle and Jarett, 1981; Saltiel *et al.*, 1981), where low concentrations of extract modulate enzyme in the direction expected for an insulin effect whereas higher concentrations of the same extract have either no effect or cause effects in the opposite direction. Larner and colleagues have proposed the existence of at least two insulin-dependent regulators that could be resolved by paper electrophoresis (Cheng *et al.*, 1980). In addition, we have observed a more reproducible difference in biological activity between extracts obtained from control versus insulin-treated cells subsequent to purification of the material by high-pressure liquid chromatography. This may be due to the presence of contaminating substances that interfere with the action of insulin-dependent enzyme regulator or to the presence of insulin-dependent factors that have opposite actions as proposed by Cheng *et al.* (1980). Similar observations have been made by Saltiel *et al.* (1982, 1983), who were able to differentially extract a stimulatory activity and an inhibitory activity on pyruvate dehydrogenase and acetyl-CoA carboxylase using solubility in absolute ethanol. The latter activity was soluble in this solvent.

In spite of the above considerations, available evidence suggests that insulin-dependent enzyme-regulator activity can be observed in several laboratories and is a real phenomenon. Multiple laboratories have published data confirming successful assay of bioactivity released from isolated liver or fat-cell membranes. Experiments by us (unpublished) and Kiechle *et al.* (1980) have also succeeded in observing insulin-dependent bioactivity in extracts of intact adipocytes. In addition, Parker *et al.* (1982) have been able to extract insulin-dependent enzyme regulator from intact H4-II-EC3′ hepatoma cells.

Results from various laboratories have increasingly extended the number of enzymes regulated by insulin-dependent bioactive material extracted from membranes or cells. Many of these enzymes are sensitive to modulation by many agents nonspecifically, and thus such effects *in vitro* must be interpreted with caution. Enzyme systems modulated similarly by insulin in intact cells and by insulin-dependent extracted bioactivity now include inhibition of adenylate cyclase (Saltiel *et al.*, 1982), stimulation of acetyl-CoA carboxylase (Saltiel *et al.*, 1983), and stimulation of cAMP phosphodiesterase (Kiechle and Jarett, 1981) as well as stimulation of the glycogen synthase complex or phosphatase and pyruvate dehydrogenase systems. It is important to note that control extracts from cells or membranes also often modulate these systems, although to a lesser extent, in the same direction as the insulin-dependent extracts.

## B. Purification of a Putative Insulin Mediator

The most problematical aspect of work on the soluble insulin-dependent bioactivities in extracts has been the failure of purification attempts despite years of intensive effort. It is generally agreed that unless complete purification and structural analysis is successful, it will not be possible to evaluate the physiological relevance of the above-described phenomena. Preliminary work devoted to attaining partial purification has been reviewed previously (Seals and Czech, 1982). Problems encountered with these approaches have also been described (Larner, 1982). The strategy used in our studies has involved the use of high-pressure liquid chromatography for purification of insulin-dependent activity from trifluoroacetic acid extracts of isolated fat cells.

Fat cells were incubated with or without insulin (5 n$M$), washed quickly, then homogenized in 1% trifluoroacetic acid containing 1 m$M$ each of EDTA and dithiothreitol. The extracts were lyophilized and tested for activity or subjected to successive high-pressure liquid chromatographic steps to purify the component possessing the activity. In all cases, activity was defined as the insulin-dependent stimulation of pyruvate dehydrogenase in isolated adipocyte mitochondria. Extracts from both control and insulin-treated cells contained stimulatory activity, but the insulin sample could be shown on serial dilution to contain up to three to four times greater activity. Purification was carried out by the following sequence of high-pressure liquid chromatographic fractionation steps: gradient anion exchange; gradient reversed phase; and isocratic anion exchange or reversed phase. The initial column resolved the crude activity into multiple peaks, which have been divided into five regions, A–E (Fig. 4). The insulin-dependent activity was concentrated in regions B, C, and D, while the greatest amount of material determined by serial dilution was found in regions B and C.

The activities from these two regions were pooled and run separately on gradient-reversed phase high-pressure liquid chromatography in 0.1% trifluoroacetic acid with a gradient of acetonitrile. A single, major peak of insulin-dependent activity was obtained from regions B and C. Region B produced a peak of activity (B1), which eluted before the start of the acetonitrile gradient; region C produced a peak (C4), which eluted between 40 and 45% acetonitrile. Each of these peaks was purified on a third column, which was designed as an isocratic modification of one of the first two columns, B1 on isocratic anion exchange, C4 on isocratic reversed phase. In each case, a single peak of activity was obtained (Fig. 5). Although the final columns were run with the combined material extracted from the adipocytes

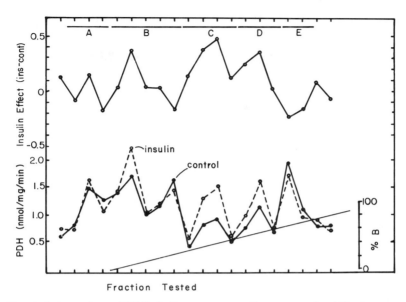

F IG. 4. Anion exchange HPLC of adipocyte extracts. Extracts were lyophilized, resuspended in $NH_4HCO_3$, pH 8.0, and injected onto a Whatman SAX column equilibrated with water, then eluted with a gradient to 2.5% trifluoroacetic acid, 50% acetonitrile, 25% isopropanol (buffer B). Fractions were collected from control and insulin samples, then tested for activity, as described in the text. The lower graph shows the results from both samples, while the upper graph plots the difference between control and insulin activities. In this experiment, untreated mitochondria possessed activity of 0.75/nmol/mg/minute. PDH-pyruvate dehydrogenase.

of 600 rats, no detectable peak of UV-absorbance (210 nM) was observed with either peak of activity. However, C4 co-eluted with a peak of o-phthaldialdehyde-reactive material on postcolumn derivatization of the insulin but not the control sample, suggesting the presence of amino groups in the insulin-dependent active component. Amino acid analysis of C4 from the insulin sample revealed a minimum composition of 32 amino acids ($M_r$ = 2979, consistent with previous estimates by exclusion chromatography). A similar composition was determined from the corresponding control fraction, but the amount was approximately one-fifth of the insulin sample. Importantly, no amino acids were found in inactive fractions from the column runs. Thus, the activity was qualitatively and approximately quantitatively associated with the occurence of a putative peptide. Current studies are underway to determine the sequence of the peptide and to determine whether it is indeed the bioactive component.

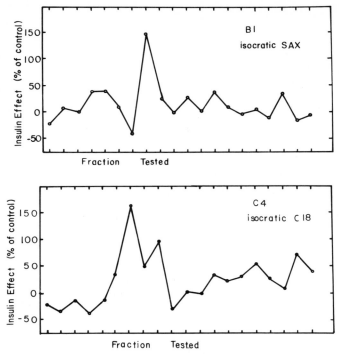

FIG. 5. Purification of insulin-dependent activities B1 and C4. Corresponding control and insulin fractions comprising insulin-dependent peaks B1 and C4 were collected from gradient reversed-phase HPLC and subjected to another step as follows. B1 was chromatographed by anion exchange HPLC in 5% buffer B (see Fig. 4). C4 was chromatographed by reversed phase HPLC in 0.1% trifluoroacetic acid/42% acetonitrile. In both cases, fractions were collected and tested for activity on pyruvate dehydrogenase activity in isolated mitochondria. The difference between each corresponding control and insulin fraction is plotted as a percentage of that control value.

## IV. SUMMARY AND CONCLUSIONS

It is clear that recent progress in understanding the effects of insulin on cellular functions has been substantial. Detailed information on the phosphorylated sites of target enzymes that are modulated (phosphorylated or dephosphorylated) by insulin is available. This information is of predictive value in formulating and assessing reasonable hypotheses on the mechanisms of these actions. In addition, new knowledge about the structure and activities of the insulin receptor are becoming available at a very rapid pace.

The discoveries made on the insulin receptor subunit structure and on its associated tyrosine kinase activity should provide a valuable framework for extending our information on its involvement in the signaling process or processes. The relevance of this kinase activity and of the insulin-generated enzyme regulatory activity found in extracts of cells and membranes to the mechanism of insulin action, if any, remains the challenge of future research.

## REFERENCES

Alexander, M. C., Kowaloff, E. M., Witters, L. A., Dennihy, D. T., and Avruch, J. (1979). *J. Biol. Chem.* **254**, 8052–8056.

Alexander, M. C., Palmer, J. L., Pointer, R. H., Kowaloff, E. M., Koumjian, L., and Avruch, J. (1982). *J. Biol. Chem.* **257**, 2049–2055.

Avruch, J., Leone, G. R., and Martin, D. B. (1976). *J. Biol. Chem.* **251**, 1511–1515.

Avruch, J., Alexander, M. C., Palmer, J. L., Pierce, M. W., Nemenoff, R. A., Blackshear, P. J., Tipper, J. P., and Witters, L. A. (1982a). *Fed. Proc., Fed. Am. Soc. Exp. Biol.* **41**, 2629–2633.

Avruch, J., Nemenoff, R. A., Blackshear, P. J., Pierce M. W., and Osthanondh, R. (1982b). *J. Biol. Chem.* **257**, 15162–15166.

Begum, N., Tepperman, H. M., and Tepperman, J. (1982). *Endocrinology (Baltimore)* **111**, 1491–1497.

Belsham, G. J., Denton, R. M., and Tanner, M. J. A. (1980). *Biochem J.* **192**, 457–467.

Benjamin, W. B., and Singer, I. (1975). *Biochemistry* **14**, 3301–3309.

Bhaumick, B., Bala, R. M., and Hollenberg, M. D. (1981). *Proc. Natl. Acad. Sci. U.S.A.* **78**, 4279–4283.

Brownsey, R. M., and Denton, R. M. (1982). *Biochem. J.* **202**, 77–86.

Brownsey, R. W., Belsham, G. J., and Denton, R. M. (1981). *FEBS Lett.* **124**, 145–150.

Cheng, K., Galasko, G., Huang, L., Kellogg, J., and Larner, J. (1980). *Diabetes* **29**, 659–661.

Chernausek, S. D., Jacobs, S., and Judson, J. V. (1981). *Biochemistry* **20**, 7345–7350.

Cohen, P. (1978). *Curr. Top. Cell. Regul.* **14**, 117–196.

Cohen, P. (1980). *Eur. J. Biochem.* **111**, 563–574.

Cohen, P. (1981). *Adv. Cyclic Nucleotide Res.* **14**, 345–359.

Cohen, P. (1982). *Nature (London)* **296**, 613–619.

Cohen, P., Nimmo, G. A., and Antoniw, J. F. (1977a). *Biochem. J.* 162, 435–444.

Cohen, P., Rylatt, D. B., and Nimmo, G. A. (1977b). *FEBS Lett.* **76**, 182–186.

Cohen, S., Carpenter, G., and King, L., Jr. (1980). *J. Biol. Chem.* **255**, 4834–4842.

Cohen, P., Yellowlees, D., Aitken, A., Donella-Deana, A., Hemmings, B. A., and Parker, P. J. (1982). *Eur. J. Biochem.* **124**, 21–35.

Corin, R. E., and Donner, D. B. (1982). *J. Biol. Chem.* **257**, 104–110.

Cuatrecasas, P. (1972). *Proc. Natl. Acad. Sci. U.S.A.* **69**, 1277–1281.

Cuatrecasas, P., and Tell, G. P. E. (1973). *Proc. Natl. Acad. Sci. U.S.A.* **70**, 485–489.

Czech, M. P. (1977). *Annu. Rev. Biochem.* **46**, 359–384.

Czech, M. P. (1981a). *In* "Handbook of Diabetes Mellitus" (M. Brownlee, ed.), pp. 117–149. Garland Press, New York.

Czech, M. P. (1981b). *Am. J. Med.* **70**, 142–150.

Czech, M. P., and Massagué, J. (1982). *Fed. Proc., Fed. Am. Soc. Exp. Biol.* **41,** 2710–2723.

Czech, M. P., Massagué, J., and Pilch, P. (1981). *Tr. Biochem. Sci.* **6,** 222–225.

DeMeyts, P., Raffaele, A., and Roth, J. (1976). *J. Biol. Chem.* **251,** 1877–1888.

Denton, R. M., and Hughes, W. A. (1978). *Int. J. Biochem.* **9,** 545–552.

DePaoli-Roach, A. A., Roach, P. J., and Larner, J. (1979). *J. Biol. Chem.* **254,** 12062–12068.

Deutsch, P. J., Wan, C. F., Rosen, O. M., and Rubin, C. S. (1983). *Proc Natl. Acad. Sci. U.S.A.* **80,** 133–136.

Ek, B., Westermark, B., Wasteson, A., and Heldin C.-H. (1982). *Nature (London)* **295,** 419–420.

Embi, N., Rylatt, D. F. B., and Cohen, P. (1979). *Eur. J. Biochem.* **100,** 339–347.

Embi, N., Rylatt, D. B., and Cohen, P. (1980). *Eur. J. Biochem.* **107,** 519–527.

Fain, J. N. (1975). *J. Cyclic Nucl. Res.* **1,** 359–369.

Fantus, I. G., Saviolakis, G. A., Hedo, J. A., and Gorden, P. (1982). *J. Biol. Chem.* **257,** 8277–8283.

Fehlmann, M., Carpentier, J. L., Van Obberghen, E., Freychet, P., Thamm, P., Derek, S., Brandenburg, D., and Orci, L. (1982). *Proc. Natl. Acad. Sci. U.S.A.* **79,** 5921–5925.

Forn, J., and Greengard, P. (1976). *Arch. Biochem. Biophys.* **176,** 721–733.

Foulkes, J. G., Jefferson, L. S., and Cohen, P. (1980). *FEBS Lett.* **112,** 21–24.

Goris, J., Dopere, F., Vandenheede, J. R., and Merlevede, W. (1980a). *FEBS Lett.* **117,** 117–121.

Goris, J., Lamps, T., Ghislain, D., and Merlevede, W. (1980b). *FEBS Lett.* **134,** 189–193.

Halestrap, A. P., and Denton, R. M. (1974). *Biochem. J.* **142,** 365–377.

Hardie, D. G., and Cohen, P. (1979). *FEBS Lett.* **103,** 333–338.

Hathaway, G. M., and Traugh, J. A. (1979). *J. Biol. Chem.* **254,** 762–768.

Hedo, J. A., Harrison, L. C., and Roth, J. (1981a). *Biochemistry* **20,** 3385–3393.

Hedo, J. A., Kasuga, M., Van Obberghen, E., Roth, J., and Kahn, C. R. (1981b). *Proc. Natl. Acad. Sci. U.S.A.* **78,** 4791–4795.

Hemmings, B. A., Yellowlees, D., Kernohan, J. C., and Cohen, P. (1981). *Eur. J. Biochem.* **119,** 443–451.

Hemmings, B. A., Aiken, A., Cohen, P., Rymond, M., and Hofmann, F. (1982a). *Eur. J. Biochem.* **127,** 473–481.

Hemmings, N. A., Resnik, T. J., and Cohen, P. (1982b). *FEBS Lett.* **150,** 319–451.

Hughes, W. A., Brownsey, R. W., and Denton, R. M. (1980). *Biochem. J.* **192,** 469–481.

Ingebritsen, T. S., Geelen, M. J. H., Parker, R. A., Evenson, K. J., and Gibson, D. M. (1979). *J. Biol. Chem.* **254,** 9986–9989.

Ingebritsen, T. S., Foulkes, G., and Cohen, P. (1980). *FEBS Lett.* **119,** 9–15.

Itarte, E., and Huang, K.-P. (1979). *J. Biol. Chem.* **254,** 4052–4057.

Itarte, E., Robinson, J. C., and Huang, K.-P. (1977). *J. Biol. Chem.* **252,** 1231–1234.

Jacobs, S., Hazum, E., Shechter, Y., and Cuatrecasas, P. (1979a). *Proc. Natl. Acad. Sci. U.S.A.* **76,** 4918–4921.

Jacobs, S., Shecter, Y., Bissell, K., Cuatrecasas, P., (1979b). *Biochem. Biophys. Res. Commun.* **77,** 981–988.

Jacobs, S., Hazum, E., and Cuatrecasas, P. (1980a). *Biochem. Biophys. Res. Commun.* **94,** 1066–1073.

Jacobs, S., Hazum, E., and Cuatrecasas, P. (1980b). *J. Biol. Chem.* **255,** 6937–6940.

Jacobs, S., and Cuatrecasas, P. (1981). *Endocrine Rev.* **2,** 251–263.

Jacobs, S., Kull, F. C., Jr., and Cuatrecasas, P. (1983). *Proc. Natl. Acad. Sci. U.S.A.* **80,** 1228–1231.

Jarett, L., Kiechle, F. L., and Parker, J. C. (1982). *Fed. Proc.* **41,** 2736–2741.

Kahn, C. R., and Baird, K. (1978). *J. Biol. Chem.* **253,** 4900–4906.

Kasuga, M., Van Obberghen, E., Nissley, S. P., and Rechler, M. M. (1981). *J. Biol. Chem.* **256**, 5305–5308.

Kasuga, M., Hedo, J. A., Yamada, K. M., and Kahn, C. R. (1982a). *J. Biol. Chem.* **257**, 10392–10399.

Kasuga, M., Karlson, F. A., and Kahn, C. R. (1982b). *Science* **215**, 185–187.

Kasuga, M., Van Obberghen, E., Nissley, S. P., and Rechler, M. M. (1982c). *Proc. Natl. Acad. Sci. U.S.A.* **79**, 1864–1868.

Kasuga, M., Zick, Y., Blithe, D. L., Crettaz, M., and Kahn, C. R. (1982d). *Nature (London)* **298**, 667–669.

Kerbey, A. L., Randle, P. J., and Kearns, A. (1981). *Biochem. J.* **195**, 51–59.

Khatra, B. S., Chiasson, J.-L., Shikama, H., Exton, J. H., and Soderling, T. R. (1980). *FEBS Lett.* **114**, 253–256.

Kiechle, F. L., and Jarett, L. (1981). *FEBS Lett.* **133**, 279–282.

Kiechle, F. L., Jarett, L., Popp, D. A., and Kotagal, N. (1980). *Diabetes* **29**, 852–855.

Kiechle, F. L., Jarett, L., Kotagal, N., and Popp, D. A. (1981). *J. Biol. Chem.* **256**, 2945–2951.

King, G. L., Kahn, C. R., Rechler, M. M., and Nissley, S. P. (1980). *J. Clin. Invest.* **66**, 130–140.

Kishimoto, A., Mori, T., Takai, Y., and Nishizuka, Y. (1978). *J. Biochem. (Tokyo)* **84**, 47–53.

Knutson, V. P., Ronnett, G. V., and Lane, D. M. (1982). *Proc. Natl. Acad. Sci. U.S.A.* **79**, 2822–2826.

Krupp, M. N., and Lane, M. D. (1982). *J. Biol. Chem.* **257**, 1372–1377.

Larner, J. (1971). *Diabetes* **21**, 428–430.

Larner, J. (1982). *J. Cyclic Nucleotide Res.* **8**, 289–296.

Larner, J., Huang, L. C., Hazen, R., Brooker, G., and Murad, F. (1975). *Diabetes* **24**, 394.

Larner, J., Galasko, G., Cheng, K., DePaoli-Roach, A. A., Huang, L., Daggy, P., and Kellogg, J. (1979). *Science* **206**, 1408–1410.

Larner, J., Cheng, K., Huang, L., and Galasko, G. (1981). *Cold Spring Harbor Conf. Cell Proliferation* **8**, 727–733.

Larner, J., Cheng, K., Schwartz, C., Kikuchi, K., Tamura, S., Creacy, S., Dubler, R., Galasko, G., Pullin, C., and Katz, M. (1982). *Fed. Proc.* **41**, 2724–2729.

Lincoln, T. M., and Corbin, J. D. (1977). *Proc. Natl. Acad. Sci. U.S.A.* **74**, 3239–3243.

Linn, T. C., Pelley, J. W., Pettit, F. H., Hucho, F., Randall, D. D., and Reed, L. J. (1972). *Arch. Biochem. Biophys.* **148**, 327–342.

Machicao, F., Urumow, T., and Wieland, O. H. (1982). *FEBS Lett.* **149**, 96–100.

Marshall, S., and Olefsky, J. M. (1979). *J. Biol. Chem.* **254**, 10153–10160.

Marshall, S., Green, A., and Olefsky, J. M. (1981). *J. Biol. Chem.* **256**, 11464–11470.

Massagué, J., and Czech, M. P. (1980). *Diabetes* **29**, 945–947.

Massagué, J., and Czech, M. P. (1982a). *J. Biol. Chem.* **257**, 5038–5045.

Massagué, J., Czech, M. P. (1982b). *J. Biol. Chem.* **257**, 6729–6735.

Massagué, J., and Czech, M. P. (1983). *In* "Frontiers in Biochemical and Biophysical Studies of Proteins," pp. 453–461. Elsevier Press, New York.

Massagué, J., Pilch, P. F., and Czech, M. P. (1980). *Proc. Natl. Acad. Sci. U.S.A.* **77**, 7137–7141.

Massagué, J., Blinderman, L. A., Czech, M. P. (1982). *J. Biol. Chem.* **257**, 13958–13963.

Massagué, J., Freidenberg, G. F., Olefsky, J. M., and Czech, M. P. (1983). *Diabetes*, **32**, 541–544.

Massagué, J., Guillette, B. J., and Czech, M. P. (1981a). *J. Biol. Chem.* **256**, 2122–2125.

Massagué, J., Pilch, P. F., and Czech, M. P. (1981b). *J. Biol. Chem.* **256**, 3182–3190.

McDonald, J. M., Bruns, D. E., and Jarett, L. (1976). *Biochem. Biophys. Res. Commun.* **71**, 114–121.

Meggio, F., Donella-Deana, A., and Pinna, L. A. (1977). *FEBS Lett.* **75**, 192–196.
Nilsen-Hamilton, M., Allen, W. R., and Hamilton, R. T. (1981). *Anal. Biochem.* **115**, 438–449.
Olefsky, J. M., Chang, H., and Stanford, M. S. (1978). *Diabetes* **27**, 946–958.
Paetzke-Brunner, I., Schon, H., and Wieland, O. H. (1978). *FEBS Lett.* **93**, 307–311.
Pang, D. T., and Shafer, J. A. (1983). *J. Biol. Chem.* **258**, 2514–2518.
Parker, J. C., Kiechle, F. L., and Jarett, L. (1982). *Arch. Biochem. Biophys.* **215**, 339–344.
Parker, P. J., Caudwell, F. B., and Cohen, P. (1983). *Eur. J. Biochem.* **130**, 227–234.
Petruzzelli, L. M., Ganguly, S., Smith, C. J., Cobb, M. H., Rubin, C. S., and Rosen, O. M. (1982). *Proc. Natl. Acad. Sci. U.S.A.* **79**, 6792–6796.
Pettit, F. H., Roche, T. E., and Reed, L. J. (1972). *Biochem. Biophys. Res. Comm.* **49**, 563–571.
Picton, C., Aitken, A., Bilham, T., and Cohen, P. (1982a). *Eur. J. Biochem.* **124**, 37–45.
Picton, C., Woodgett, J., Hemmings, B., and Cohen, P. (1982b). *FEBS Lett.* **150**, 191–196.
Pilch, P. F., and Czech, M. P. (1979). *J. Biol. Chem.* **254**, 3375–3381.
Pilch, P. F., and Czech, M. P. (1980a). *Science* **210**, 1152–1153.
Pilch, P. F., and Czech, M. P. (1980b). *J. Biol. Chem.* **255**, 1722–1731.
Pilch, P. F., Axelrod, J. D., Colello, J., and Czech, M. P. (1981). *J. Biol. Chem.* **256**, 1570–1575.
Proud, C. G., Rylatt, D. B., Yeaman, S. J., and Cohen, P. (1977). *FEBS Lett.* **80**, 435–442.
Reed, B. C., and Lane, M. D. (1980). *Proc. Natl. Acad. Sci. U.S.A.* **77**, 285–289.
Rinderknecht, E., and Humbel, R. E. (1978). *J. Biol. Chem.* **253**, 2769–2776.
Risnik, V. V., Dobrovolskii, A. B., Gusev, N. B., and Severin, S. E. (1980). *Biochem. J.* **191**, 851–854.
Roach, P. J., Depaoli-Roach, A. A., and Larner, J. (1978). *J. Cyclic Nucleotide Res.* **4**, 245–257.
Ronnett, G. V., and Lane, M. D. (1981). *J. Biol. Chem.* **256**, 4704–4707.
Ronnett, G. V., Knutson, V. P., and Lane, M. D. (1982). *J. Biol. Chem.* **257**, 4285–4291.
Ronnett, G. V., Tennekoon, G., Knutson, V. P., and Lane, M. D. (1983). *J. Biol. Chem.* **258**, 283–290.
Roth, R. A., and Cassell, D. J. (1983). *Science* **219**, 299–301.
Rylatt, D. B., Aitken, A., Bilham, T., Condon, G. D., Noor, E., and Cohen, P. (1980). *Eur. J. Biochem.* **107**, 529–537.
Saltiel, A., Jacobs, S., Siegel, M., and Cuatrecasas, P. (1981). *Biochem. Biophys. Res. Commun.* **102**, 1041–1047.
Saltiel, A. R., Siegel, M. I., Jacobs, S., and Cuatrecasas, P. (1982). *Proc. Natl. Acad. Sci. U.S.A.* **79**, 3513–3517.
Saltiel, A. R., Doble, A., Jacobs, S., and Cuatrecasas, P. (1983). *Biochem. Biophys. Res. Commun.* **110**, 789–795.
Schlender, K. K., Beebe, S. J., Willey, J. C., Lutz, S. A., and Reimann, E. M. (1980). *Biochim. Biophys. Acta* **615**, 324–340.
Schlessinger, J., Shechter, Y., Willingham, M. C., and Pastan. I. (1978). *Proc. Natl. Acad. Sci. U.S.A.*, **75**, 2659–2663.
Seals, J. R., and Czech, M. P. (1980). *J. Biol. Chem.* **255**, 6529–6531.
Seals, J. R., and Czech, M. P. (1981). *J. Biol. Chem.* **256**, 2894–2898.
Seals, J. R., and Czech, M. P. (1982). *Fed. Proc.* **41**, 2730–2735.
Seals, J. R., and Jarett, L. (1980). *Proc. Natl. Acad. Sci. U.S.A.* **77**, 77–81.
Seals, J. R., McDonald, J. M., and Jarett, L. (1978). *Biochem. Biophys. Res. Commun.* **83**, 1365–1372.
Seals, J. R., McDonald, J. M., and Jarett, L. (1979). *J. Biol. Chem.* **254**, 6991–6996.
Sheorain, V. S., Khatra, B. S., and Soderling, T. R. (1981). *FEBS Lett.* **127**, 94–96.
Sheorain, V. S., Khatra, B. S., and Soderling, T. R. (1982). *Fed. Proc.* **41**, 2618–2622.

Shia, M. A., and Pilch, P. F. (1983). *Biochemistry* **22**, 717–721.

Smith, C. J., Wejksnora, P. J., Warner, J. R., Rubin, C. S., and Rosen, O. M. (1979). *Proc. Natl. Acad. Sci. U.S.A.* **76**, 2725–2729.

Sobrino, F., and Hers, H. G. (1980). *Eur. J. Biochem.* **109**, 239–246.

Soderling, T. R. (1979). *Mol. Cell. Endocrinol.* **16**, 157–179.

Soderling, T. R., Jett, M. F., Hutson, N. J., and Khatra, B. S. (1977). *J. Biol. Chem.* **252**, 7517–7524.

Stansbie, D., Denton, R. M., Bridges, B. J., Pask, H. T., and Randle, P. J. (1976). *Biochem. J.* **154**, 225–236.

Stewart, A., Ingebritsen, T. S., Manalan, A., Klee, C. B., and Cohen, P. (1982). *FEBS Lett.* **137**, 80–84.

Takio, K., Smith, S. B., Krebs, E. G., Walsh, K. A., and Titani, K. (1982). *Proc. Natl. Acad. Sci. U.S.A.* **79**, 2544–2548.

Teague, W. M., Pettit, F. H., Wu, T. L., Silberman, S. R., and Reed, L. J. (1982). *Biochemistry* **21**, 5585–5592.

Tipper, J. P., and Witters, L. A. (1982). *Biochim. Biophys. Acta* **715**, 162–169.

Van Obberghen, E., and Kowalski, A. (1982). *FEBS Lett.* **143**, 179–182.

Van Obberghen, E., Rossi, B., Kowalski, A., Gazzano, H., and Ponzio, G. (1983). *Proc. Natl. Acad. Sci. U.S.A.* **80**, 945–949.

Van Obberghen-Schilling, E. E., Rechler, M. M., Romanus, J. A., Knight, A. B., Nissley, S. P., and Humbel, R. E. (1981). *J. Clin. Invest.* **68**, 1356–1365.

Vila, J., Salavert, A., Itarte, E., and Guinovart, J. J. (1982). *Arch. Biochem. Biophys.* **218**, 1–7.

Walkenbach, R. J., Hazen, R., and Larner, J. (1980). *Biochim. Biophys. Acta* **629**, 421–430.

Walsh, D. A., Perkins, J. P., and Krebs, E. G. (1968). *J. Biol. Chem.* **243**, 3763–3765.

Wieland, O. H. (1983). *Rev. Physiol. Biochem. Pharmacol.* **96**, 123–170.

Wisher, M. H., Baron, M. D., Jones, R. H., and Sonksen (1980). *Biochem. Biophys. Res. Commun.* **92**, 492–498.

Witters, L. A. (1981). *Biochem. Biophys. Res. Commun.* **100**, 872–878.

Woodgett, J. R., Tonks, N. K., and Cohen, P. (1982). *FEBS Lett.* **148**, 5–11.

Yang, S. D., Vandenheede, J. R., and Merleveda, W. (1981). *J. Biol. Chem.* **256**, 10231–10234.

Yeaman, S. J., Hutcheson, E. T., Roche, T. E., Pettit, F. H., Brown, J. R., Reed, L. J., Watson, D. C., and Dixon, G. H. (1978). *Biochemistry* **17**, 2364–2369.

Yip, C. C., Yeung, C. W. T., and Moule, M. L. (1978). *J. Biol. Chem.* **253**, 1743–1745.

Yip, C. C., Yeung, W. T., and Moule, M. L. (1980). *Biochemistry* **19**, 70–76.

Yu, K. T., and Czech, M. P. (1983). (Submitted for publication.)

Zapf, J., Schoenle, E., and Froesch, E. R. (1978). *Eur. J. Biochem.* **87**, 285–296.

Zick, Y., Kasuga, M., Kahn, C. R., and Roth, J. (1983). *J. Biol. Chem.* **258**, 75–80.

# CHAPTER 5

# Antibodies to the Insulin Receptor: Studies of Receptor Structure and Function

## C. Ronald Kahn

Research Division
Joslin Diabetes Center, and Department of Medicine
Brigham and Women's Hospital
Harvard Medical School
Boston, Massachusetts


## José A. Hedo*

Diabetes Branch
National Institute of Arthritis, Diabetes, and Digestive and Kidney Diseases
National Institutes of Health
Bethesda, Maryland


## Masato Kasuga†

Research Division
Joslin Diabetes Center, and Department of Medicine
Brigham and Women's Hospital
Harvard Medical School
Boston, Massachusetts


*Present address: Department of Experimental Endocrinology, Universidad Autónoma de Madrid, Clínica Puerta de Hierro, San Martín de Porres, 4, Madrid-35, Spain.
†Present address: The Third Department of Internal Medicine, Faculty of Medicine, University of Tokyo, 7-3-1 Hongo, Bunkyo-ku, Tokyo, Japan 113.

BIOCHEMICAL ACTIONS OF HORMONES, VOL. XI

## I. INTRODUCTION

Antibodies have provided important probes for studies of both the structure and the function of many biologically active molecules. In the area of endocrinology, the unique specificity and sensitivity of the antigen–antibody interaction has been extensively exploited in the radioimmunoassay, which has allowed not only for measurements of plasma levels of circulating hormones but also for analysis of the heterogeneity of hormones, analysis of metabolic clearance of hormones, and analysis of structure–function relationships of hormones.

Since the techniques have become available to study directly receptors for various hormones and neurotransmitters, attempts have been made to produce antibodies to these biologically active molecules. In most cases, however, both the amount and the purity of antigen (receptor) available are quite limited, and thus these approaches have been slow to develop. For peptide hormone receptors, the first useful antibodies came through the study of diabetic patients with a rare form of insulin resistance characterized by existence of autoantibodies to the insulin receptor (Flier *et al.*, 1975; Kahn *et al.*, 1976). Using these human autoantibodies, it has been possible to elucidate the structure of the insulin receptor, study its turnover, develop receptor radioimmunoassays and immunoradioassays, and, most recently, characterize the protein kinase activity of the receptor. In this chapter, we will review some of our work in this area.

## II. ANTIBODIES TO THE INSULIN RECEPTOR

Antibodies to the insulin receptor were first discovered during evaluation of patients with insulin resistance, hyperinsulinemia, glucose intolerance, and the skin disorder acanthosis nigricans. In 1975, Flier *et al.* found that sera from these patients inhibited the binding of insulin to a variety of normal tissues. Subsequently, about 30 patients have been described with this autoimmune syndrome. Titers of the antibody vary over a wide range and tend to correlate with the clinical severity of disease; some sera are active at dilutions of 1:5000 or more (Kahn and Harrison, 1981). In all cases, the antibody activity is predominately of the IgG class and is polyclonal (Flier *et al.*, 1976). Some patients also have IgM antibodies, but these have been less extensively characterized. The antireceptor activity of these antibodies has been shown to be due to the Fab$_2$ rather than the Fc portions of the molecule.

In addition to inhibiting insulin binding, the autoantibodies to the insulin receptor can immunoprecipitate the solubilized insulin receptors quantitatively (Harrison *et al.*, 1979). This feature of the antibody has led to most of the structural studies described later. Furthermore, the antireceptor antibodies mimic most of insulin's biological effects on cells (see Section VII). Both the binding inhibition and the insulin-like effects of the antireceptor antibody can be demonstrated in a wide variety of tissues from species as diverse as man, mice, birds, and fish. This suggested that insulin receptors were well conserved throughout nature, and thus these polyclonal antibodies can be used successfully in a wide variety of systems.

Recently, two groups have succeeded in raising polyclonal antibodies in rodents (Jacobs *et al.*, 1978, 1980; Roth *et al.*, 1982) and making monoclonal antibodies by the hybridoma technique (Jacobs *et al.*, 1983; Roth *et al.*, 1982). While there are some differences between these antibodies and the autoantibodies, these relate primarily to domains of the receptor that they recognize rather than their basic usefulness in studies of receptor structure and function. Although we have used the human autoantibodies as the primary tool in our studies of receptor structure and function, similar observations can and have been made using these rodent-derived and monoclonal antibodies.

## III. INSULIN RECEPTOR STRUCTURE

### A. PURIFICATION

The insulin receptor, like the receptors for other peptide hormones, is a very minor component of the cell membrane. In rat liver and human placental membranes, which have relatively high concentrations of insulin receptors as compared to most tissues, about 0.01% of the protein is receptor. Thus, purification has been difficult.

Using sequential chromatography on lectin–affinity columns and insulin–sepharose columns, Jacobs *et al.* (1977), Siegel *et al.* (1981), and Fujita-Yamaguchi *et al.* (1983) have succeeded in making substantial progress in purification of the insulin receptor. Based on insulin-binding activity, the preparation by Fujita-Yamaguchi *et al.* (1983) is over 80% pure, if one assumes two insulin-binding sites per 350,000 molecular weight receptor.

The structure of these purified insulin-receptor preparations has been analyzed using SDS-gel electrophoresis and has yielded similar results. With Comassie staining, a major band of $M_r = 135,000$ is found on gels run under reducing conditions (Fig. 1). Using more sensitive methods of protein detection, such as silver staining or iodination, proteins of $M_r$ about 95,000 and 45,000–60,000 are also found. The $M_r = 135,000$ and 95,000 proteins have been termed the α and β subunits of the receptor, respectively. Peptide mapping suggests that the 45–60K material is a degradation product of the 95K protein (Y. Fujita-Yamaguchi, personal communication). On nonreducing gels, the α and β subunits appear to be disulfide linked to form one or more complexes of $M_r > 300,000$ (see Section I,C). Using a combination of lectin chromatography and affinity chromatography on antireceptor antibody-Sepharose, Harrison and Itin (1980) have identified the same pattern of subunits.

### B. AFFINITY LABELING

Since one of the primary functions of the insulin receptor is to bind the hormone specifically, another approach to the study of insulin receptor structure has been to covalently link [125I]insulin to its receptor and to analyze these complexes after denaturation of SDS. In the past several years, a great deal of information concerning insulin receptor structure has occurred with the development of photoaffinity probes (Yip *et al.*, 1978, 1980;

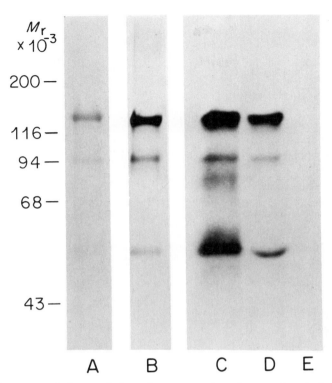

FIG. 1. Structure of the purified insulin receptor from human placenta by SDS-poly-acrylamide-gel electrophoresis under reducing conditions. Lane A is stained with Coomassie blue; lane B with silver stain; lanes C and D are autoradiograms of iodinated receptor without (C) or with immunoprecipitation by antireceptor antibody (D) or a control serum (E). [From Kasuga *et al.* (1983).]

Jacobs *et al.*, 1979; Wisher *et al.*, 1980; Wang, 1983) and the use of bifunctional cross-linking agents (Pilch and Czech, 1980; Massagué *et al.*, 1981a; Kasuga *et al.*, 1981a) to covalently link radiolabeled insulin to its receptor. With both of these approaches, autoradiograms after SDS-gel electrophoresis in the presence of reducing agents reveal heavy labeling of the α subunit of the receptor ($M_r = 135,000$) suggesting that this subunit contains the insulin-binding site. Labeling of this band is specific as judged by the ability of both insulin and antireceptor antibody to inhibit binding (Fig. 2). In addition, some investigators have found lighter and variable labeling of the β subunit and a protein of 45K, but the intensity of these bands is usually < 10% than that of the α subunit. On nonreduced SDS gels, the apparent

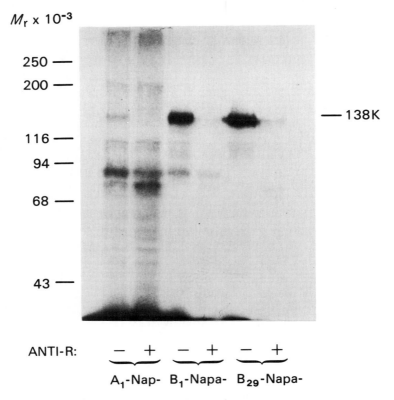

$M_r \times 10^{-3}$

250 —

200 —

— 138K

116 —

94 —

68 —

43 —

ANTI-R:     − +     − +     − +

A₁-Nap-  B₁-Napa-  B₂₉-Napa-

Fig. 2. Effect of antireceptor antibody on photoaffinity labeling of the insulin receptor in isolated adipocytes. The three pairs of lanes represent autoradiograms after SDS-gel electrophoresis of the insulin receptor labeled with three different iodinated-photoreactive insulin derivatives ($A_1$– nitroazidophenyl-insulin; $B_1$– nitroazidophenylacetyl-insulin; $B_{29}$– nitroazidophenylacetyl-insulin). In each pair of lanes, the lane on the left is cello treated with tracer insulin only and on the right with tracer insulin in the presence of an autoantibody to the insulin receptor. [From Wang *et al.* (1982). Reproduced with permission from the American Diabetes Association, Inc.]

molecular weight of the receptor is 350K, again suggesting oligomers of the α and β subunits. Unfortunately, since the labeling of the β subunit by affinity techniques is low, most of the information regarding this β subunit using affinity approaches has been inferential, i.e., based on changes in the electrophoretic mobility of the receptor under nonreduced or only partially reduced conditions. In addition, since many of the reagents used for these studies are bifunctional, there is an additional risk of artifacts due to cross-linking of membrane proteins.

## C. Studies Using Antireceptor Antibodies

### 1. Biosynthetic and Surface Labeling

As an alternative to direct purification or affinity labeling, we have taken advantage of the antireceptor antibody to study the structure of the insulin receptor (Lang *et al.*, 1980; Van Obberghen *et al.*, 1981; Hedo *et al.*, 1981a; Kasuga *et al.*, 1981b, 1982a). The basic principle for the method is shown in Fig. 3 and may be applied to cells in which the receptors have been biosynthetically labeled or labeled using surface labeling techniques. For biosynthetic labeling, the cells are cultured in medium containing either radioactive amino acids, such as [$^{35}$S]methionine, or tritiated sugars. For the surface labeling, proteins may be iodinated by the Na$^{125}$I/lactoperoxidase method or glycoproteins may be labeled by reduction of the sugars with Na$^3$H$_4$ after either galactose oxidase or peroxidate oxidation. The biosynthetic labeling procedure may be modified to study total cellular insulin receptors or plasma membrane receptors only, by adding a membrane fractionation step, or may be used to study only the various glycosylated forms of the receptor by adding a lectin purification step before immunoprecipitation. In

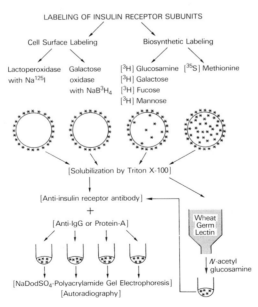

Fig. 3. Schematic protocol for identification of insulin receptor subunits using antireceptor antibodies.

the case of the insulin receptor, purification on wheat germ agglutinin has proven especially useful since it provides a 20-fold purification of the receptor and reduces nonspecifically immunoprecipitated material simultaneously (Hedo, 1982b). Other lectins may also be used to study other glycosylated forms (Hedo, 1981b).

The results of both biosynthetic and surface labeling using cultured human lymphocytes are shown in Fig. 4. When these cells are labeled as described above and the solubilized labeled glycoproteins are immunoprecipitated with serum from a normal individual, a few minor bands ranging from 25K to 70K are observed. Immunoprecipitation with sera containing autoantibodies against the insulin receptor reveals two major additional bands of apparent molecular weight 135,000 and 95,000 and a minor band of molecular weight 210,000 molecular weight. The 135,000 and 95,000 correspond to the α and β subunits observed in the purified receptor; the

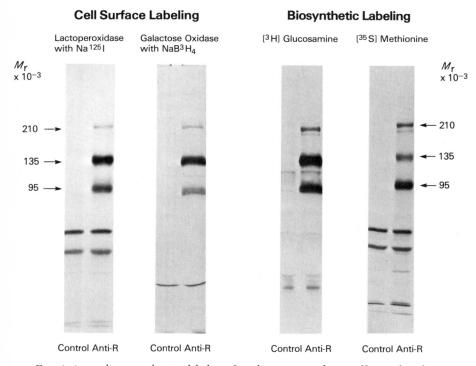

FIG. 4. Autoradiograms showing labeling of insulin receptor subunits of human lymphocytes by SDS-gel electrophoresis after biosynthetic or surface labeling. Each pair of lanes represents a control immunoprecipitate (left) and antireceptor antibody immunoprecipitate (right).

TABLE I

COMPARISON OF RADIOACTIVE PRECURSORS INCORPORATED INTO
INSULIN RECEPTOR SUBUNITS[a]

| | Radioactivity incorporated (dpm) | | |
| | α Subunit | β Subunit | Ratio |
|---|---|---|---|
| [$^3$H]Fucose | 7,420 | 3,958 | 1.9:1 |
| [$^3$H]Galactose | 17,970 | 15,426 | 1.2:1 |
| [$^3$H]Glucosamine | 18,525 | 10,148 | 1.8:1 |
| [$^3$H]Mannose | 6,414 | 3,198 | 2.0:1 |
| [$^{35}$S]Methionine | 677 | 2,167 | 0.3:1 |

[a]The data were obtained by cutting the gels, eluting the slices, and measuring radioactivity in a scintillation counter. dpm loaded per lane: [$^3$H]fucose, 33,370; [$^3$H]galactose, 148,690; [$^3$H]glucosamine, 120,034; [$^3$H]mannose, 30,580.

nature of the 210K band will be discussed in Section IV. Similar patterns are observed by all four labeling methods, although the 210K band is more prominent when cells are biosynthetically labeled rather than surface labeled. Interestingly, the ratio of activity in the α and β subunits differs with the different labeling methods (Table I). For example, [$^{35}$S]methionine preferentially labels the β subunit, whereas [$^3$H]mannose preferentially labels the α subunit.

Evidence that these bands are in fact subunits of the insulin receptor includes not only their molecular weights and immunoprecipitation by antireceptor antibody but also the fact that their immunoprecipitation is blocked by unlabeled insulin, consistent with previous studies showing that insulin at high concentration inhibited antireceptor antibody binding (Van Obberghen *et al.*, 1981). In addition, most of the radioactivity in these bands is lost after "down-regulation" of cells, which markedly decreases insulin-receptor number (Kasuga *et al.*, 1981b; Van Obberghen *et al.*, 1981). Sera from four different patients with antireceptor antibodies all precipitate the same two major bands of $M_r = 135,000$ and $95,000$ (Van Obberghen *et al.*, 1981; Hedo *et al.*, 1981a), as does an anti-insulin receptor antibody, which had been raised against purified insulin receptor by immunization of rabbits (kindly provided by S. Jacobs). More recently, Roth and Cassell (1983) have prepared monoclonal antibodies to the insulin receptor and have been able to immunoprecipitate these two major subunits. Thus, the autoantibodies are directed against the same insulin-receptor subunits that can be identified by all other existing methods.

## 2. Proteolysis: Fact and Artifact

An important caveat in all studies of receptor structure is the possible effect that endogenous proteases may play in interpretation of data. Thus, most preparations of "purified" receptor contain a 40–60K protein, which appears to be a degradation product of the β subunit. Likewise, in the initial studies from our laboratory (Lang *et al.*, 1980) the major subunit of the receptor was identified as a 90K protein, with smaller subunits of 67K, 56K, and 35K. Recently, these studies have been repeated, using high concentrations of protease inhibitors (Kasuga *et al.*, 1981b, 1982d), and under these conditions, the major subunit has a molecular weight of 135,000 with decreased amounts of the smaller proteins. This suggests that the previous observation may have been, at least in part, spurious due to receptor degradation.

In contrast to peptides derived by artifactual proteolysis of the receptor, the 95K β subunit appears distinct from the 135K α subunit. Thus, peptide mapping using *Staphylococcus aureus* protease or papain to produce limited proteolysis in SDS gels clearly indicates that the major peptides of the 95K subunit are different from those of the 135K subunit, indicating that the 95K protein is not derived from the 135K protein (Kasuga *et al.*, 1982a). We have also conducted tryptic peptide "fingerprinting" of the 135K and 95K subunits, and again distinct peptides can be identified (Fig. 5) (Hedo *et al.*,

**135K**                              **95K**

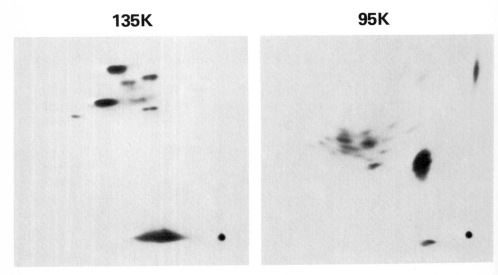

FIG. 5. Two-dimensional tryptic fingerprint of the iodinated α (135K) and β (95K) subunits of the insulin receptor after tryptic digestion.

TABLE II
PROPERTIES OF THE SUBUNITS OF THE INSULIN RECEPTOR

| Properties | α Subunit | β Subunit |
|---|---|---|
| Molecular weight | 135,000 | 95,000 |
| Chemical nature | Glycoprotein | Glycoprotein |
| Predominant terminal sugars | Galactose | Sialic acid |
| Isoelectric point | 6.0 | 5.4 |
| Trypsin sensitivity | +++ | Minimal |
| Membrane orientation | External | Transmembrane |
| Function | Insulin-binding subunit | Effector (kinase) subunit |

1983). A number of peptides of similar mobility do occur in both subunits. Whether this suggests domains of homology in the two subunits or is a result of the chance occurrence of peptides with similar properties is unknown.

### 3. Properties of Receptor Subunits

In addition to molecular weight, the α and β subunits differ in a number of other properties (Table II). As already noted, both subunits are glycoproteins and are expressed on the external surface of the cell. Surface labeling with the galactose oxidase/$NaB^3H_4$ method preferentially labels the α subunit (Hedo *et al.*, 1981a), whereas $NaB^3H_4$ preferentially labels the β subunit after periodate oxidation. These findings suggest that there are more terminal galactose and $N$-acetylgalactosamine residues present in the α subunit, whereas β subunit has more exposed sialic acid residues. The results of two-dimensional electrophoresis showed that the β subunit is a more acidic protein than the α subunit (Kasuga *et al.*, 1982a), consistent with a higher content of sialic acid.

The role of the carbohydrate in receptor function is uncertain. Treatment of cells with neuraminidase does not alter insulin binding or receptor turnover rate (J. A. Hedo and C. R. Kahn, unpublished observation). Sequential treatment of cells with neuraminidase and β-galactosidase has been reported to decrease insulin binding (Cuatrecasas, 1982), but this has not been confirmed in other studies (L. C. Harrison, personal communication).

The exact topography of the receptor subunits in the membrane is unknown, but preliminary data suggest that the α subunit is primarily externally oriented, while the β subunit may be a transmembrane protein. Thus, the α subunit is preferentially labeled by insulin-affinity labeling techniques (Section III,B) and is sensitive to proteolysis when the intact cell is treated with trypsin. The β subunit, on the other hand, is relatively resistant to

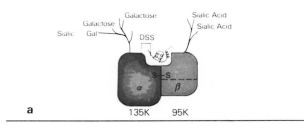

a    135K    95K

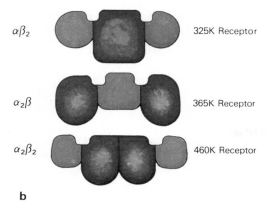

$\alpha\beta_2$    325K Receptor

$\alpha_2\beta$    365K Receptor

$\alpha_2\beta_2$    460K Receptor

b

FIG. 6. Model for structure of the insulin receptor subunits. The upper panel (a) shows the basic α-β heterodimer. The lower panel (b) indicates other possible disulfide oligomers of these two subunits.

proteolysis when the intact cell is treated with trypsin (M. Fehlmann and C. R. Kahn, unpublished observation). Hedo *et al.* (1982) have found that the β subunit of the insulin receptor can be labeled on the inside-out membrane vesicles, which occur when insulin receptors are internalized, whereas the β subunit does not label under these conditions. Finally, in intact cells, the β subunit but not the α subunit of the insulin receptor undergoes an insulin-stimulated phosphorylation, again suggesting that it has access to the intracellular ATP pool (Section VI). Thus, we believe that the α subunit is the insulin-binding subunit and is externally oriented, whereas the β subunit is transmembrane and may be involved in signal transmission. A tentative model of these two subunits is shown in Fig. 6.

### 4. The Unreduced Insulin Receptor

Some information concerning the state of the insulin-receptor subunits in the native receptor can be made by studying the labeled, immunoprecipitated receptor with SDS-gel electrophoresis in the absence of reduction. Under this condition, six major bands are observed with apparent molecular weights of 520,000, 350,000, 230,000, 190,000, 120,000, and 90,000 (Fig. 7). To characterize these proteins, we used a two-dimensional gel technique in which the immunoprecipitates were analyzed in the first dimension in SDS-polyacrylamide-gel electrophoresis without reduction. Then the entire lane of interest was cut out, placed horizontally on a second SDS-polyacrylamide gel, and was analyzed by electrophoresis with disulfide bond reduction by dithiothreitol (Kasuga *et al.*, 1982a). When culture human lymphocytes were used, the highest molecular-weight band ($M_r = 520,000$) was separated into three spots of $M_r = 210,000$, 135,000, and 95,000, with the relative intensity of label being $210,000 > 95,000 > 135,000$ (Table III). The 210K protein is believed to be a proreceptor (see Section IV). Thus, in lymphocytes this 520K receptor appears to be an oligomer of α and β subunits with some uncleaved proreceptor. The band of molecular weight 350,000 gave predominantly two spots of $M_r = 135,000$ and 95,000 on reduction, suggesting

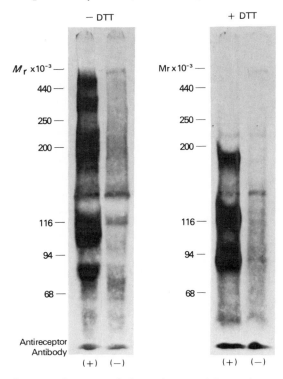

FIG. 7. Autoradiograms after SDS-gel electrophoresis of the insulin receptor from human lymphocytes under nonreducing (left) and reducing (right) conditions. Each pair of lanes shows an antireceptor antibody and control immunoprecipitate.

TABLE III
The Structure and Function of the Insulin Receptor in Human Lymphocytes

| Unreduced form | Bands after reduction[a] | Tentative identification |
|---|---|---|
| 520K | 210K>95K>135K | Partialy cleaved pro-receptor and $\alpha_x\beta_y$ oligomers |
| 350K | 135K, 95K | $\alpha_x\beta_y$ oligomers |
| 230K | 135K | $\alpha$-$\alpha$ dimer |
| 210K | 135K, 95K | $\alpha$-$\beta$ heterodimer |
| 190K | 210K | Proreceptor |
| 115K | 135K | Free $\alpha$ subunit |
| 85K | 95K | Free $\beta$ subunit |

[a]The apparent change in molecular weight and lack of perfect additivity may be due to differences in subunit mobility after reduction and differences in apparent molecular weight in 7.5% gels (after reduction) versus 5% gels (prior to reduction).

that it is an oligomer of $\alpha$ and $\beta$ subunits. The 230,000 band on reduction yielded only the 135,000 protein, suggesting that this is an $\alpha$-$\alpha$ disulfide dimer. On reduction, the 190,000, 120,000, and 90,000 spots migrated as the 210,000 protein, $\alpha$ and $\beta$ subunits, respectively, suggesting that the cell also has "free" subunits and free proreceptor. The difference in apparent molecular weight for the free $\alpha$ subunit and proreceptor on reduction suggests that these may contain intramolecular disulfide bonds, which when reduced cause an increase in apparent molecular weight. Although the amounts of these free subunits differ from experiment to experiment, we have observed free subunits in a variety of different cell types, including cultured human lymphocytes (IM-9), hepatoma cells, and freshly isolated adipocytes; we also observed these using different labeling methods, including affinity labeling and surface labeling with immunoprecipitation. Thus, we believe that free subunits exist and are present, at least in part, on the surface of the cell, as well as internally.

## IV. BIOSYNTHESIS OF THE INSULIN RECEPTOR

In addition to their use in elucidation of the structure of the insulin receptor, the antibodies to the insulin receptor can be used to reveal the dynamic aspects of insulin receptor, that is, biosynthesis and degradation of insulin receptor, as well as the time course of posttranslational modifications.

Glycoproteins can be divided into two groups based on the nature of the sugar linkage to the amino acid backbone: N-linked glycoproteins, where the sugars are on asparagine residues and O-linked glycoproteins, where the sugars are on serine residues. Furthermore, $N$-linked glycoproteins can be divided into two groups: one is a high-mannose type of sugar side chain and the other is a more complex type of sugar side chain. The biosynthesis of $N$-linked glycoproteins is thought to occur via an elaborate process. High-mannose oligosaccharide chains are transferred co-translationally from a lipid carrier to the nascent polypeptide chain (Struck and Lennarz, 1980). Subsequently, in the case of the complex-type glycoprotein, this precursor is modified through the action of a series of glycosidases and glycosyl trans-ferases, which remove the glucose and some of the mannose residues and add the distal sugars (Schacter and Roseman, 1980). Almost all of the $N$-linked glycoproteins in the plasma membrane are of the complex type. In general, the amount of these complex type side chains is less and the amount of high-mannose type side chain more when the glycoprotein is still in the process of synthesis, i.e., in the smooth and rough endoplasmic reticulum.

From the results of biosynthetic labeling with H-monosaccharides and cell surface labeling of galactose and sialic acid residues, we can conclude that both $\alpha$ and $\beta$ subunits of insulin receptor are glycoproteins containing carbo-hydrate chains of the complex, $N$-linked type (Hedo *et al.*, 1981a). This is supported by the fact that tunicamycin, an inhibitor of N-glycosylation, decreases the expression of insulin receptors on the cell surface (Rosen *et al.*, 1979). We might also predict that the intracellular precursor of the insulin receptor would contain primarily the high-mannose type of $N$-linked oligosaccharide chains, since these are precursors of all $N$-linked oligosac-charides. To better elucidate the nature of the receptor carbohydrate, cultured human lymphocytes were biosynthetically labeled with either [$^3$H]glucosamine, [$^3$H]mannose, [$^3$H]galactose, or [$^3$H]fucose, and the in-sulin receptors were isolated as described above (Hedo, 1983). All four sugars labeled the $\alpha$ and $\beta$ subunits, as well as the $M_r = 210,000$ proreceptor (Fig. 8). In addition, a $M_r = 190,000$ band was labeled by [$^3$H]glucosamine and [$^3$H]mannose but not by [$^3$H]galactose or [$^3$H]fucose (Fig. 8), suggesting that this receptor component has only high-mannose type oligosaccharide chains. The $M_r = 190,000$ protein cannot be labeled by surface labeling techniques and is resistant to the trypsin treatment, consistent with the notion that $M_r = 190,000$ protein is probably an intracellular precursor of the insulin receptor. This notion was also supported by the fact that all the [$^3$H]mannose label of $M_r = 190,000$ component was sensitive to endo-glycosidase-H treatment, which will remove high-mannose oligosaccharide chains, whereas the [$^3$H]mannose label in $\alpha$ and $\beta$ subunits and the 210K precursor was only partially sensitive to endoglycosidase-H treatment (Hedo *et al.*, 1983).

To test the possibility that this high-mannose type glycoprotein of $M_r = 190,000$ may be the precursor of the insulin receptor, the time course of

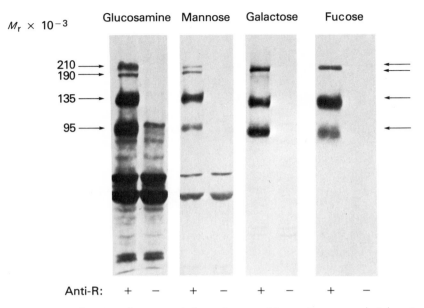

FIG. 8. Autoradiograms after SDS-gel electrophoresis of the insulin receptor on human lymphocytes labeled with [³H]glucosamine, [³H]mannose, [³H]fucose. The left lane in each pair shows the specific antireceptor immunoprecipitate. [Adapted from Hedo et al. (1983).]

pulse-chase labeling of the receptor by [³H]mannose was studied using the immunoprecipitation method (Fig. 9). The earliest component to be labeled was the $M_r = 190,000$ band (Hedo et al., 1983). Labeling of this component was maximum at 30–60 minutes and then decreased rapidly and progressively with a $t_{1/2}$ of 2.5 hours. Concomitantly, the radioactivity in α and β subunits and the 210K protein increased. The $M_r = 210,000$ glycoprotein, on the other hand, contains carbohydrate chains of both complex and high-mannose type and is at least partially expressed on the plasma membrane. In the pulse-chase experiment, this protein appears after the 190K precursor and slightly before the α and β subunits. Peptide mapping by both partial proteolysis in the gel (Kasuga et al., 1982a), exhaustive digestion with trypsin, and two-dimension separation (Hedo et al., 1983) suggest that the $M_r = 210,000$ component contains peptides of both the α and β subunits (Fig. 5).

From these data, we propose that $M_r = 190,000$ component is the initial precursor of the insulin receptor, which is converted to the $M_r = 210,000$ "fully glycosylated" form. The $M_r = 210,000$ component can be proteolytically cleaved to generate the two major subunits of the insulin receptor. However, at present, we cannot rule out an alternative order of events. For example, proteolytic cleavage of the proreceptor may occur prior to terminal

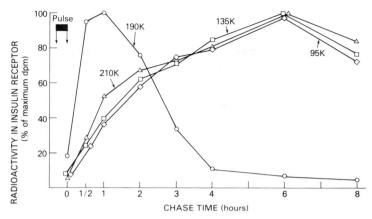

F<small>IG</small>. 9. Time course of labeling of insulin receptor in human lymphocytes after a 15-minute pulse with [³H]mannose. [Adapted from Hedo *et al.* (1983).]

glycosylation, and formation of the 210K protein may represent glycosylation of precursor that escapes cleavage.

## V. INSULIN RECEPTOR TURNOVER AND THE MECHANISM OF DOWN-REGULATION

### A. M<small>EASUREMENT OF</small> D<small>EGRADATION</small> R<small>ATE</small>

All proteins of the cell, including the insulin receptor, appear to be in a state of continual turnover. Thus, in addition to synthesis, there must also be a process of receptor degradation. In the case of membrane proteins, degradation may occur via several pathways, including shedding to outside of the cell or internalization and proteolysis inside the cell. The observation that the number of the insulin receptors in the plasma membrane can be regulated in physiologic and pathologic states suggests a dynamic equilibrium between these processes.

Estimates of the turnover rate of the insulin receptor have been made using a variety of techniques. Loss of insulin-binding activity in cells treated with inhibitors of protein synthesis (Gavin *et al.*, 1974; Shimizu *et al.*, 1980) or glycosylation (Rosen *et al.*, 1979) have suggested that the turnover rate of the insulin receptor is of the order of 12–24 hours. Using heavy-isotope labeling, Reed and Lane (1980) reported $t_{1/2}$ of 7 hours for insulin receptors in 3T3-L1 adipocytes. All of these methods, however, depend on measurement of insulin-binding activity and not recognition of receptor protein. Furthermore, in experiments with inhibitors of protein synthesis and glycosylation, it is well recognized that these agents may affect multiple processes that are involved in the regulation of a single protein, such as the insulin receptor.

We have developed a technique to study insulin-receptor turnover, taking advantage of specific immunoprecipitation by antibodies to insulin receptor. In cultured human lymphocytes, we have been able to measure the half-life of the receptor in cells that have been labeled with [$^{35}$S]methionine or Na$^{125}$I and lactoperoxidase by the isolation of labeled receptor by specific immunoprecipitation with antireceptor antibody at several points after labeling or during a chase (Kasuga $et\ al.$, 1981b). From the rate of loss of radioactivity from [$^{35}$S]methionine prelabeled-receptor subunits, the half-lives of the $\alpha$ and $\beta$ subunit of the insulin receptor were calculated as 10–11 hours under normal growth conditions (Fig. 10). Since one of the problems of pulse-chase experiments using metabolic labeling is possible reutilization of radioactive amino acid or sugar, a similar experiment was performed after the lymphocytes were surface labeled by lactoperoxidase and Na$^{125}$I. Using this method, again the half-lives of the insulin-receptor subunits were between 10 and 11 hours under normal growth conditions. These data suggest not only that the reutilization of [$^{125}$S]methionine is very low in our experimental condition but also suggest that intracellular pool of insulin receptor in the lymphocytes is small.

"Down-regulation" is a basic mechanism by which a ligand may regulate the concentration of its own receptor. This process was first recognized $in\ vivo$ as a decreased number of insulin receptors in animals and patients with various states of hyperinsulinemia (Bar $et\ al.$, 1979). Subsequently, regulation was also observed by culturing cells in medium supplemented with high concentrations of insulin (Gavin $et\ al.$, 1974; Kosmakos and Roth, 1980). Using biosynthetic and surface labeling and immunoprecipitation, we have studied the mechanism of down-regulation (Kasuga $et\ al.$, 1981b). When the labeled lymphocytes were cultured with 1 $\mu M$ insulin, the radioactivity in the receptor subunits was lost more rapidly than in control cells. The half-lives of both subunits after either biosynthetic or surface labeling were decreased to about 3 hours, indicating an accelerated rate of degradation (Fig. 10). This occurred in the absence of a change in the overall rate of protein turnover, as estimated by precipitation of labeled proteins with 5% trichloroacetic acid. The increase in degradation rate was dependent on the insulin concentration and correlated well with the ability to down-regulate the receptor (Kasuga $et\ al.$, 1981b). Guinea pig insulin was about 2% as active as porcine insulin in accelerating degradation, and human growth hormone was without effect. The acceleration of receptor degradation in-

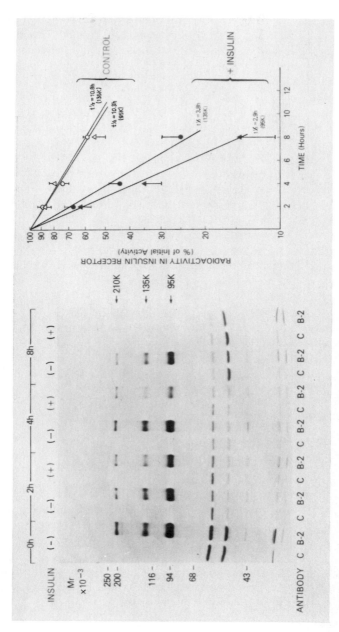

Fig. 10. Degradation of the biosynthetically labeled insulin receptor of human lymphocytes under normal conditions and down-regulation with $10^{-6}$ M insulin. [Adapted from Kasuga et al. (1981b).]

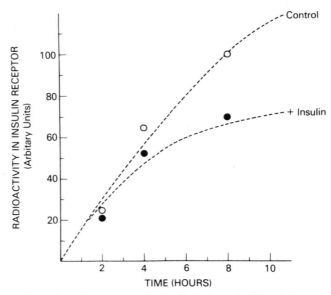

FIG. 11. Synthesis of insulin receptors during normal growth (○) and down-regulation (●). The open and closed circles are the experimental data. The dashed lines are calculated theoretically as described in the text, assuming that the only change is in the rate of receptor degradation. [From Kasuga *et al.* (1981b).]

duced by insulin was partially blocked by 100 μ*M* cycloheximide, suggesting that there is some short half-life protein that is important for regulation of the degradation rate of receptor.

## B. MEASUREMENT OF BIOSYNTHETIC RATE

Since the concentration of insulin receptors is a function of both synthesis and degradation, it is also desirable to measure the effect of insulin on the rate of receptor synthesis. Assuming a simple model for receptor turnover,

$$dR/dt = K_S - K_D R \tag{1}$$

in which $R$ is the receptor concentration, $K_S$ is a zero-order synthesis rate, and $K_D$ is a first-order degradation rate. The kinetics of receptor synthesis can then be described by

$$R_t = \frac{K_S}{K_D}(1 - e^{-K_D t}) + R_0 e^{-K_D t} \tag{2}$$

in which $R_t$ is the receptor concentration at time $t$ and $R_0$ is the concentration at zero time. $K_D$ can be calculated from the measured $t_{1/2}$ of degradation according to

$$t_{1/2} = \ln 2/K_D \qquad (3)$$

Since at steady state $dR/dt = 0$,

$$K_S = K_D R \qquad (4)$$

Although it is difficult to measure directly $K_S$, as a first approximation we can assume that $K_S$ is not changed in the presence of insulin, and we thus see if the predicted time course of insulin-receptor labeling from Eq. (2) and the $K_D$ values obtained from Eq. (3) actually match experimental data. Figure 11 shows a plot of the theoretical rate of receptor synthesis under control and down-regulation conditions and of experimental data obtained using [$^{35}$S]methionine labeling. In both control and insulin-treated cells, the experimental data agree well with the theoretical curves (Kasuga *et al.*, 1981b). These data suggest that our assumption is probably correct and that insulin does not alter the rate of synthesis of its receptor in cultured lymphocytes. From these data, several parameters concerning the biosynthesis and degradation of human cultured lymphocytes can be calculated (Table IV).

Krupp and Lane (1981) have reported that during down-regulation in primary cultures of chicken hepatocytes, there is an apparent translocation of receptors from the plasma membranes to an intracellular compartment with no change in either synthesis or degradation rate as measured by heavy-isotope labeling. Also, in this case, there is no change in Triton X-100 extractable total insulin receptor content. This type of mechanism is clearly not present in cultured human lymphocytes, since in down-regulation there is a loss of total cellular receptor extractable with Triton X-100. We believe that the difference of mechanism in down-regulation is mostly explained by the difference of cell type studied. Recently, Lane and his co-workers, using heavy-isotope techniques, have reported that insulin-dependent regulation

TABLE IV
Turnover of Insulin Receptors on Cultured Lymphocytes

|  | Normal growth conditions | Down-regulation |
|---|---|---|
| Receptor half-life, $t_{1/2}$ | 10 hr | 3 hr |
| Degradation rate, $K_D$ | 0.065 hr$^{-1}$ | 0.231 hr$^{-1}$ |
| Synthesis rate, $K_S$ | 1300 hr$^{-1}$ | 1300 hr$^{-1}$ |
| Receptor concentration, $R$ | 120,000/cell | 5600/cell |

of insulin receptor level in 3T3-L1 adipocytes involves a change in the rate of receptor degradation without changing the rate of receptor synthesis (Ronnet *et al.*, 1982).

Although the exact intracellular pathway necessary for the degradation of insulin receptor protein is unknown, Hedo *et al.* (1982), using surface labeling and specific immunoprecipitation, have shown that in isolated adipocytes both α and β subunits of the insulin receptor are internalized into a Golgi-enriched membrane fraction and that insulin stimulates this internalization process. At present, we have not performed such studies during the degradation of insulin receptor in IM-9 human cultured lymphocytes; however, it has been reported that with this cell line some insulin receptors can be shed into the medium (Berhanu and Olefsky, 1982).

## VI. INSULIN RECEPTOR PHOSPHORYLATION

### A. *In Vivo* STUDIES

Phosphorylation reactions produce a rapid covalent modification of proteins and are well known to change the activity of many enzymes. Considerable evidence has been accumulated to show that phosphorylation and dephosphorylation of proteins may play an important role in insulin action. Furthermore, phosphorylation has also been shown to occur for some receptors, such as EGF receptor, acetylcholine receptor, rhodopsin, etc. These findings prompted us to study the possibility that the insulin receptor might undergo phosphorylation, again taking advantage of the antireceptor antibody as a tool to isolate the receptor.

To study phosphorylation, a well-differentiated hepatoma cell line (Fao) derived from the Reuber H-35 hepatoma was labeled with either [$^{35}$S]methionine or [$^{33}$P]orthophosphate. The insulin receptor was then isolated from the cell by sequential solubilization, lectin chromatography, immunoprecipitation, and gel electrophoresis, as described above. An autoradiogram of gels of these experiments is shown in Fig. 12. With [$^{35}$S]methionine, peptides of $M_r = 135,000$ and $95,000$ were labeled corresponding to the α and β subunits of the receptor. When cells were prelabeled with [$^{32}$P]orthophosphate, only the $M_r = 95,000$ band was labeled (Kasuga *et al.*, 1982b). If the cells were treated with $10^{-7}$ $M$ insulin at 37° C for 15 minutes after labeling the cell either by [$^{35}$S]methionine or [$^{32}$P]orthophosphate but before isolation of the insulin receptor, there was no change in the labeling of the α and β subunits by [$^{35}$S]methionine; however, the labeling of $M_r = 95,000$ peptide by [$^{32}$P]phosphate was increased about threefold.

All data suggest that this 95K phosphoprotein is the β subunit of insulin

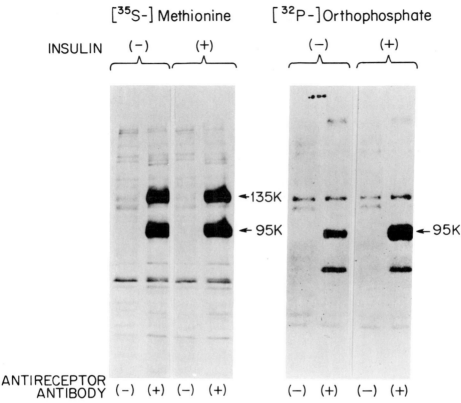

FIG. 12. Labeling of insulin receptor subunits in rat hepatoma cells by [32S]methionine and [32P]orthophosphate. Cells were labeled with [35S]methionine for 16 hours or [32P]ortho-phosphate for 2 hours, then insulin $(10^{-7}\ M)$ was added for 15 minutes at 37° C. Insulin receptors were extracted with Triton X-100 and immunoprecipitated with control or antirecep-tor antiserum. The precipitates were then subjected to SDS-gel electrophoresis and auto-radiography.

receptor. First, the protein migrates in the same position in SDS-PAGE as the β subunit of the receptor under both nonreduced and reduced condi-tions. Second, this phosphoprotein can be immunoprecipitated by a panel of antireceptor antibodies according to their titers for precipitation of the in-sulin receptor (Kasuga *et al.*, 1982c). Third, when the solubilized materials are exposed to an excess of unlabeled insulin during immunoprecipitation, there is a significant decrease in the precipitation of $M_r = 95,000$ phos-phoprotein (Kasuga *et al.*, 1982c), consistent with our previous observation that high concentrations of insulin block receptor immunoprecipitation. Finally, although it is well known that the structure of the receptor for insulin and for IGF-I is very similar, this $M_r = 95,000$ phosphoprotein cannot be the β subunit of IGF-I receptor, because this cell line has negligible amounts of type I IGF receptors (C. R. Kahn and M. Kasuga, unpublished observation). Thus, we can conclude that insulin stimulates the phosphorylation of the β subunit of its own receptor in intact cells.

The phosphorylation of the β subunit of the insulin receptor is stimulated by insulin in dose-dependent fashion and with an analog specificity that is identical to that for insulin binding to its receptor (Kasuga et al., 1982b). Furthermore, when the bound insulin is dissociated from its receptor in hepatoma cells, the phosphorylation of β subunit is decreased. These results suggest not only that the bound insulin molecule is important for stimulation of phosphorylation but also that there are cellular phosphatases that can act to dephosphorylate the phosphorylated β subunit of the insulin receptor when insulin is removed. Phosphorylation of β subunit of insulin receptor has been confirmed in the variety of cell types, including cultured human lymphocytes (Kasuga et al., 1982b), transformed human B lymphocytes (J. A. Whittaker, personal communication), freshly isolated rat hepatocytes (Van Obberghen and Kowalski, 1982), isolated rat adipocytes (Häring et al., 1982), 3T3-L1 adipocytes (Petruzzelli et al., 1982), and mouse melanoma cells in culture (Häring et al., 1983).

## B. *In Vitro* STUDIES

Although studies in the intact cell are useful for determining the possible physiological role of receptor phosphorylation, they are not convenient for elucidating the underlying molecular mechanism of the phenomenon. Thus, it was useful to further explore receptor phosphorylation in *in vitro* systems. For these studies, insulin receptors of the hepatoma cells (Fao) were partially purified by solubilization with Triton X-100 and chromatography on wheat germ agglutinin-affinity columns, then incubated with [γ-$^{32}$P]ATP in the presence of $Mn^{2+}$. The receptor subunits were isolated by immunoprecipitation and SDS-PAGE. Autoradiogram of these gels again revealed that the β subunit of insulin receptor was phosphorylated (Kasuga et al., 1982d) (Fig. 13). Furthermore, when $10^{-7}$ $M$ insulin was added *in vitro* to this partially purified receptor fraction and phosphorylation was studied, there was about a 10-fold increase in the $^{32}$P incorporated β subunit. Thus, insulin stimulates the phosphorylation of the β subunit of its own receptor in this broken cell system. Furthermore, these results indicate that the insulin receptor accepts the phosphate from $^{32}$P-labeled ATP in the broken cell system, suggesting that ATP is the source of phosphate in the intact cell system.

Phosphorylation of the β subunit of the insulin receptor in a solubilized

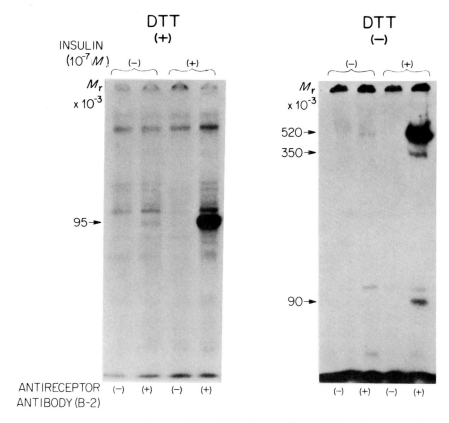

FIG. 13. *In vitro* phosphorylation of the solubilized, partially purified insulin receptor from rat hepatoma cells. The insulin receptor was extracted with Triton X-100 and partially purified by chromatography on wheat germ agglutinin-sepharose. Phosphorylation was then conducted *in vitro* with 50 μM [γ$^{32}$P]-ATP and 5 mM MnCl$_2$. The insulin receptor was then precipitated with control or antireceptor serum and subjected to SDS-gel electrophoresis under reducing (DTT+) or nonreducing (DTT−) conditions. [Reprinted by permission from Kasuga *et al.* (1982d), *Nature (London)* **298**, 667. Copyright © 1982 Macmillan Journals Limited.]

fraction was first described in rat liver and subsequently has been confirmed in a wide variety of cells. These include cultured human lymphocytes, transformed human B lymphocytes (J. A. Whittaker, personal communication), freshly isolated rat hepatocytes (Van Obberghen *et al.*, 1982), adipocytes (Häring *et al.*, 1982), 3T3-L1 adipocytes (Petruzzelli *et al.*, 1982), melanoma cells (Häring *et al.*, 1982), human placental membranes (Avruch *et al.*, 1982), and human erythrocytes (Grigorescu *et al.*, 1983). These studies also indicate that at least one of the protein kinases that catalyzes the phosphorylation of β subunit of insulin receptor also exists in the wheat germ agglutinin-purified receptor (see Section VI,D for identification of the kinase).

## C. Phosphoamino Acid Determination

In general, protein kinases catalyze the transfer of phosphate from the position of ATP to the hydroxyl groups of serine or threonine residues of the protein. However, recently, a new group of protein kinase has been identified which catalyzes the transfer of phosphate to tyrosine residues of proteins. The latter occurrences are rare reactions, and thus the amount of phosphotyrosine in cells is about 1/3000 of the amounts of phosphoserine and phosphothreonine combined (Hunter and Sefton, 1980). However, interestingly, the phosphotyrosine content of cells is increased after transformation by RNA-tumor viruses and in cells stimulated to grow by epidermal growth factor (EGF), suggesting some relationship to growth control (Hunter and Cooper, 1981). Furthermore, a tyrosine-specific protein kinase activity has now been found to be closely associated with many oncogene products of RNA-tumor virus (Hunter and Sefton, 1980; Collett *et al.*, 1980; Witte *et al.*, 1980) and the receptor for EGF (Cohen *et al.*, 1982; Ushiro and Cohen, 1980; Buhrow *et al.*, 1982; Avruch *et al.*, 1982). Since insulin also has a growth-promoting effect, we were prompted to investigate the phosphoamino acids of β subunit of the insulin receptor.

In the intact cell, there are multiple sites of phosphorylation; insulin stimulates an increase in phosphoserine (and possibly phosphothreonine) and in the appearance of phosphotyrosine (Fig. 14) (Kasuga *et al.*, 1982c). However, in broken cell systems, only phosphotyrosine was found (Kasuga *et al.*, 1982d). These results suggest that the tyrosine phosphorylation of the β subunit may be the initial reaction that occurs on insulin binding and that phosphorylation of serine residue requires other components, which were lost in lectin purification step. Similar differences of phosphoamino acids composition between intact cells and cell-free systems have been observed in the phosphorylation of RNA-tumor virus oncogene products and the receptor for EGF.

## D. Identification of the Kinase

To determine if the tyrosine kinase that catalyzes the phosphorylation of β subunit of insulin receptor is the receptor itself, we performed experiments with a preparation of purified receptor prepared by Fujita-Yamaguchi *et al.*, (1983). They have developed a method for eluting the insulin receptor from the insulin-affinity column with full binding activity using a mild acidic

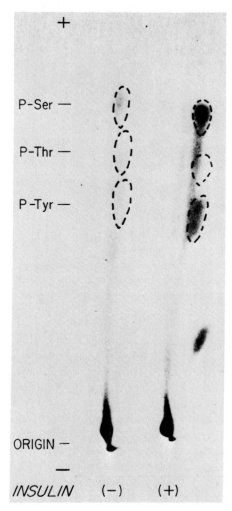

Fig. 14. Phosphoamino acid determination of the β-subunit of the insulin receptor after *in vivo* phosphorylation.

condition. The method depends on sequential affinity chromatography on wheat germ agglutinin coupled to agarose and insulin-succinyl di-aminodipropyl agarose. The final preparation obtained from a solubilized human placental membrane fraction by this method has an insulin-binding activity of 4700 pmol/mg protein and represents a 2500-fold purification. Based on a molecular weight of 300,000–350,000 for the insulin receptor complex, this purified insulin receptor can bind about 1.7 molecules of

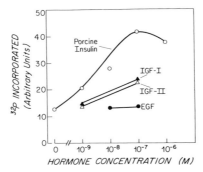

Fɪɢ. 15. Dose-response curves for phosphorylation of the purified insulin receptor from human placenta *in vitro.* [From Kasuga *et al.* (1983).]

[$^{125}$I]insulin per receptor complex. The purity of the receptor using this method was shown by staining and iodination (Fig. 1). As previously noted, there are three major bands: the α and β subunits and a peptide of $M_r$ = 52,000, which is a degradation product of β subunit. All of the three peptides are immunoprecipitated by antiinsulin receptor antibodies (Kasuga *et al.*, 1983).

When the purified receptor is incubated with $Mn^{2+}$ and [γ-$^{32}$P]ATP and directly analyzed by SDS-PAGE and autoradiography, the β subunit ($M_r$ = 95,000) is labeled (Kasuga *et al.*, 1983). As in the intact cell, insulin increases the $^{32}$P incorporation into this peptide in dose-dependent fashion. Both IGF-I and IGF-II are about 5% as potent as insulin (Fig. 15). These results again suggest that this phosphoprotein is the β subunit of insulin receptor, not the IGF receptor. Furthermore, insulin stimulation of phosphorylation of the 95K subunit of the receptor was also observed by adding [γ-$^{32}$P]ATP to the immunoprecipitate of this, purified by anti-insulin receptor antibodies. These data suggest that the tyrosine-specific kinase activity is present in the insulin receptor itself. This notion has been further supported by the finding that protein kinase activity is found in the immunoprecipitate of insulin–insulin receptor complex produced by insulin antibody (Zick *et al.*, 1983b) and the recent reports that the β subunit of insulin receptor can be labeled by components ATP affinity-labeling methods (Roth and Cassell, 1983; Van Obberghen *et al.*, 1983).

## E. Summary Model

From these results, we conclude that insulin receptor is the membrane protein that has two function components: the α subunit, which binds the

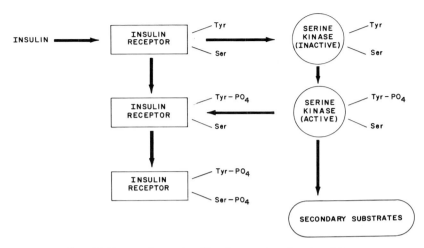

F<small>IG</small>. 16. Proposed cascade of insulin receptor phosphorylation.

insulin molecule, and the β subunit, which is an insulin-stimulated, membrane-bound tyrosine protein kinase. Although the natural substrates for the insulin receptor kinase are not known, these findings suggest that some or all of the insulin actions may be transmitted from the insulin receptor by activating insulin receptor kinase through a cascade of phosphorylation– dephosphorylation reactions (Fig. 16). Further studies will be required to elucidate the nature of this cascade, if indeed it exists.

## VII. INSULIN-LIKE ACTIVITY OF ANTIRECEPTOR ANTIBODIES

### A. E<small>FFECT ON</small> I<small>NSULIN</small> B<small>INDING</small>

When cells are exposed to sera containing autoantibodies to the insulin receptor, there is a blockade of insulin binding similar to that seen by the addition of unlabeled insulin. This is due primarily to a decrease in the affinity of the insulin receptor for insulin (Flier *et al.*, 1977; Kahn *et al.*, 1977). By contrast to the autoantibodies, most polyclonal antibodies raised in animals will immunoprecipitate the solubilized receptor but do not block insulin binding (Jacobs *et al.*, 1978). This finding suggests that the autoantibodies bind to domains of the receptor near the insulin-binding site, whereas the antibodies induced by immunization of rodents bind to other sites on the receptor. Interestingly, both types of antibodies induce an insulin-like response in cells, and this biological effect has been the subject of a number of studies.

## B. Insulin-Like Bioeffects

The insulin-like bioeffect of antireceptor antibodies was first noted by Kahn et al. (1977) in rat adipocytes. In these cells, antireceptor antibodies mimic all of insulin's acute metabolic effects; these include stimulation of glucose oxidation and glucose transport, inhibition of lipolysis, stimulation of leucine incorporation into protein, and stimulation of a number of enzymes, including pyruvate dehydrogenase, acetyl-CoA carboxylase, and glycogen synthase (Kahn et al., 1977; Kasuga et al., 1978a,b; Jacobs et al., 1978; Lawrence et al., 1978; Belsham et al., 1980). In addition, in other cell types, the antibodies can mimic some of the more chronic metabolic effects of insulin. For example, antireceptor antibody can stimulate tyrosine aminotransferase activity in hepatoma cells (Fig. 17), activate lipoprotein lipase in the cultured 3T3-L1 fatty fibroblasts (Van Obberghen et al., 1979), increase sulfate incorporation into protoglycans in chondrosarcoma chondrocytes (Foley et al., 1982), and stimulate thymidine incorporation into DNA in a well-differentiated hepatoma cell line (Koonitz, 1980). In contrast, antireceptor antibody cannot mimic insulin's effect on DNA synthesis in cultured diploid cells such as human fibroblasts, presumably be-

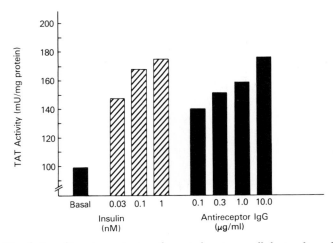

Fig. 17. Stimulation of tyrosine aminotransferase in hepatoma cells by insulin and antireceptor antibody.

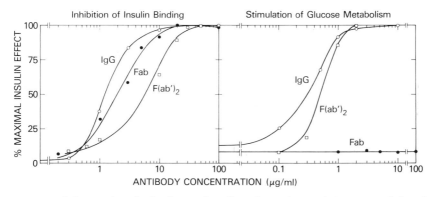

FIG. 18. Inhibition of insulin binding in fat cells and stimulation of glucose metabolism by antireceptor IgG, F(ab')₂, and Fab. [Reproduced from King *et al.* (1980), *The Journal of Clinical Investigation* **66**, 130–140, by copyright permission of The American Society for Clinical Investigation.]

cause this effect is mediated via one of the receptors for the insulin-like growth factors (IGF-II) (King *et al.*, 1980).

Both the binding inhibition and the bioactivity of the antireceptor antibodies are due to IgG and can be bound to protein A-Sepharose. The IgG's are polyclonal in nature, since precipitation with both specific anti-Kappa and anti-Lambda antisera is needed in order to remove all of the biological effect or blocking activity from a single antiserum (Kahn *et al.*, 1977). The antireceptor antibodies bind via the Fab combining site and require bivalency for biological activity (Fig. 18). Thus, when (Fab)₂ and Fc fragments are made from the IgG by digestion with pepsin, both the biological activity and the blocking effects of the IgG are found to be with the (Fab)₂ fragments (Kahn *et al.*, 1978). However, if monovalent Fab is prepared by papain digestion and reduction with cysteine, there is a loss of the insulin-like bioactivity, although the Fab retains the ability to inhibit insulin binding to the receptor (Kahn *et al.*, 1978; King *et al.*, 1980). Addition of a second anti-Fab antibody will restore the biological activity of the monovalent Fab fragment. These data indicate that the simple occupation of the insulin receptor is not enough for the transmission of the biological signal and that aggregation of the hormone-receptor complex induced by the antibody is important to its biological effects.

The monovalent Fab fragments of the antireceptor antibody have the property of being able to block insulin binding without inducing biological activity and are therefore competitive antagonists of insulin at the receptor level (Fig. 19). If isolated adipocytes are treated with the Fab fragments of the antibody, there is a blockade of insulin binding and a rightward shift of the dose–response curves for insulin stimulation of glucose oxidation (King

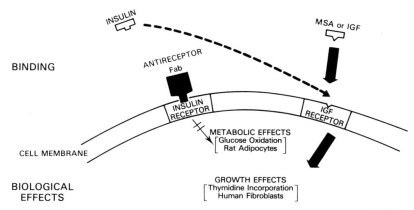

FIG. 19. Model of insulin receptor blockade by monovalent antireceptor antibody.

*et al.*, 1980). The Fab also blocks the metabolic effect of the insulin-like growth factor MSA (multiplication stimulating activity) but does not block the effects of vitamin $K_5$ or spermine, which stimulate glucose oxidation through a postreceptor mechanism. These data indicate that both insulin and IGF's mediate their acute metabolic effects through the insulin receptor. By contrast, the ability of insulin and MSA to stimulate thymidine incorporation into the DNA of human fibroblasts, a growth-promoting effect, is not impaired when the insulin receptors are blocked by the monovalent Fab, again indicating that this effect is not mediated via the insulin receptor (King *et al.*, 1980).

## C. DESENSITIZATION BY ANTIBODY

The ability of the antireceptor antibody to produce an insulin-like effect *in vitro* seems rather paradoxical in light of the clinical finding of an insulin-resistance state in patients bearing these antibodies. This apparent discrepancy can be partially explained by differences between the acute and the chronic effects of the antibody. Thus, when 3T3-L1 cells are exposed to antireceptor antibody, there is a biphasic response (Karlsson *et al.*, 1979). Initially, the antibody is insulin-like, stimulating glucose uptake and metabolism and lipoprotein lipase. However, if the antibody is incubated with the cells for more than 1 hour, the insulin-like effect begins to decrease, and by 6 hours the antibody has lost its biological effect (Fig. 20). Accompanying the decrease in antibody response is a decrease in insulin response. This process of desensitization occurs without any changes in insulin binding. Only bivalent antibody will produce an insulin-like effect and only bivalent anti-

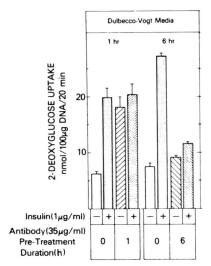

FIG. 20. Desensitization of insulin action induced by chronic exposure of 3T3-L1 cells to antireceptor antibody. 3T3-L1 cells were exposed to normal medium or medium containing antireceptor antibody for 1 or 6 hours and 2-deoxyglucose uptake was measured in the absence (−) or presence (+) of insulin. Note that at 1 hour the antibody effect is equal to that of insulin. At 6 hours, the antibody has lost its insulin-like effect and the cells no longer respond to insulin, i.e., are desensitized. [Reproduced from Grunfeld *et al.* (1980), *The Journal of Clinical Investigation* **66,** 1124–1134, by copyright permission of The American Society for Clinical Investigation.]

body will produce desensitization. The exact site of the desensitization is unknown but appears to be at steps beyond insulin binding. The desensitization process requires that the medium for the cells contain a source of energy such as glucose, pyruvate, and glucose analogs that are capable of being phosphorylated (Grunfeld *et al.*, 1980). Currently, studies are under way in our laboratory to determine if this could involve the kinase activity of the receptor.

## VIII. CONCLUSIONS

Although we have been able to review only studies using antireceptor antibodies to study insulin action, we believe that these studies illustrate the importance of such antibodies as experimental probes of the insulin receptor. Antibodies to receptors provide sensitive and specific assays useful for the study of both receptor structure and function. Using antibodies to the insulin receptor structure, we have been able to elucidate the structure of this protein, demonstrate its protein kinase activity, and study its synthesis and degradation. Because cell surface receptors exist for most peptide hormones, neurotransmitters, drugs, and antigens, the techniques described here should prove applicable to a wide variety of systems.

## ACKNOWLEDGMENTS

The authors wish to thank Barbara Cornell for excellent secretarial assistance. This work was supported in part by NIH Grant AM 31036.

## REFERENCES

Avruch, J., Nemenoff, R. A., Blackshear, P. J., Pierce, M. W., and Osathanondh, R. (1982). *J. Biol. Chem.* **257**, 15162–15166.

Bar, R. S., Harrison, L. C., Muggeo, M., Gorden, P., Kahn, C. R., and Roth, J. (1979). *Adv. Intern. Med.* **24**, 23.

Belsham, G. J., Brownsey, R. W., Hughes, W. A., and Denton, R. M. (1980). *Diabetologia* **18**, 307.

Berhanu, P., and Olefsky, J. N. (1982). *Diabetes* **31**, 410.

Buhrow, S. A., Cohen, S., and Staros, J. V. (1982). *J. Biol. Chem.* **257**, 4019.

Cohen, S., Ushiro, H., Stoscheck, C., and Chinkers, M. (1982). *J. Biol. Chem.* **257**, 1523.

Collett, M. S., Purchio, A., and Erikson, R. L. (1980). *Nature (London)* **285**, 167.

Cuatrecasas, P. (1972). *In* "Insulin Action" (L. B. Fritz, ed.), pp. 137–169. Academic Press, New York.

Flier, J. S., Kahn, C. R., Roth, J., and Bar, R. S. (1975). *Science* **190**, 63.

Flier, J. S., Kahn, C. R., Jarrett, D. B., and Roth, J. (1976). *J. Clin. Invest.* **58**, 1442.

Flier, J. S., Kahn, C. R., Jarrett, D. B., and Roth, J. (1977). *J. Clin. Invest.* **60**, 784.

Foley, T. P., Nissley, S. P., Stevens, R. L., King, G. L., Hascall, V. C., Hunibel, R. E., Short, P. A., and Rechler, M. M. (1982). *J. Biol. Chem.* **257**, 663.

Fujita-Yamaguchi, Y., Choi, S., Sakamoto, Y., and Itakura, K. (1983). *J. Biol. Chem.* **258**, 5045–5049.

Gavin, J. R., III, Roth, J., Neville, D. M., Jr., DeMeyts, P., and Buell, D. N. (1974). *Proc. Natl. Acad. Sci. U. S. A.* **71**, 84.

Grigorescu, F., White, M. S., and Kahn, C. R. (1983). *J. Biol. Chem.*, in press.

Grunfeld, C., Van Obberghen, E., Karlsson, F. A., and Kahn, C. R. (1980). *J. Clin. Invest.* **66**, 1124.

Häring, H. U., Kasuga, M., and Kahn, C. R. (1982). *Biochem. Biophys. Res. Commun.* **108**, 1538.

Harrison, L. C., and Itin, A. (1980). *J. Biol. Chem.* **255**, 12066.

Harrison, L. C., Flier, J. S., Kahn, C. R., and Roth, J. (1979). *J. Clin. Endocrinol.* **48**, 59.

Hedo, J. A., Kasuga, M., Van Obberghen, E., Roth, J., and Kahn, C. R. (1981a). *Proc. Natl. Acad. Sci. U. S. A.* **78**, 4791.

Hedo, J. A., Harrison, L. C., and Roth, J. (1981b). *Biochemistry* **20**, 3385.

Hedo, J. A., Cushman, S. W., and Simpson, I. A. (1982). *Diabetes, Suppl.* 2, **31**, 2A.

Hedo, J. A., Kahn, C. R., Hayashi, M., Yamada, K., and Kasuga, M. (1983). *J. Biol. Chem.*, **258**, 10020–10026.

Hunter, T., and Sefton, B. M. (1980). *Proc. Natl. Acad. Sci. U. S. A.* **77**, 1311.

Hunter, T., and Cooper, J. A. (1981). *Cell* **24**, 741–752.

Jacobs, S., Schechter, Y., Bissell, K., and Cuatrecasas, P. (1977). *Biochem. Biophys. Res. Commun.* **77**, 981.
Jacobs, S., Chang, K.-J., and Cuatrecasas, P. (1978). *Science* **200**, 1283.
Jacobs, S., Hazum, E., Schechter, Y., and Cuatrecasas, P. (1979). *Proc. Natl. Acad. Sci. U. S. A.* **76**, 4918.
Jacobs, S., Hazum, E., and Cuatrecasas, P. (1980). *J. Biol. Chem.* **255**, 6937.
Jacobs, S., Kull, F. C., Jr., and Cuatrecasas, P. (1983). *Proc. Natl. Acad. Sci. U. S. A.* **80**, 1228.
Kahn, C. R., and Harrison, L. C. (1981). *In* "Carbohydrate Metabolism and Its Disorders" Vol. 3. Academic Press, New York.
Kahn, C. R., Flier, J. S., Bar, R. S., Archer, J. A., Gorden, P., Martin, M. M., and Roth, J. (1976). *N. Engl. J. Med.* **294**, 739.
Kahn, C. R., Baird, K., Flier, J. S., and Jarrett, D. B. (1977). *J. Clin. Invest.* **60**, 1094.
Kahn, C. R., Baird, K. L., Jarrett, D. B., and Flier, J. S. (1978). *Proc. Natl. Acad. Sci. U. S. A.* **75**, 4209.
Karlsson, F. A., Van Obberghen, E., Grunfeld, C., and Kahn, C. R. (1979). *Proc. Natl. Acad. Sci., U. S. A.* **76**, 809.
Kasuga, M., Akanuma, Y., Tsushima, T., Suzuki, K., Kosaka, K., and Kibata, M. (1978a). *J. Clin. Endocrinol. Metab.* **47**, 66.
Kasuga, M., Akanuma, Y., Tsushima, T., Iwamoto, Y., Kosaka, K., Kibata, M., and Kawanishi, K. (1978b). *Diabetes* **27**, 938.
Kasuga, M., Van Obberghen, E., Yamada, K. M., and Harrison, L. C. (1981a). *Diabetes* **30**, 354.
Kasuga, M., Kahn, C. R., Hedo, J., Van Obberghen, E., and Yamada, K. M. (1981b). *Proc. Natl. Acad. Sci. U. S. A.* **78**, 6917.
Kasuga, M., Hedo, J. A., Yamada, K. M., and Kahn, C. R. (1982a). *J. Biol. Chem.* **257**, 10392.
Kasuga, M., Karlsson, F. A., and Kahn, C. R. (1982b). *Science* **215**, 185.
Kasuga, M., Zick, Y., Blithe, D. L., Karlsson, F. A., Haring, H. U., and Kahn, C. R. (1982c). *J. Biol. Chem.* **257**, 9891.
Kasuga, M., Zick, Y., Blithe, D. L., Crettaz, M., and Kahn, C. R. (1982d). *Nature (London)* **298**, 667.
Kasuga, M., Fujita-Yamaguchi, Y., Blithe, D. L., and Kahn, C. R. (1983). *Proc. Natl. Acad. Sci. U. S. A.*, **80**, 2137–2141.
*King, G. L., Kahn, C. R., Rechler, M. M., and Nissley, J. P. (1980). J. Clin. Invest.* **66**, 130.
Koonitz, J. (1980). *J. Supramol. Struct., Suppl.* 4, **15**, 171.
Kosmakos, F. C., and Roth, J. (1980). *J. Biol. Chem.* **255**, 9860.
Krupp, M., and Lane, M. D. (1981). *J. Biol. Chem.* **256**, 1689.
Lang, U., Kahn, C. R., and Harrison, L. C. (1980). *Biochemistry* **19**, 64.
Lawrence, J. C., Jr., Larner, J., Kahn, C. R., and Roth. (1978). *Mol. Cell. Biochem.* **22**, 153.
Massague, J., Pilch, P. F., and Czech, M. P. (1981a). *J. Biol. Chem.* **256**, 3182.
Massague, J., Pilch, P. F., and Czech, M. P. (1981b). *Proc. Natl. Acad. Sci. U. S. A.* **77**, 7137.
Petruzzelli, L. M., Ganguly, S., Smith, C. J., Cobb, M. H., Rubin, C. S., and Rosen, O. M. (1982). *Proc. Natl. Acad. Sci. U. S. A.* **79**, 6792.
Pilch, P. F., and Czech, M. P. (1980). *J. Biol. Chem.* **255**, 1722.
Reed, B. C., and Lane, M. D. (1980). *Proc. Natl. Acad. Sci. U. S. A.* **77**, 285.
Ronnett, G. V., Knutson, V. P., and Lane, M. D. (1982). *J. Biol. Chem.* **257**, 4285.
Rosen, O. M., China, G. H., Fung, C., and Rubin, C. S. (1979). *J. Cell. Physiol.* **99**, 37.
Roth, R. A., and Cassell, D. J. (1983). *Science* **219**, 299.
Roth, R. A., Wong, K. Y., and Goldfine, I. D. (1982). *64th Annu. Meet. Endocr. Soc.*, p. 377.
Schachter, H., and Roseman, S. (1980). *In* "The Biochemistry of Glycoproteins and Proteoglycans" (W. J. Lennarz, ed.), pp. 85–160. Plenum, New York.

Shimizu, F., Hooks, J. J., Kahn, C. R., and Notkins, A. L. (1980). *J. Clin. Invest.* **66**, 1144.

Siegel, T. W., Ganguly, S., Jacobs, S., Rosen, O. M., and Rubin, C. S. (1981). *J. Biol. Chem.* **256**, 9266.

Struck, D. K., and Lennarz, W. (1980). *In* "The Biochemistry of Glycoproteins and Proteoglycans" (W. J. Lennarz, ed.), pp. 35–83. Plenum, New York.

Ushiro, H., and Cohen, S. (1980). *J. Biol. Chem.* **255**, 8363.

Van Obberghen, E., and Kowalski, A. (1982). *FEBS Lett.* **143**, 179.

Van Obberghen, E., Spooner, P. M., Kahn, C. R., Chernick, S. S., Garrison, M. M., Karlsson, F. A., and Grunfeld, C. (1979). *Nature (London* **280**, 500.

Van Obberghen, E., Kasuga, M., Le Cam, A., Itin, A., Hedo, J. A., and Harrison, L. C. (1981). *Proc. Natl. Acad. Sci. U. S. A.* **78**, 1052.

Van Obberghen, E., Rosse, B., Kowalski, A., Gazzone, H., and Ponzio, G. (1983). *Proc. Natl. Acad. Sci. U. S. A.* **80**, 945.

Wang, C. C., Hedo, J. A., Kahn, C. R., Saunders, D. T., Thamm, P., and Brandenburg, D. (1982). *Diabetes* **31**, 1068.

Wisher, M. H., Baron, M. D., Jones, R. H., Sonksen, P. H., Saunders, D. J., Thamm, P., and Brandenburg, D. (1980). *Biochem. Biophys. Res. Commun.* **92**, 492.

Witte, O. M., Dasgupta, A., and Baltimore, D. (1980). *Nature London* **283**, 826.

Yip, C. C., Yeung, C. W. T., and Moule, M. L. (1978). *J. Biol. Chem.* **253**, 1743.

Yip, C. C., Yeung, C. W. T., and Moule, M. L. (1980). *Biochemistry* **19**, 70.

Zick, Y., Kasuga, M., Kahn, C. R., and Roth, J. (1983a). *J. Biol. Chem.* **258**, 75.

Zick, Y., Whittaker, J., and Roth, J. (1983b). *J. Biol. Chem.*, in press.

# CHAPTER 6

# Insulin Biology from the Perspective of Studies on Mammary Gland Development*

*Yale J. Topper, Kevin R. Nicholas,† Lakshmanan Sankaran, and Jerzy K. Kulski***

Laboratory of Biochemistry and Metabolism
National Institute of Arthritis, Diabetes, and Digestive and Kidney Diseases
National Institutes of Health
Bethesda, Maryland

*Abbreviations: MSA, multiplication-stimulating activity; EGF, epidermal growth factor; NGF, nerve growth factor; FGF, fibroblast growth factor; PDGF, platelet-derived growth factor; SmC, somatomedin C; BSA, bovine serum albumin; AIB, α-aminoisobutyric acid; $mRNA_{csn}$, casein mRNA.

†Present address: Division of Wildlife and Rangelands Research, CSIRO, P.O. Box 84, Lyneham, Canberra, ACT 2602, Australia.

**Present address: Department of Microbiology, University of Western Australia, The Queen Elizabeth II Medical Centre, Nedlands, Western Australia 6009, Australia.

BIOCHEMICAL ACTIONS OF HORMONES, VOL. XI
Copyright © 1984 by Academic Press, Inc.
All rights of reproduction in any form reserved.
ISBN 0-12-452811-2

# I. INTRODUCTION

## A. TERMINAL DIFFERENTIATION OF MAMMARY EPITHELIUM

This is an account of observations on insulin biology made in the course of studies on mammary development. The mammary system is an unexpected source of information on the biology of insulin for two reasons. First, mammary tissue has not been a popular target for study of the hormone. Second, even among investigators whose primary interests relate to hormone-dependent mammary development, insulin has not been a primary focal point. Nevertheless, delineation of the hormonal determinants for phenotypic expression of mammary epithelium has yielded significant information about the biological properties of insulin.

Organogenesis includes two major types of developmental change: (1) Morphogenetic, i.e., the multiplication of the various cellular elements and their characteristic juxtaposition in relation to one another; (2) terminal differentiation, i.e., the phenotypic expression of the cellular components of the tissue elicited by a number of kinds of stimuli, including hormones. This report is not concerned with the control of morphogenesis. Rather, it is restricted to a discussion of aspects of the terminal differentiation of the epithelial cells in the mammary gland under the influence of hormones. As indicated by the title, the emphasis here is on insulin.

The mammary epithelial cell is one of the few cell types that is not yet in a mature functional state in the adult, nonpregnant animal. Maturity is attained only during pregnancy and lactation. After weaning of the suckling young, the cells revert to a condition resembling that found in the mature virgin. Two markers of the fully developed, mammary epithelial cell are the caseins and α-lactalbumin. Both types of protein appear to be synthesized only by these cells. Caseins comprise a group of phosphoproteins; α-lactalbumin is one of the two protein components of the lactose-synthetase system. The present report deals primarily with these two markers. Most of the studies to be described concern the determination of the minimal hormone requirements for the premature expression of the casein and α-lactalbumin genes in mouse and rat mammary epithelial cells. Of the several hormones required, insulin is the major point of emphasis.

## B. The Experimental System

The experimental system used was first described by Elias (1957). Small mammary explants are supported at the surface of Medium 199 containing various combinations of several hormones, and the system is incubated for some days at 37°C. Usually, no macromolecules other than the hormones are added. Tissue from both virgin and pregnant animals has been employed. After incubation, the premature presence of casein and α-lactalbumin in the tissue and media and the premature accumulation of the corresponding mRNA's in the tissue are determined.

## C. Assays for Casein Synthesis

Even though the caseins and α-lactalbumin are synthesized in the same cell, their hormonal requirements are not identical. For this reason it is useful to consider them separately; studies on casein will be presented first. Newly synthesized caseins can be identified and quantified in two ways. They can be precipitated from cell extracts in the presence of $Ca^{2+}$ ions and rennin and then separated from noncasein phosphoproteins and identified individually on the basis of their electrophoretic mobility (Juergens *et al.*, 1965; Turkington *et al.*, 1965). In this context, the tissue is first pulse labeled with either radioactive inorganic phosphate or [$^3$H]amino acids to permit quantification of the newly synthesized caseins. Alternatively, the newly synthesized caseins can be precipitated and quantitated in tissue extracts by addition of appropriate casein antisera. The $Ca^{2+}$-rennin method detects only caseins that have been phosphorylated posttranslationally. The immunoprecipitation method can detect both phosphorylated caseins and casein polypeptides that have not yet undergone phosphorylation.

## D. Hormonal Requirements for Induction of Casein Synthesis

The premature phenotypic expression of the casein genes in isolated mouse and rat mammary tissue requires insulin, glucocorticoid, prolactin, and estrogen. Before beginning a detailed discussion of insulin in this system, it is of interest to provide a brief account of the other hormones needed for this aspect of mammary development. Using tissue from intact, immature mice (Voytovich and Topper, 1967) and mice in midpregnancy (Turkington *et al.*, 1965), it was demonstrated that all four caseins can be induced in the presence of exogenous insulin, glucocorticoid, and prolactin. No incomplete complement of these three hormones is effective (Juergens *et al.*, 1965). Furthermore, the coordinate pattern of induction of the four mouse caseins that occurs *in vitro* is similar to that which takes place throughout mammary gland development *in vivo* (Lockwood *et al.*, 1966). In the *in vitro* conditions described, the need for estrogen is not apparent. However, an estrogen requirement can be demonstrated using tissue from ovariectomized mice (Bolander and Topper, 1980) and rats (L. Sankaran and Y. J. Topper, unpublished data). This tissue does not synthesize casein *in vitro* in response to insulin, glucocorticoid, and prolactin. Also, it does not accumulate casein mRNA in these conditions (Bolander and Topper, 1981). While addition of estrogen during culture does not correct the problem, estrogen replacement therapy *in vivo* does restore the responsiveness of the tissue as tested *in vitro*. Apparently, mammary tissue isolated from intact animals can retain endogenous estrogen, or its effects, for an extended period, thus making it appear that the tissue is independent of the steroid. Long-term retention of estrogen by a mammary cell line has been demonstrated directly (Strobl and Lippman 1979).

It is clear that prolactin is required not only for the formation of caseins but is also essential for premature accumulation of the corresponding mRNA's (Guyette *et al.*, 1979) in rat mammary tissue. Similar observations have been reported (Ganguly *et al.*, 1980; Nagaiah *et al.*, 1981) in regard to the relationship between glucocorticoid and isolated mouse tissue. However, other reports (Hobbs *et al.*, 1982) have suggested that glucocorticoid is not essential but is merely potentiative for the accumulation of casein mRNA's in rat mammary explants. This is incorrect, at least in terms of certain rat casein mRNA's. Depletion of endogenous glucocorticoids by adrenalectomy of virgin rats 2 weeks prior to isolation of the tissue renders the tissue completely dependent on exogenous glucorticoid for accumulation of certain casein mRNA species (Kulski *et al.*, 1983). Tissue survival *in vitro* is not compromised by absence of the steroid. Long-term retention of glucocorticoid by the rat tissue has been demonstrated directly (Bolander *et al.*, 1979).

These observations on the relationships of estrogen and glucocorticoid to mammary tissue reemphasize an important general consideration. Isolated tissue may not be devoid of the humoral factors to which it has been exposed *in vivo*.

## E. Assays for α-Lactalbumin

While α-lactalbumin has been long recognized as a major milk protein, its function as a component of the lactose-synthetase complex was discovered more recently (Brodbeck *et al.*, 1967). This complex between galactosyl-transferase and α-lactalbumin, present in the Golgi apparatus (Brew, 1969), produces lactose, a disaccharide. The molecular interaction between the two proteins has been discussed in a number of reports (Brew *et al.*, 1968; Klee and Klee, 1972; Ebner and Schambacher, 1974). The ability of α-lactalbumin to promote lactose formation by the transferase is the basis for a commonly used assay of the milk protein (Ip and Dao, 1978; Nagamatsu and Oka, 1980). Radioimmunoassay is also employed for this purpose (Nagamatsu and Oka, 1980).

## F. Hormonal Requirements for Induction of α-Lactalbumin

It was stated above that a minimum of four hormones, insulin, glucocorticoid, prolactin, and estrogen, is essential for phenotypic expression of casein genes in mouse and rat mammary tissue *in vitro*. The essential hormonal determinants for the premature induction of α-lactalbumin in this tissue *in vitro* are less rigid. Under some circumstances, particularly when the prolactin concentration is high, glucocorticoid may not be essential. Mammary cells from rats also appear to possess a prolactin-independent pathway leading to α-lactalbumin synthesis (Nicholas and Topper, 1980). However, no conditions are known in which the induction of α-lactalbumin in murine cells *in vitro* can occur in the absence of insulin and estrogen. In this respect, the hormonal requirements for casein and α-lactalbumin are the same.

## II. INSULIN RESISTANCE

### A. Mammary Epithelium Experiences Cyclic Changes in Insulin Responsiveness during Ontogeny

We said in the previous section that insulin is essential for casein and α-lactalbumin expression in isolated mouse and rat mammary tissue. Actually, in virtually all studies on milk-protein gene expression in murine mammary tissue *in vitro* carried out over a span of almost 20 years, insulin has been an indispensable component of the culture media. The reason is that in the absence of this hormone, premature induction of the milk proteins does not occur. Even 20% fetal calf serum cannot substitute for insulin (Majumder and Turkington, 1971). Nevertheless, while the roles of other hormones in this system have been discussed frequently, that of insulin has been rarely articulated. Although it is recognized as essential *in vitro*, insulin has been regarded merely as a factor required for cell maintenance. It has been considered not to be an authentic member of the lactogenic hormone complex. Evidence will be presented later which is contrary to this view. However, it is propitious to present first some observations on cyclic changes in general insulin responsiveness of murine mammary epithelium during ontogeny.

As pointed out above, unlike most tissues, mammary epithelium does not begin to develop fully until the onset of pregnancy. Furthermore, whereas some degree of systemic resistance to insulin is manifested during pregnancy (Burt, 1956), mammary epithelium in the mouse and rat experiences the reverse pattern. That is, mammary cells in virgin animals show very little biological response to the hormone, while the cells in pregnant animals are responsive (Friedberg *et al.*, 1970). Responsiveness is retained throughout lactation, but the cells revert to an insulin-resistant state after cessation of lactation (Oka *et al.*, 1974). The parameters of insulin action examined in this context were the accumulation of α-aminoisobutyric acid, combined activities of glucose-6-phosphate dehydrogenase and gluconate-6-phosphate dehydrogenase, activity of reduced NAD dehydrogenase, and RNA synthesis.

A critical question arises at this point. If insulin is essential for casein and α-lactalbumin gene expression *in vitro* and if the mammary epithelial cells in nonpregnant animals are insulin resistant, how can premature differentiation of the cells in explants from virgin mice be effected? The answer is illustrated in Fig. 1 (Friedberg *et al.*, 1970) in terms of the accumulation of α-aminoisobutyric acid. Virtually no response to insulin occurs during the first 24 hours of culture in the explants from virgin mice (explants from pregnant mice respond immediately; data not shown). However, at the beginning of

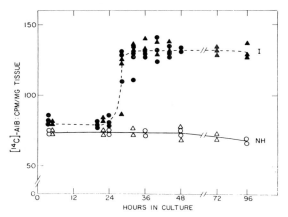

FIG. 1. Time course of AIB accumulation by mammary explants derived from mature virgin mice. Explants from two mice were cultured separately in the absence (NH) or in the presence (I) of insulin. The accumulation of AIB was measured after pulsing with [$^{14}$C]AIB (0.1 μCi/ml) for 3 hours, ending at the time indicated. Each point represents a single determination. (○) and (●) represent values from one animal and (△) and (▲) from another. [From Friedberg *et al.* (1970).]

the second day of culture the cells rapidly manifest the ability to respond to the insulin which had been added at the start of the incubation. In these experiments the insulin level was $10^{-9}$ M. Figure 2 (Friedberg *et al.*, 1970) demonstrates that the presence of exogenous insulin during the first day of culture is not required for the acquisition of insulin sensitivity. Similar phenomenology has been observed in regard to reduced-NAD dehydrogenase activity and the combined activities of glucose-6-phosphate dehydrogenase and gluconate-6-phosphate dehydrogenase (Friedberg *et al.*, 1970).

The resolution of the apparent paradox alluded to above is now clear. Although mammary tissue isolated from the virgin animal is quite insulin resistant initially, it acquires the capacity to respond to the hormone some time after explantation. This makes it possible for insulin then to exert its vital influence on the induction of casein synthesis and α-lactalbumin activity.

Insulin sensitivity of mammary epithelium develops by the second or third day of pregnancy in the mouse (Oka *et al.*, 1974) and somewhat later in pregnancy in the rat (Oka and Topper, 1972). Precocious sensitization of the epithelium to insulin can be effected by administration of prolactin for a few days to virgin mice (Oka and Topper, 1972). It is not known if prolactin exerts this influence *in vivo* during pregnancy, but a reported (Morishige *et al.*, 1973) early spike in prolactin levels is consistent with this possibility. A third way to convert insulin-resistant into insulin-responsive mammary cells,

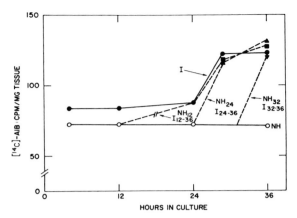

Fig. 2. Effect of culture in the absence of insulin on the subsequent insulin-stimulated accumulation of AIB by virgin explants. During culture in the absence (NH) of insulin, virgin explants were transferred to insulin (I) medium at the indicated times. AIB accumulation was measured after pulsing with [$^{14}$C]AIB (0.1 μCi/ml) for 3 hours, ending at the times shown. Each point represents the average of three determinations. [From Friedberg *et al.* (1970).]

as we have seen, is simply to explant virgin mammary tissue. The mechanism by which the cells acquire the ability to respond to the hormone is not understood in any of these instances. It does appear, however, that insulin itself does not have a role in determining the insulin responsiveness of mammary epithelial cells.

## B. Insulin Resistance in Pathological Conditions

It appears that insulin resistance in certain pathological conditions is related to the insulin receptors. Kahn (1979) has provided a summary of these relationships as they were understood at that time (cf. Section II,D). Insulin resistance associated with obesity in the animal models studied, with the exception of the Zucker fatty rat, and in human obesity can apparently be fully accounted for by a decrease in the number of insulin receptors. The remaining receptors have a normal affinity for insulin. In these cases it appears that the depressed receptor number is a consequence of down-regulation caused by elevated basal levels of circulating insulin. By contrast, with insulin resistance associated with these instances of obesity, that which is associated with excess glucocorticoid seems to be due to a marked decrease in the affinity of the insulin receptor for insulin. Conversely, the enhanced insulin sensitivity that develops after adrenalectomy is related to an increase in insulin binding due to elevated affinity of the insulin receptor.

## C. Insulin Resistance in Normal Mammary Epithelium

Unlike the instances of insulin resistance described earlier, the insulin resistance of mammary epithelium in nonpregnant animals (see Section II,A) is not pathological. Rather, it is a normal condition related to a particular stage of ontogeny. Speculation about a possible role for the cyclic changes in insulin responsiveness, which mammary epithelium experiences during development, will be presented later.

Another major difference between the insulin resistance associated with obesity and excess glucocorticoid and that observed in mammary epithelium of nonpregnant animals is related to insulin receptors. In the first instance the resistance was thought to be due to a decreased number of receptors, while in the second it is due to a depressed affinity of the receptors for insulin (Kahn, 1979). Insulin-resistant mammary cells from virgin mice have neither derangement. Thus, although it was confirmed (O'Keefe and Cuatrecasas, 1974) that cells from the virgin animal are biologically unresponsive while those from pregnant mice are biologically responsive to insulin, no difference was observed in the number of specific insulin-binding sites or in the dissociation constant of binding. Similar results were reported recently (Inagaki and Kohmoto, 1982).

It may be concluded that the virtual inability of murine mammary epithelial cells from nonpregnant animals to respond biologically to insulin is not a reflection of impaired binding of the hormone. In this case, the cellular insufficiency appears to lie distal to the formation of the insulin–receptor complex. This is one of the earliest known examples of another type of insulin resistance, one which recurs normally during ontogeny and which is unrelated to the binding of the hormone.

## D. Other Instances of Insulin Resistance Unrelated to Insulin Binding

Since the demonstration that the insulin unresponsiveness of mammary epithelial cells in nonpregnant mice and rats is linked to postbinding events other instances of insulin resistance unrelated to insulin binding have been reported. Kasuga *et al.* (1978) demonstrated that streptozotocin-induced diabetes in the rat is associated with a marked reduction in the ability of insulin to stimulate glucose metabolism in the isolated adipose cells, despite an increase in the number of insulin receptors. Kobayashi and Olefsky (1979) observed that such insulin-resistant adipocytes manifest both an increased capacity and affinity of insulin binding. They concluded that the cellular defect resides distal to the insulin receptor. Karnieli *et al.* (1981) concur and suggest that the insulin-resistant glucose transport is a consequence of a depletion of glucose transport systems in the intracellular pool. Hissin *et al.*

(1982) draw a similar conclusion in relation to insulin-resistant glucose transport in adipose cells from rats fed a high-fat/low-carbohydrate diet. Foley *et al.* (1981) and Cushman *et al.* (1981) have demonstrated that the insulin-resistant glucose transport activity in enlarged adipose cells from the aged, obese rat is not related to deficient insulin binding.

Insulin postbinding defects have been reported in certain instances of human insulin resistance also. Kobayashi *et al.* (1978) concluded that the insulin resistance in a patient with leprechaunism was due to an inherited cellular defect in the coupling mechanism between occupied insulin receptors and the plasma membrane glucose-transport system. The insulin resistance in terms of glucose disposal by peripheral tissue in obese human subjects is heterogeneous. In those obese patients with mild insulin resistance and hyperinsulinemia, decreased insulin binding entirely accounted for the reduced glucose disposal. However, as the hyperinsulinemia became more severe a postreceptor defect in insulin action emerged, and in the most severe hyperinsulinemic patients the postreceptor defect was the predominant cause of the peripheral insulin resistance (Ciaraldi *et al.*, 1981). The mechanisms of insulin resistance in patients with Type II noninsulin-dependent diabetes are also heterogeneous (Kolterman *et al.*, 1981). In patients with the mildest disorders of carbohydrate homeostasis, the insulin resistance can be accounted for solely on the basis of decreased insulin receptors. In patients with fasting hyperglycemia, insulin resistance is due to both decreased insulin receptors and a postreceptor defect in the glucose disposal mechanisms. As the hyperglycemia worsens, the postreceptor defect in peripheral glucose disposal increases progressively.

It is clear, then, that as more information becomes available the earlier notion (Kahn, 1979) that most instances of insulin resistance of fat cells are related to deficient binding of the hormone to its receptor requires revision. It now appears that postbinding defects are implicated in some of these pathological states. One of the first examples of such defects was observed in the course of studies on the insulin resistance of mammary cells from nonpregnant mice (Friedberg *et al.*, 1970). It should be reemphasized that in this instance no pathology is involved. The insulin resistance accompanies normal cyclic changes in the physiological state of the mammary gland.

## III. INSULIN AS A DEVELOPMENTAL HORMONE

In the previous section, insulin resistance in relation to peripheral glucose intolerance was discussed. This aspect of insulin biology is of great clinical importance in relation to diabetes. Insulin, of course, exerts other acute effects on its target tissues. In addition, insulin is known to elicit growth responses and to evoke other "late" or long-term biological effects. For example, insulin treatment of 3T3-L1 fatty fibroblasts increases the activity of lipoprotein lipase maximally after 2–4 days but is without effect during the first 4 hours (Spooner *et al.*, 1979). Such late effects have occasionally been termed "chronic metabolic" responses to insulin (Van Obberghen *et al.*, 1979). Other instances of such "late" effects will be presented later. Here we wish to suggest that it might be useful to regard at least some so-called chronic metabolic responses to insulin as developmental effects of the hormone. More particularly, we wish to suggest that insulin may be essential for selective gene expression in certain cells at particular stages of ontogeny. Regardless of whether or not such functions of insulin are critical in relation to diabetes, they are probably significant in terms of general developmental biology. In this section the role of insulin as an essential developmental agent for the terminal differentiation of murine mammary epithelial cells will be discussed. This system may serve as a prototype for similar studies on other systems.

### A. PHYSIOLOGICAL LEVELS OF INSULIN SUFFICE FOR MILK-PROTEIN GENE EXPRESSION IN MURINE MAMMARY EPITHELIUM *in Vitro*

It was stated earlier that glucocorticoid and prolactin, in the absence of insulin, do not support the induction of casein or α-lactalbumin in murine mammary tissue *in vitro*. Supporting evidence is provided in Figs. 3 and 4,

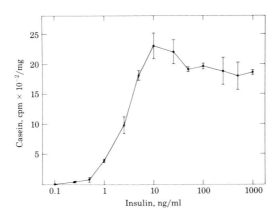

FIG. 3. Insulin dose–response relationship for casein synthesis in mammary gland explants from midpregnant mice. Explants were cultured for 44 hours in Medium 199 containing cortisol (1 μg/ml), prolactin (1 μg/ml), and insulin and then pulsed for 4 hours with $^{33}P_i$ (10 μCi/ml). Casein was determined by immunoprecipitation; results (radioactivity per mg of tissue) are mean ± SEM of three pools of tissue. [From Bolander *et al.* (1981).]

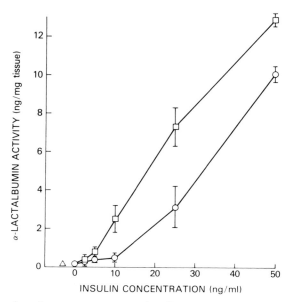

FIG. 4. Effect of insulin concentration on α-lactalbumin activity in pregnant rat mammary-gland explants. Tissue was cultured for 96 hours in media containing hydrocortisone (0.05 μg/ml), prolactin (1 μg/ml), and insulin (concentrations indicated) in the presence (1 mg/ml) (□) or absence (○) of BSA. △ indicates the α-lactalbumin activity in the mammary gland prior to culture. Each value represents mean ± SEM for 3 rats.

respectively. However, a physiological level of insulin, in the presence of cortisol and prolactin, does support the induction of casein synthesis by mouse mammary explants (Fig. 3) (Bolander *et al.*, 1981) and does promote the induction of α-lactalbumin activity in cultured rat mammary tissue (Fig. 4). These effects of insulin do not require the presence of glucose in the medium; similar responses are observed when the Medium 199 contains fructose instead. It was pointed out previously that, although the mammary cells in nonpregnant mice and rats are insulin resistant, they can avail themselves of the essential contribution of insulin *in vitro* since they acquire insulin responsiveness after explantation. Although insulin is not essential for milk-protein gene expression in rabbit mammary gland, it appears to be required for other aspects of the terminal differentiation of this tissue (L. Sankaran and Y. J. Topper, unpublished data).

## B. Specificity of Insulin for Milk-Protein Synthesis and mRNA Accumulation

In an effort to determine whether insulin is unique in its ability to support milk-protein induction, other factors have been tested in the culture system containing cortisol and prolactin. In the experiment depicted in Fig. 5, relating to rat α-lactalbumin activity, each factor was tested at 0.25 μg/ml, a concentration considerably above their physiological level (Cohen and Savage, 1974; Antoniades and Scher, 1977; Jaffe and Behrman, 1979; Wilde and Kuhn, 1979; Moses *et al.*, 1980); the blood level of FGF has not been reported. In addition, both MSA and EGF were tested at a concentration of 1 μg/ml, with similar results (data not shown). MSA, EGF, and FGF are less than 10% as active as insulin, while proinsulin, PDGF, and NGF have no detectable activity. Figure 6 shows that insulin is also far more effective than the other factors in promoting the induction of casein synthesis in the isolated rat tissue; proinsulin and MSA are less than 10% as effective. The low activity of proinsulin suggests that the effects elicited by insulin involve interaction between the hormone and its own receptor.

A prolactin-independent pathway leading to the induction of α-lactalbumin activity in rat mammary explants was alluded to in the introduction. This pathway, which is not found in mammary tissue from mice or rabbits, requires both insulin and glucocorticoid (Nicholas and Topper,

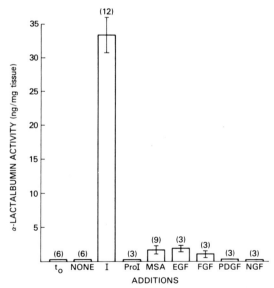

FIG. 5. Comparison of insulin, proinsulin, and several growth factors for their ability to support accumulation of α-lactalbumin activity in pregnant rat mammary explants. All culture media contained hydrocortisone (0.05 μg/ml) and prolactin (1 μg/ml). Tissue was cultured for 96 hours with these two hormones only or together with one of the following factors (each at 0.25 μg/ml): insulin (I), proinsulin (proI), MSA, EGF, FGF, PDGF, or NGF. $t_0$ indicates the α-lactalbumin activity in the mammary gland prior to culture. Each value represents mean ± SEM for the number of rats shown in parenthesis.

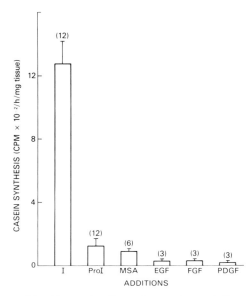

FIG. 6. Comparison of insulin, proinsulin, and several growth factors for their ability to induce casein synthesis in pregnant rat mammary-gland explants. Explants from 14-day pregnant rats were cultured for 72 hours in medium containing hydrocortisone and prolactin, each at 1 μg/l, and either insulin (I), proinsulin (proI), or the growth factors, each at 0.25 μg/ml. The explants were pulsed with 20 μCi/ml of [³H]L-amino acid mixture during the last 16 hours of incubation and the amount of casein formed was measured by immunoprecipitation using sheep, anti-rat casein serum. Values are mean ± SEM for the number of rats shown, each analyzed separately.

1980; Nicholas *et al.*, 1981). Furthermore, the pathway is enhanced by addition of bovine serum albumin (BSA); the latter does not function by virtue of a prolactin contamination (K. R. Nicholas and Y. J. Topper, unpublished data). This system, also, has a specificity for insulin. Neither EGF nor MSA is effective in the presence of cortisol and BSA (Fig. 7).

Actually, the only substance found capable of substituting for insulin in the induction of murine milk protein is anti-insulin-receptor antibody. Its effect on the induction of mouse casein synthesis is depicted in Fig. 8. The implications of such a "late" effect in terms of insulin biology have been discussed by Van Obberghen *et al.* (1979).

Insulin is not only specifically required for the formation of milk proteins but is also essential for the accumulation of mouse $mRNA_{csn}$. Culture for 48 hours in the presence of cortisol and prolactin alone results in an 80% loss of the $mRNA_{csn}$ present in the freshly isolated tissue (Table I) (Bolander *et al.*, 1981). Addition of epidermal growth factor or somatomedin C maintains the

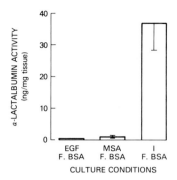

FIG. 7. Essentiality of insulin for induction of α-lactalbumin activity in pregnant rat mammary explants in the presence of hydrocortisone and BSA. Mammary explants were cultured for a total of 4 days in Medium 199 containing hydrocortisone (F, 1 μg/ml) and BSA (2 mg/ml) together with either insulin (I, 0.1 μg/ml), EGF (1 μg/ml), or MSA (1 μg/ml). α-Lactalbumin was determined in tissue extracts in the presence of galactosyltransferase. Each value represents mean ± SEM for 3 rats.

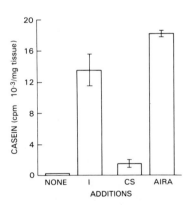

FIG. 8. Capacity of insulin and anti-insulin-receptor antibodies to induce casein synthesis in pregnant mouse mammary explants. Mammary explants from 12-day pregnant mice were cultured for 2 days in Medium 199 containing hydrocortisone (1 μg/ml) and prolactin (1 μg/ml) or in media containing hydrocortisone and prolactin together with either insulin (0.02 μg/ml), anti-insulin-receptor antibodies (AIRA, 1:50 dilution of serum), or control serum (CS, 1:50 dilution of normal adult serum). A mixture of [³H]amino acids (20 μCi/ml) was added to the media for the final 24 hours of culture and casein synthesis in explants determined by immunoprecipitation. Each value represents mean ± SEM for 3 groups of mice (3–4 mice/group).

*Yale J. Topper et al.*

TABLE I

EFFECT OF GROWTH FACTORS ON mRNA$_{csn}$ ACCUMULATION AND
RER FORMATION[a]

| Addition | mRNA$_{csn}$% | RNA in RER ($\mu g/100$ mg) |
|---|---|---|
| None ($t_0$) | $0.099 \pm 0.011$ | $2.2 \pm 0.2$ |
| None (cultured) | $0.020 \pm 0.004$ | $2.0 \pm 0.4$ |
| Insulin | $1.39 \pm 0.16$ | $9.9 \pm 0.5$ |
| Epidermal growth factor | $0.093 \pm 0.008$ | $8.8 \pm 0.5$ |
| Somatomedin C | $0.103 \pm 0.011$ | $9.1 \pm 0.3$ |

[a]Mammary gland explants from midpregnant mice were either assayed immediately ($t_0$) or cultured for 48 hours in Medium 199 containing growth factor (50 ng/ml) and cortisol (1 μg/ml). When mRNA$_{csn}$ was to be assayed, prolactin (1 μg/ml) was also present. mRNA$_{csn}$ was determined by RNA excess hybridization (Nagaiah *et al.*, 1981) and RNA in RER was measured in an epithelial cell-enriched fraction (Oka and Topper, 1971). Results are mean ± SEM of three pools of tissue, except for somatomedin C which, because of limited supplies, was assayed twice and is average ± range.

initial level of the messenger but does not enhance its level. By contrast, insulin evokes a 14-fold increase in the accumulation of mRNA$_{csn}$.

## C. CELL MAINTENANCE *in Vitro*

Barnawell (1965) reported that the epithelial cells in rat mammary explants lose viability during culture in the absence of exogenous insulin. The observation (Table I) that much of the mRNA$_{csn}$ present in freshly isolated mouse mammary tissue is lost during culture in the absence of insulin is consistent with this conclusion. A critical question, then, is whether the unique ability of insulin to promote milk-protein gene expression reflects a unique ability of the hormone to maintain the cells or whether, in addition to its cell maintenance function, it also participates more directly in casein and α-lactalbumin gene expression. An approach to this question is to determine whether any of the factors found to be ineffective in such gene expression can, nevertheless, maintain the cells.

Table I (Bolander *et al.*, 1981) demonstrates that cortisol alone does not produce an increment in the rough endoplasmic reticulum (RER) of cultured mouse mammary epithelium. When insulin is also present a four- to fivefold increase in RER accumulation occurs. Despite the fact that neither EGF nor

SmC elicited any increase in the accumulation of $mRNA_{csn}$, they were as effective as insulin in promoting enhanced accumulation of the RER. Epidermal growth factor is also as effective as insulin in maintaining general cellular responsiveness to prolactin (Bolander *et al.*, 1981). The results suggest that although both EGF and SmC can maintain the cells as well as insulin, only insulin has the additional capacity to participate in milk-protein gene expression.

Similarly, Table II shows that hydrocortisone alone does not maintain the initial level of rat mammary epithelial NADH-cytochrome *c* reductase activity in culture. Addition of insulin, MSA, or EGF does result in maintenance of the initial enzyme activity, which denotes maintenance of cellular responsiveness to hydrocortisone (Oka and Topper, 1971). Again, it appears that while MSA and EGF can sustain the cells as well as insulin, only insulin can function in the production of the milk proteins (cf. Figs. 5–7).

Although the type of evidence presented above is consistent with the possibility that other factors can sustain murine mammary epithelial cells as well as insulin, it might be argued that the particular activities selected do not adequately represent cell maintenance as required for the complex processes involved in the induction of the milk proteins. A more direct experimental approach to this issue is presented in Fig. 9. Here it is apparent that although MSA in the presence of glucocorticoid and prolactin has little

TABLE II

CAPACITY OF INSULIN, MSA, AND EGF TO MAINTAIN NADH-CYTOCHROME *c* REDUCTASE ACTIVITY IN PREGNANT RAT MAMMARY GLAND EXPLANTS[a]

| Culture conditions | NADH-cytochrome *c* reductase ($\Delta A_{550nm}$/min/g tissue) |
|---|---|
| Uncultured | $0.377 \pm 0.08$ (2) |
| Hydrocortisone | $0.119 \pm 0.01$ (5) |
| Insulin + hydrocortisone | $0.400 \pm 0.07$ (4) |
| MSA + hydrocortisone | $0.373 \pm 0.03$ (5) |
| EGF + hydrocortisone | $0.344 \pm 0.02$ (2) |

[a]Tissue was cultured for 96 hours in media containing hydrocortisone ($0.05$ $\mu$g/ml) alone or a combination of hydrocortisone and either insulin, MSA, or EGF (each at a concentration of $0.25$ $\mu$g/ml). NADH-cytochrome *c* reductase was measured (Oka and Topper, 1971) in epithelial cell enriched fractions following collagenase digestion of the explants (Freeman and Topper, 1978). Values represent mean $\pm$ SEM or mean $\pm$ range with the number of observations shown in parenthesis.

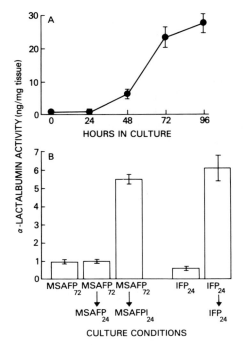

FIG. 9. Capacity of MSA to maintain hormone-responsive mammary epithelial cells. (A) Explants from pregnant rat mammary glands were cultured in media containing insulin (0.25 μg/ml), hydrocortisone (0.05 μg/ml), and prolactin (1 μg/ml), and the α-lactalbumin activity in tissue extracts determined at daily intervals. Each value represents mean ± SEM for 3 groups of rats (2 rats/group). (B) Explants were cultured in media containing hydrocortisone (F, 0.05 μg/ml), prolactin (P, 1 μg/ml) and MSA (0.25 μg/ml) for 72 hours, and then the media were changed to fresh MSAFP medium or MSAFPI medium (I, 0.25 μg/ml); culture was continued for an additional 24 hours. α-Lactalbumin activity was determined in tissue extracts. The values shown for the IFP system correspond to those shown in (A). Each value represents mean ± SEM for 3 groups of rats (2 rats/group).

ability to promote the induction of α-lactalbumin activity, it does maintain, during 3 days of culture, the cells' potential for prompt response to the delayed addition of insulin. More specifically, the presence of insulin for 1 day following 3 days with MSA, glucocorticoid, and prolactin resulted in approximately as much induction as that which occurred during a 1-day period in a system containing insulin from the start.

Although an attractive feature of the mammary system as a model for the study of hormone-dependent development is its ability to respond in chemically defined media, fetal calf serum (FCS) has been useful recently in the segregation of maintenance and inductive effects. It was stated (Section II,A) that 20% FCS cannot substitute for insulin in terms of milk-protein gene expression. However, data in Fig. 10 demonstrate that FCS is an effective maintenance agent (Kulski *et al.*, 1983). Note that while hydrocortisone and prolactin alone do not sustain the ability of the tissue to respond to the delayed addition of insulin, FCS, in addition, does sustain this ability. This maintenance property of FCS was exploited to learn more about the hormonal requirements for the accumulation of rat casein mRNA. Several observations are recorded in Fig. 11: (1) The high initial level of 25K casein mRNA present in tissue from the pregnant rat falls during culture with FCS, hydrocortisone, and prolactin and also falls during culture with FCS, insulin, and hydrocortisone. (2) The delayed addition of insulin to the FCS-hydrocortisone-prolactin system leads to an enhanced level of 25 K mRNA, but the delayed addition of MSA or EGF does not; this again points up the specificity of insulin. (3) The delayed addition of prolactin to the FCS-insulin-hydrocortisone system produces about the same effect as the delayed addition of insulin. Similar results were obtained in relation to the 42K casein mRNA (data not shown). It is clear that both insulin and prolactin are required for the accumulation of rat casein mRNA and that the hormone added last cannot account for the entire response. For this reason, previous attribution

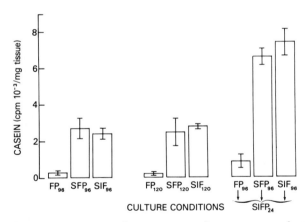

FIG. 10. Effect of fetal calf serum on the maintenance of rat mammary explants. The explants were cultured for 96 hours with F and P; fetal calf serum (S), F, and P; or S, I, and F; they were then cultured for an additional 24 hours with S, I, F, and P. The cultures were pulsed with [³H]amino acids (30 μCi/ml) during the last 4 hours of culture, and newly synthesized casein was determined by immunoprecipitation. The concentration of S was 20% (v/v) and the concentrations of I, F, and P were 25, 50, and 1000 ng/ml, respectively. Each value represents mean ± SEM for three groups of day-13 pregnant rats, with two animals per group.

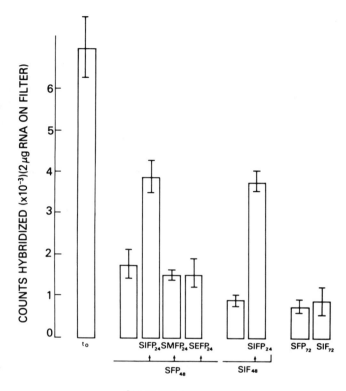

FIG. 11. Effect of insulin or prolactin on the accumulation of 25K casein mRNA. Explants were cultured for 48 hours with fetal calf serum (S), F, and P and then for an additional 24 hours with (S, I, F, and P), (S, MSA, F, and P), or (S, EGF, F, and P). Alternatively, the explants were first cultured with S, I, and F and then with S, I, F, and P. The concentrations of I, EGF (E), MSA (M), F, and P were 10, 100, 100, 50, and 1000 ng/ml, respectively. RNA (1 or 2 µg) was bound to DBM paper for the hybridization assay. Each value represents mean ± SEM for three groups of day-13 pregnant rats with two animals per group. $t_o$ represents the amount of casein mRNA present in the freshly isolated tissue.

(Guyette *et al.*, 1979) of changes in transcription rate and half-life of casein mRNA to prolactin alone must be reconsidered.


### D. Cell Maintenance *in Vivo*

It has been reported (Walters and McLean, 1968; Baldwin and Louis, 1975) that lactating mammary cells do not survive in animals with diabetes.

However, it is not known whether this lability is due to the absence of insulin *per se* or to the systemic pathology associated with this disease. By contrast, mammary epithelial cells in normal nonpregnant mice and rats exist in the functional absence of insulin (cf. Section II,A). Under these circumstances, of course, no pathology exists and other circulating factors are presumably implicated in maintenance of the cells. Similarly, other factors can maintain the cells *in vitro* in the absence of insulin under normal culture conditions, including controlled glucose concentration, as we have seen.

### E. Conclusions Concerning Insulin as a Developmental Hormone in the Mammary System

The explant system used in these studies has made it possible to demonstrate a unique role of insulin in the phenotypic expression of murine mammary epithelial cells unrelated to its function in cell maintenance. The biological events involved in this role are virtually completely dependent on insulin. By contrast, the events related to the acute metabolic functions of the hormone, such as transport of substrates, general protein synthesis, etc., generally do not show such total dependency.

Cyclic changes in insulin responsiveness during ontogeny, experienced by murine mammary epithelial cells, were discussed earlier. The physiological purpose of such changes is certainly not obvious. One possibility is that insulin resistance of the cells in nonpregnant animals is one device by which premature differentiation of the cells can be obviated, while acquisition of responsiveness during pregnancy permits insulin to play its critical developmental role during this stage of rapid mammary differentiation.

### F. Other Systems in Which Insulin May Function as a Developmental Hormone

There have been sporadic reports in the literature which suggest that insulin may play a role in selective gene expression in other cell types also. Some of these studies were carried out in the whole animal, nondiabetic and diabetic, with the usual attendant difficulties of interpretation. Others demonstrate a direct effect of insulin on isolated tissues or cells, but the specificity of the hormone has not been established.

Administration of insulin to adrenalectomized rats increases the accumulation of mRNA for tyrosine aminotransferase in the liver (Hill *et al.*, 1981). This may not be a unique response to insulin, since glucocorticoid can induce the corresponding enzyme in isolated rat hepatoma cells (Tomkins *et al.*, 1966). The pancreas of diabetic rats manifests a selective reduction in the level of mRNA for amylase (Korc *et al.*, 1981), and the livers of mildly diabetic rats show a selective reduction in the level of mRNA for $\alpha_{2\mu}$-globulin (Roy *et al.*, 1980). It is not clear, however, whether the defects are the result of deprivation of insulin *per se* or of the systemic derangements of diabetes.

Insulin can induce $\delta$-crystallin mRNA in cultures of chicken lens epithelial cells (Milstone and Piatigorsky, 1977). Serum is also effective in this system, but the active component of serum has not been identified. Lipoprotein lipase activity in 3T3-L1 fibroblasts is stimulated to maximum levels after 4 days of culture in the presence of insulin (Spooner *et al.*, 1979), as mentioned earlier, and insulin can effect the determination of preadipocytes (Sager and Kovac, 1981).

We suggest that such effects, variously termed "late," "long-term," and "chronic metabolic," and which we have referred to as developmental effects, probably represent a category of biological activity distinct from the more commonly studied acute effects of the hormone. More particularly, they may represent important influences of insulin at the level of gene expression and warrant greater attention than they have received heretofore. It will be of great interest to determine whether the isolated systems cited above are similar to the mammary system, i.e., whether they, too, have a unique requirement for insulin unrelated to its efficacy in cell maintenance.

## IV. CONCLUSIONS

Mammary epithelial cells in nonpregnant mice and rats are insulin resistant, despite the fact that they have the same number of insulin receptors with the same affinity for insulin as the insulin-responsive mammary cells in pregnant animals. This is one of the earliest known instances of insulin resistance related to a postbinding defect. Since then, other instances of insulin resistance, initially thought to be due to receptor deficiency, have been shown to be related to postbinding defects.

It has been demonstrated that insulin has a unique and critical role in murine milk-protein gene expression. This role is independent of insulin's efficacy in cell maintenance. The hormone is also able to evoke certain types of gene expression in other cells. It will be of interest to determine whether insulin's role is unique and unrelated to cell maintenance in these systems, too. We suggest that in addition to its more commonly studied acute metabolic effects and growth-promoting properties, insulin may be important in differentiative processes at particular stages of ontogeny.

# REFERENCES

Antoniades, H. N., and Scher, C. D. (1977). *Proc. Natl. Acad. Sci. U. S. A.* **74,** 1973–1977.

Baldwin, R. L., and Louis, S. (1975). *J. Dairy Sci.* **58,** 1033–1041.

Barnawell, E. B. (1965). *J. Exp. Zool.* **160,** 189–206.

Bolander, F. F., Jr., and Topper, Y. J. (1981). *Endocrinology (Baltimore)* **108,** 1649–1653.

Bolander, F. F., Jr., Nicholas, K. R., and Topper, Y. J. (1979). *Biochem. Biophys. Res. Commun.* **91,** 247–252.

Bolander, F. F., Jr., and Topper, Y. J. (1980). *Endocrinology (Baltimore)* **107,** 1281–1285.

Bolander, F. F., Jr., Nicholas, K. R., Van Wyk, J. J., and Topper, Y. J. (1981). *Proc. Natl. Acad. Sci. U. S. A.* **78,** 5682–5684.

Brew, K. (1969). *Nature (London)* **222,** 671–672.

Brew, K., Vanaman, T. C., and Hill, R. L. (1968). *Proc. Natl. Acad. Sci. U. S. A.* **59,** 491–497.

Brodbeck, U., Denton, W. L., Tanahashi, N., and Ebner, K. E. (1967). *J. Biol. Chem.* **242,** 1391–1397.

Burt, R. L. (1956). *Obstet. Gynecol.* **7,** 658–664.

Ciaraldi, T. P., Kolterman, O. G., and Olefsky, J. M. (1981). *J. Clin. Invest.* **68,** 875–880.

Cohen, S., and Savage, C. R. (1974). *Recent Prog. Horm. Res.* **30,** 551–574.

Cushman, S. W., Noda, D., and Salans, L. B. (1981). *Am. J. Physiol.* **240,** E166–E174.

Ebner, K. E., and Schambacher, F. L. (1974). *In* "Lactation: A Comprehensive Treatise" (B. L. Larson and V. R. Smith, eds.), Vol. II, pp. 77–113. Academic Press, New York.

Elias, J. J. (1957). *Science* **126,** 842–844.

Foley, J. E., Laursen, A. L., Sonne, E., and Gliemann, J. (1981). *Diabetologia* **19,** 234–241.

Freeman, C. S., and Topper, Y. J. (1978). *Endocrinology (Baltimore)* **103,** 186–192.

Friedberg, S. H., Oka, T., and Topper, Y. J. (1970). *Proc. Natl. Acad. Sci. U. S. A.* **67,** 1493–1500.

Ganguly, R., Ganguly, N., Mehta, N. M., and Banerjee, M. R. (1980). *Proc. Natl. Acad. Sci. U. S. A.* **77,** 6003–6006.

Guyette, W. A., Matusik, R. J., and Rosen, J. M. (1979). *Cell* **17,** 1013–1023.

Hill, R. E., Lee, L. L., and Kenney, F. T. (1981). *J. Biol. Chem.* **256,** 1510–1513.

Hissin, P. J., Karnieli, E., Simpson, I. A., Salans, L. B., and Cushman, S. W. (1982). *Diabetes* **31,** 589–592.

Hobbs, A. A., Richards, D. A., Kessler, D. J., and Rosen, J. M. (1982). *J. Biol. Chem.* **257,** 3598–3605.

Inagaki, Y., and Kohmoto, K. (1982). *Endocrinology (Baltimore)* **110,** 176–182.

Ip, C., and Dao, T. L. (1978). *Cancer Res.* **38,** 2077–2083.

Jaffe, B. M., and Behrman, H. R. (1979). "Methods of Hormone Radioimmunoassay," Appendix 3, pp. 1005–1014. Academic Press, New York.

Juergens, W. G., Stockdale, F. E., Topper, Y. J., and Elias, J. J. (1965). *Proc. Natl. Acad. Sci. U. S. A.* **54,** 629–634.

Kahn, C. R. (1979). *Proc. Soc. Exp. Biol. Med.* **162,** 13–21.

Karnieli, E., Hissin, P. J., Simpson, I. A., Salans, L. B., and Cushman, S. W. (1981). *J. Clin. Invest.* **68,** 811–814.

Kasuga, M., Akanuma, Y., Iwamoto, Y., and Kosaka, K. (1978). *Am. J. Physiol.* **235,** E175–E182.

Klee, W. A., and Klee, C. B. (1972). *J. Biol. Chem.* **247,** 2336–2344.

Kobayashi, M., and Olefsky, J. M. (1979). *Diabetes* **28,** 87–95.

Kobayashi, M., Olefsky, J. M., Elders, J., Mako, M. E., Given, B. D., Schedwie, H. K., Fiser, R. H., Hintz, R. L., Horner, J. A., and Rubenstein, A. H. (1978). *Proc. Natl Acad. Sci. U. S. A.* **75,** 3469–3473.

Kolterman, O. G., Gray, R. S., Griffin, J., Burstein, P., Insel, J., Scarlett, J. A., and Olefsky, J. M. (1981). *J. Clin. Invest.* **68**, 957–969.

Korc, M., Owerbach, D., Quinto, C., and Rutter, W. J. (1981). *Science* **213**, 351–353.

Kulski, J. K., Topper, Y. J., Chomczynski, P., and Qasba, P. (1983). *Biochem. Biophys. Res. Commun.* **114**, 380–387.

Lockwood, D. H., Turkington, R. W., and Topper, Y. J. (1966). *Biochim. Biophys. Acta* **130**, 493–501.

Majumder, G. C., and Turkington, R. W. (1971). *Endocrinology (Baltimore)* **88**, 1506–1510.

Milstone, L. M., and Piatigorsky, J. (1977). *Exp. Cell Res.* **105**, 9–14.

Morishige, W. K., Pepe, G. J., and Rothchild, I. (1973). *Endocrinology (Baltimore)* **92**, 1527–1535.

Moses, A. C., Nissley, S. P., Short, P. A., Rechler, M. M., White, R. M., Knight, A. B., and High, O. Z. (1980). *Proc. Natl. Acad. Sci. U. S. A.* **77**, 3649–3653.

Nagaiah, K., Bolander, F. F., Jr., Nicholas, K. R., Takemoto, T., and Topper, Y. J. (1981). *Biochem. Biophys. Res. Commun.* **98**, 380–387.

Nagamatsu, Y., and Oka, T. (1980). *Biochem. J.* **185**, 227–237.

Nicholas, K. R., and Topper, Y. J. (1980). *Biochem. Biophys. Res. Commun.* **94**, 1424–1431.

Nicholas, K. R., Sankaran, L., and Topper, Y. J. (1981). *Endocrinology (Baltimore)* **109**, 978–980.

Oka, T., and Topper, Y. J. (1971). *J. Biol. Chem.* **246**, 7701–7707.

Oka, T., and Topper, Y. J. (1972). *Proc. Natl. Acad. Sci. U. S. A.* **69**, 1693–1696.

Oka, T., Perry, J. W., and Topper, Y. J. (1974). *J. Cell. Biol.* **62**, 550–556.

O'Keefe, E., and Cuatrecasas, P. (1974). *Biochim. Biophys. Acta.* **343**, 64–77.

Roy, A. K., Chatterjee, B., Prasad, M. S. K., and Unaker, N. J. (1980). *J. Biol. Chem.* **255**, 11614–11618.

Sager, R., and Kovac, P. (1981). *Proc. Natl. Acad. Sci. U. S. A.* **79**, 480–484.

Spooner, P. M., Chernick, S. S., Garrison, M. M., and Scow, R. O. (1979). *J. Biol. Chem.* **254**, 1305–1311.

Strobl, J. S., and Lippman, M. E. (1979). *Cancer Res.* **39**, 3319–3327.

Tomkins, G. M., Thompson, E. B., Hayashi, S., Gelehrter, T., Granner, D., and Peterkofsky, B. (1966). *Cold Spring Harbor Symp. Quant. Biol.* **31**, 349–360.

Turkington, R. W., Juergens, W. G., and Topper, Y. J. (1965). *Biochim. Biophys. Acta.* **111**, 573–576.

Van Obberghen, E., Spooner, P. M., Kahn, C. R., Chernick, S. S., Garrison, M. M., Karlsson, F. A., and Grunfeld, C. (1979). *Nature (London)* **280**, 500–502.

Voytovich, A. E., and Topper, Y. J. (1967). *Science* **158**, 1326–1327.

Walters, E., and McLean, P. (1968). *Biochem. J.* **109**, 407–417.

Wilde, C. J., and Kuhn, N. J. (1979). *Biochem. J.* **182**, 287–294.

# CHAPTER 7

# Steroid Hormone Action Interpreted from X-Ray Crystallographic Studies

*William L. Duax, Jane F. Griffin, Douglas C. Rohrer, Charles M. Weeks*

Molecular Biophysics Department
Medical Foundation of Buffalo, Inc.
Buffalo, New York


*Richard H. Ebright*

Department of Microbiology and Molecular Genetics
Harvard Medical School
Boston, Massachusetts

## I. INTRODUCTION

The characteristic responses of steroidal hormones require that they bind to specific receptor proteins in target tissue (Jensen and Jacobson, 1962).

BIOCHEMICAL ACTIONS OF HORMONES, VOL. XI

While response clearly depends on the interaction of the receptor–steroid complex and nuclear chromatin, the precise details of this interaction and the role played by the steroid in this process remain undetermined (King and Mainwaring, 1974; O'Malley and Birnbaumer, 1978; Milgrom, 1981). Structural details undoubtedly have a direct bearing on receptor affinity and will directly or indirectly influence receptor activation, transport, and nuclear interaction. The existence of antagonists that compete for the steroid-binding site of the receptor with high affinity demonstrates that the phenomena of binding and activity are at least partially independent. If agonists and antagonist compete for the same site on a receptor, a comparison of their structures should make it possible to identify which structural features are responsible for binding and which control activity.

Crystallographic data on over 400 steroids (Duax and Norton, 1975; Griffin *et al.*, 1983) provide information concerning preferred conformations, relative stabilities, and substituent influence on the interactive potential of steroid hormones. The analysis of subsets of these data (Duax *et al.*, 1976, 1981a, 1983b) suggests strongly that the conformations (three-dimensional shapes) observed in the solid state are at or near the global minimum energy position for the isolated molecules. In some cases two or more conformationally distinct isomers (molecules of identical composition but different three-dimensional shape) cocrystallize in the same lattice (Campsteyn *et al.*, 1979; Duax *et al.*, 1982). This cocrystallization indicates that these conformers may be of nearly equal energy and that they were in equilibrium in the solvent from which the crystals were grown.

If the receptor-bound steroid is in its minimum energy conformation, then it should be possible to compare the crystallographically observed structures of a series of steroids that compete for a specific binding site and determine what structural features of the steroid are essential for binding, how tight a fit exists between the steroid and the receptor, and to what extent the binding site of the receptor protein is flexible. If a conformation of the steroid differing from that seen in the crystals is required for binding, this will place an additional energy requirement on the binding process. Certain steroids that exhibit exceptionally high affinity for the receptor might be expected to be in their minimum energy conformation when bound, thus eliminating the need for the additional energy of activation.

On the basis of an examination of the data on molecular structure, receptor binding, and biological activity of a series of estrogen, progestin, and corticoid agonists and antagonists, we have proposed a model for hormone action in which the A-ring end of the steroid is primarily responsible for initiating receptor binding while the D-ring end controls the subsequent molecular interactions governing biological response (Duax *et al.*, 1978a;

Duax and Weeks, 1980). A description of that model, the data supporting it, and its further implications are the subject of this review.

## II.  PROGESTIN BINDING

Examination of the chemical structures of steroids whose affinity for the progesterone receptor in rabbit, mouse, sheep, or human uterus is equal to or higher than that of progesterone itself (Smith *et al.*, 1974; Raynaud *et al.*, 1973; Terenius, 1974; Kontula *et al.*, 1975) indicates that extensive structural variation is compatible with high-affinity binding (Duax *et al.*, 1978a). The 17β-progesterone side chain is not essential (norgestrel); removal of the 19-methyl group enhances binding; and additional hydrophobic bulk at the 10α, 16α, and 18 positions is not essential but can enhance binding. The only structural feature common to all compounds with high affinity for the progesterone receptor is the steroid ring system and 4-en-3-one composition.

These observations suggest that tight receptor-steroid contacts involve only the A ring of the steroid. Thus we propose a classical lock-and-key relationship between the receptor and the steroid's 4-en-3-one A ring. However, it is true that many steroids that have the 4-en-3-one composition have little or no affinity for the uterine progesterone receptor (i.e., testosterone). Since a 4-en-3-one A ring appears to be required but not sufficient for high-affinity binding to the progesterone receptor, we examined the conformations (three-dimensional shapes) of the 4-en-3-one A rings of the highest affinity binders in search of some unusual electronic, geometric, or stereochemical feature that might explain their enhanced binding.

In 141 of the 182 4-en-3-one containing structures for which x-ray data are available, the A rings have conformations similar to that shown in Fig. 1a. The A rings of all of the naturally occurring 4-en-3-one steroids that have been studied crystallographically have this normal conformation in which C-1 is below and C-2 is above the plane of the en-one system. In Fig. 2, the displacement of the C-2 atom from the plane is plotted versus a measure of

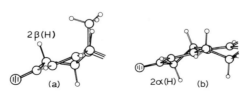

FIG. 1. Of 182 steroids having 4-en-3-one composition, 141 have the normal A-ring conformation (a). The unusual 1β,2α inverted half-chair conformation (b) is observed in 6 4-en-3-one structures, 16 4,9-dien-3-one structures and 4 4,9,11-trien-3-one structures.

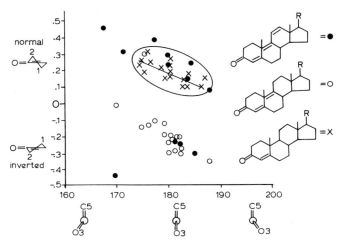

FIG. 2. A-ring conformation as a function of the distance of the C-2 atom from the plane of the atoms C-3, C-4, C-5, and C-10 versus the conjugation of the 4-en-3-one system as measured by the torsion angle τ (O-3–C-3–C-4–C-5). The distinct conformational patterns of the 4-en-3-one (x), 4,9-dien-3-one (○), and 4,9,11-trien-3-one (●) structures are compared.

4-en-3-one conjugation (the O-3/C-3/C-4/C-5 torsion angle). The conformations of the A rings of structures that have no other substituent on the all-*trans* steroid backbone vary in a range centered about the point of perfect conjugation of the 4-en-3-one (180°), as shown within the ellipse of Fig. 2.

In 41 of the 4-en-3-one steroids studied crystallographically, the A ring is observed in the "inverted" conformation (Fig. 1b). In this unnatural conformation C-1 is above and C-2 is below the plane of the en-one group. The inverted A ring has only been observed in semisynthetic steroids that have unnatural chirality, unusual substitution, or certain types of bond unsaturation. Many of these compounds of unnatural composition and unusual conformation exhibit enhanced affinity for the progesterone receptor.

Introduction of a double bond at the 9–10 position induces A-ring inversion in 16 of the 17* structures for which x-ray analysis has been undertaken. The conformations of these molecules and the planarity of their 4-en-3-one systems are contrasted against the range observed for the A rings of naturally occurring hormones in Fig. 2. The observed conformation of 17α-methyl-19-nor-4,9-pregnadiene-3,20-dione (R5020) (Courseille *et al.*, 1975), one of the most potent competitors for the progesterone receptor, is illustrated in Fig.

*The sole observation of a normal conformation of a 4,9-dien-3-one structure occurs in a disordered molecule in a crystal having two molecules in the crystallographic repeat unit. Consequently, even in this crystal only one molecule in four has the normal conformation.

3a. Many of the 4,9-dien-3-one structures exhibit a very high affinity for the progesterone receptor (Raynaud *et al.*, 1979). The remarkable correspondence between the consistency of inverted conformation and of high affinity for the receptor suggests that the key to receptor binding is the presence of a 4-en-3-one ring *in the inverted conformation.*

Addition of a third double bond at C-11/C-12 destabilizes the inverted A ring and produces a molecule able to exist in a number of conformations (Mornon *et al.*, 1977). The flexibility is probably the result of an effort to balance three forces: the constraints of planarity to increase conjugation throughout the system from O-3 to C-12, unfavorable interactions in two regions (1–3 hydrogen interactions at C-4 and C-6), and 1–4 hydrogen in-

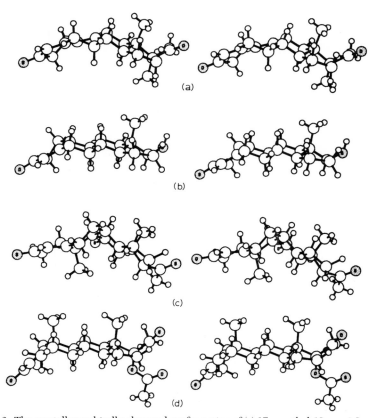

FIG. 3. The crystallographically observed conformation of (a) 17α-methyl-19-nor-4,9-pregnadiene-3,20-dione, (b) nortestosterone, (c) retroprogesterone, and (d) medroxyprogesterone acetate illustrating the similarity in the inverted conformations of their A rings. The stereo illustrations were prepared using the program ORTEP (Johnson, 1965).

teractions at C-1 and C-11. It is worth noting that while these steroids generally have lower affinity than the 4,9-diene steroids for the progesterone receptor, they exhibit more effective competition for other steroid receptors than do the 4,9-dienes (Raynaud *et al.*, 1979). This suggests that different conformers of the more flexible 4,9,11-trien-3-one structures satisfy the requirements of different receptors.

Another structure for which the inverted A-ring conformation appears to be relatively stable is 19-nortestosterone (Precigoux *et al.*, 1975). In one of four crystallographic observations of 19-nortestosterone (Fig. 3b), its A ring is observed in the inverted conformation. In contrast, testosterone in six crystallographically distinct determinations (Roberts *et al.*, 1973; Busetta *et al.*, 1972; Cooper *et al.*, 1968, 1969) is observed in the normal conformation without exception. This is consistent with data showing 19-nortestosterone to have much higher affinity for the progesterone receptor than testosterone (Kontula *et al.*, 1975). Molecular mechanics calculations using a modified version of the Allinger program MM2 (Duax *et al.*, 1983b) indicate that the inverted conformations of testosterone and progesterone have 1.3 kcal/mol higher energy than the normal forms. Removal of the 19-methyl group reduces this energy difference to 0.3 kcal/mol in the case of 19-nortestosterone.

The most remarkable case in which the 4-en-3-one A ring is observed to be inverted is that of medroxyprogesterone acetate, a compound exhibiting very high affinity for the progesterone receptor (Smith *et al.*, 1974). This is the only 19-methyl steroid (other than 2β-acetoxy compounds*) observed to have the inverted A ring (Fig. 3d). We attribute the A-ring inversion to a combination of a long-range effect of the 17α-acetate substitution and the proximal influence of the 6α-methyl substituent (Duax *et al.*, 1978b). Removal of either of these substituents leads to a restoration of the normal A-ring conformation (Duax *et al.*, 1978c, 1979) *and* a significant reduction in affinity for the receptor (Smith *et al.*, 1974).

The remaining 11 crystallographic observations of the inverted A ring occur in 9β,10α-retro steroids. The chiral change generates the conformational change and, in some cases, an enhancement of progesterone receptor-binding affinity (Kontula *et al.*, 1975). The conformation of an 11α-hydroxy derivative of retroprogesterone is illustrated in Fig. 3c.

The high progesterone receptor affinities of steroids having the inverted

---

*The reason for A-ring inversion in four 2β-acetoxy compounds can be readily deduced from examination of models in which the diaxial interaction between the 2β-acetate and the 19-methyl can be seen to induce the inversion. These compounds fail to bind to the progesterone receptor, despite the A-ring inversion, because the acetate substituent interferes with close approach of the A ring to the receptor binding site.

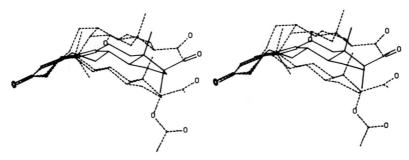

FIG. 4. A stereo diagram illustrating superposition of the nearly identical A rings of high-affinity binders R5020, retroprogesterone, and medroxyprogesterone acetate suggests a progestin receptor site that provides intimate, specific contact with the A ring but far less specific contact with the remainder of the steroid.

A-ring conformation suggest that this conformation is optimal for binding. The most potent progestins appear to be constrained to the conformation that permits strongest association with the receptor, and consequently, they are observed in this conformation in the solid state. Compounds with lower affinity for the receptor, including progesterone itself, are not constrained. In three different crystal forms, including a complex with resorcinol (Campsteyn *et al.*, 1972; Dideberg *et al.*, 1975; Foresti Serantoni *et al.*, 1975), progesterone is observed in the normal conformation. If there is 1.5 kcal/mol difference between the normal and inverted forms of the A ring of progesterone, 1 molecule in 10 would be predicted to have the inverted form suited to receptor binding. Compounds such as R5020 in which most, if not all, molecules are in the inverted form would be expected to have 10 times higher affinity for the receptor (Raynaud *et al.*, 1973).

In summary, examination of the compositions, configurations, and conformations of steroids with high affinity for the progesterone receptor suggests that there is highly stereospecific association between the receptor and the A-ring region that is best satisfied by a 4-en-3-one ring in the inverted conformation. Association between the receptor and the D-ring end of the steroids either does not occur or is far less stereospecific (Fig. 4).

## III. ESTROGEN BINDING

Compounds that bind to the estrogen receptor exhibit remarkable variability in composition and stereochemistry (Fig. 5). They include nonsteroidal compounds, semisynthetic steroids having unnatural chirality, clinically useful anticancer agents, suspected carcinogens, and simple one- or two-ring

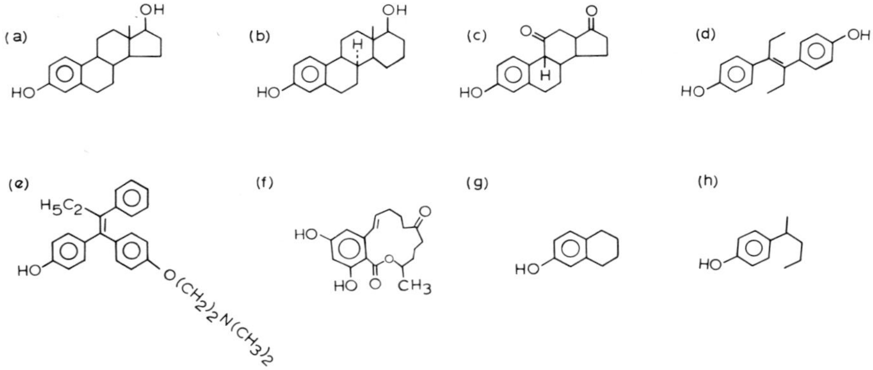

FIG. 5. Compounds that bind to the estrogen receptor with varying degrees of affinity include (a) estradiol, (b) 8α-D-homoestradiol, (c) 11-keto-9β-estrone, (d) diethylstilbestrol (DES), (e) monohydroxy-*trans*-tamoxifen, (f) *trans*-zearalenone, (g) tetrahydronaphthol and, (h) *p-sec*-amylphenol.

compounds. The structural features first proposed as being essential to estrogen activity are two hydroxyl groups separated by a specific distance ($\approx 11.5$ Å) from one another at either end of a flat, hydrophobic molecule (Keasling and Schueler, 1950). However, recent structural and biochemical studies have raised serious questions about the need for a flat molecular and for a highly specific distance between the functional groups.

Despite its twisted shape, *rac*-D-homo-8α-estra-1,3,5(10)-triene-3,17a-diol has a higher affinity for the estrogen receptor than does the flatter isomer with the natural 8β configuration (Duax *et al.*, 1981b). When the A rings of the crystallographically observed structures are superimposed (Fig. 6b), the D-ring bulk and hydroxyl group are observed to lie below the α-face of estradiol. Likewise, the twisted 11-keto-9β-estrone has higher estrogenic activity than the flat 9α-epimer (Segaloff *et al.*, 1980). The functional D-ring oxygens are displaced 8.4 Å from one another (Fig. 6c) when the A rings of 11-keto 9β-estrone and estradiol are superimposed.

When the crystallographically observed structure of the micotoxin *trans*-zearalenone is compared with estradiol (Fig. 6d), there is a surprisingly good fit of the hydrophobic bulk despite the dissimilarity between the two estrogens. In order to achieve this fit, the phenol rings of zearalenone and estradiol must be superimposed, as shown in Fig. 7. Although the phenol hydroxyls are not overlapping, their locations are close enough to one another to allow hydrogen bond formation to the same site (Duax and Weeks, 1980).

The differences in relative binding affinities of the catechol estrogens, 2-hydroxyestradiol and 4-hydroxyestradiol (Merriam *et al.*, 1980), suggest fur-

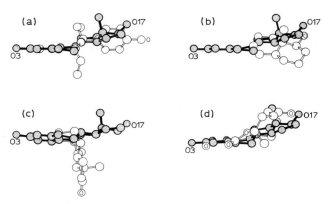

FIG. 6. Comparison of the crystallographically observed conformation of estradiol (darker) with those of (a) DES, (b) 8α-D-homoestradiol, (c) 11-keto-9β-estrone, and (d) *trans*-zearalenone.

ther details concerning the topology of the A-ring binding site (Duax *et al.*, 1983a). The reduced affinity of 2-hydroxyestradiol for the estrogen receptor may be due to a combination of steric interactions and interference with hydrogen bond formation in the direction implied by the estradiol zearalenone comparision of Fig. 7. The fact that the affinity of 4-hydroxyestradiol for the estrogen receptor is comparable to that of estradiol itself indicates that substitution at the 4 position does not interfere with receptor interaction. In addition, the 4-hydroxy substituent restricts the 3-hydroxyl hydrogen to an orientation compatible with that indicated in the estradiol zearalenone comparison.

Simple one-and two-ring structures such as tetrahydronaphthol and *p-sec*-amylphenol have been shown to inhibit binding of estradiol to the receptor and to displace prebound estradiol (Mueller and Kim, 1978). In short, if any structural feature is essential for high-affinity binding to the estrogen recep-

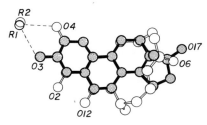

FIG. 7. Superposition drawings of estradiol (stippled) and *trans*-zearalenone illustrating similarities in overall conformation and possible hydrogen bonding to the same receptor site (R).

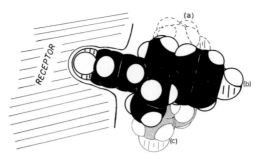

Fig. 8. Model for estrogen receptor binding in which the phenolic ring has an intimate association with the receptor and differences in the D ring are tolerated: (a) *trans*-zearalenone, (b) diethylstilbestrol, and (c) 11-keto-9β-estrone.

tor, it must be the A ring of steroidal estrogens or the analogous ring in nonsteroidal compounds.

When the phenol rings of diethylstilbestrol, zearalenone and 17-keto-9β-estrone are superimposed on the A ring of estradiol, very significant differences in the D-ring region of the molecules are observed (Fig. 8). Hence, as with the progestins, tight contact between the estrogens and receptor would appear to be limited to the A and possibly to the B rings. The observation that estradiol can be enzymatically converted to estrone while bound to the receptor (Brooks *et al.*, 1980) suggests that the D ring must be exposed. Since the 3-hydroxyl of estradiol can serve as a donor or acceptor in hydrogen bonds (Duax and Weeks, 1980), it can account for 6 kcal/mol of binding energy (Duax *et al.*, 1981b). This energy, plus the energy from possible stacking interactions involving the phenol ring, could easily account for the observed binding energy of 13 kcal/mol, and no binding to the D-ring hydroxyl need be postulated.

It should be noted that the binding of steroids to specific binding proteins in the blood (corticoid-binding globulin, progesterone-binding globulin, etc.) appears to be very different. Whereas the receptor is able to accommodate extensive structural variation and to have greatly enhanced affinity for synthetic steroids and nonsteroidal compounds, the binding globulins allow fewer structural variations in any region of the steroid and have the highest affinity for a specific natural hormone (Westphal *et al.*, 1977, 1978; Mickelson and Westphal, 1980). These observations are, perhaps, surprising in that steroids are more tightly bound by receptors than by binding globulins. One possible explanation for this difference would be that the binding to the receptor may have a stronger electronic contribution. The association between A ring and receptor may involve the formation of an interaction approaching a covalent linkage or a charge transfer interaction.

## IV. AGONISTS AND ANTAGONISTS

Antagonists of hormone action can act by interfering with the synthesis or metabolism of a specific steroid or with any of the proteins that are essential to the expression of its physiological response. In those cases where the antagonist acts by direct competition for the hormone-binding site on the receptor, it should be possible to identify which structural features are responsible for binding to that site and which control agonist versus antagonist responses. Examples consistent with the hypothesis of A-ring binding to the receptor are cited below for the estrogens, mineralocorticoids, and glucocorticoids.

Both *trans*-tamoxifen and its principal phenolic metabolite (Fig. 5e) are potent estrogen antagonists (Binart *et al.*, 1979; Borgna and Rochefort, 1981; Robertson *et al.*, 1982). This phenol has much higher affinity for the estrogen receptor and is a stronger antagonist than *trans*-tamoxifen itself. It is reasonable to suppose that the phenol ring of the tamoxifen metabolite binds to the estrogen receptor in one of the two ways illustrated in Fig. 9. In either case, the absence of an oxygen substitution comparable to estradiol O-17 accounts for the observed inactivity or antagonistic properties. In addition, the amino-substituted ring may sterically interfere with some event (e.g., a conformational change in the receptor or a genomic interaction) that is essential to hormone action.

When the structures of aldosterone and its antagonists spironolactone (Hoffman, 1974) and canrenone (Karmin and Brown, 1972) are compared

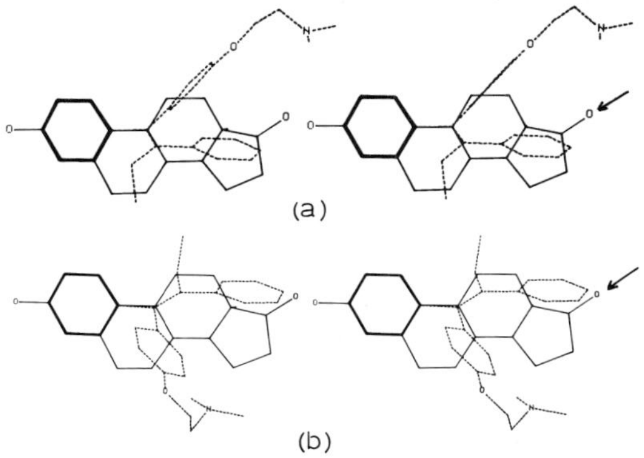

(a)

(b)

FIG. 9. Comparison of the crystallographically observed conformation and hydrogen bonding of estradiol (solid line) with that of tamoxifen (dashed line). The A ring of estradiol is superimposed on the phenyl ring of tamoxifen that is hydroxylated *in vivo*. The two possible superpositions of these rings are illustrated in (a) and (b). Arrows indicate the 17β-OH of estradiol, which is not present in the antiestrogen, tamoxifen.

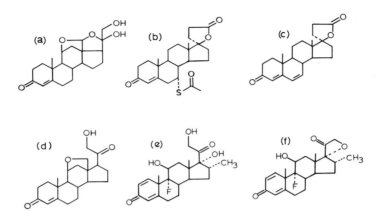

FIG. 10. (a) The natural mineralocorticoid aldosterone, its antagonists (b) spironolactone and (c) canrenone, and (d) the mixed agonist antagonist 18-deoxyaldosterone. (e) The potent synthetic glucocorticoid dexamethasone and (f) its antagonist dexamethasone oxetanone.

(Fig. 10), the only common feature is 4-en-3-one composition and conformation (Fig. 11). The antagonist behavior of spironolactone and canrenone probably results from the absence of hydrogen bond-donating groups capable of mimicing the function of the aldosterone O-20 and O-21 hydroxyls. Whereas the aldosterone hydroxyls can act either as hydrogen bond donors or acceptors, the lactone oxygens of canrenone and spironolactone can only be hydrogen bond acceptors.

18-Deoxyaldosterone (21-hydroxy-11β,18-oxido-4-pregnene-3,20-dione) is a derivative of aldosterone in which the aldehyde hemiacetal is replaced by an 11β,18-oxide ring (Fig. 10d). The 18-deoxy derivative possesses one-third of the binding affinity of aldosterone for the cytoplasmic aldosterone receptor but exhibits a 2:1 antagonist to agonist ratio (Ulick *et al.*, 1979). Crystals of 18-deoxyaldosterone contain two crystallographically independent molecules that differ significantly from one another in the orientation of

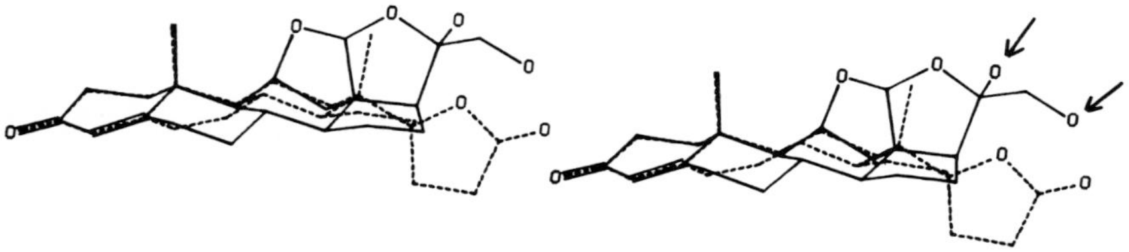

FIG. 11. Comparison of the conformation and possible hydrogen bonds of aldosterone (solid line) and of the aldosterone antagonist canrenone (dashed line). Arrows indicate H-bonding centers of aldosterone absent in the antagonist.

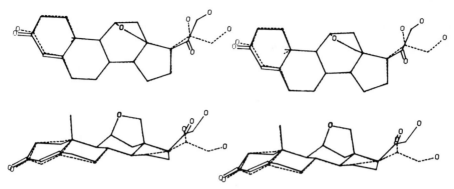

FIG. 12. Stereo views of the two molecules of 18-deoxyaldosterone, illustrating differences in 17β-side chain orientation. The lower view is obtained by a 77° rotation about the horizontal axis. Molecule I is drawn in dashed lines and molecule II is drawn in solid lines.

the 17β side chain (Fig. 12). These two conformers are of approximately equal energy and in equilibrium in solution. Both 18-deoxyaldosterone molecules resemble aldosterone in the overall shape of the A, B, C and E rings and thus would be expected to compete successfully for the aldosterone receptor. In the aldosterone crystal, the two F-ring hydroxyls, O-20 and O-21, each donate and accept a hydrogen bond. Similarly, the O-21 hydroxyl

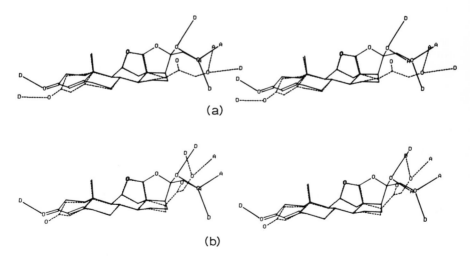

FIG. 13. Comparison of crystallographically observed conformations of 18-deoxyaldosterone and aldosterone (solid line) after least-squares fitting of the C and E rings of (a) molecule I and aldosterone and (b) molecule II and aldosterone. The locations of hydrogen bond donors (D) and acceptors (A) in the crystal are indicated.

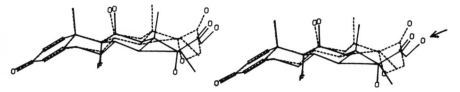

FIG. 14. Comparison of the conformation and hydrogen bonding potential of dexamethasone (solid line) and the glucocorticoid antagonist dexamethasone oxetanone (dashed line). The arrow indicates the hydrogen bond donor in dexamethasone that is absent in the antagonist.

of 18-deoxyaldosterone (both conformations) donates and accepts a hydrogen bond.* The similarity between the O-21 hydrogen bond orientations of aldosterone and molecule I of 18-deoxyaldosterone (Fig. 13a) suggests that this 18-deoxyaldosterone conformer is responsible for the partial agonism exhibited by the molecule. On the other hand, molecule II appears to have a side-chain orientation that would elicit little or no subsequent activity (Fig. 13). Thus, this conformer may account for the antagonist properties of the molecule.

Dexamethasone oxetanone (Fig. 10f) is a potent glucocorticoid antagonist (Pons and Simons, 1981). When its x-ray crystal structure is compared with the potent glucocorticoid dexamethasone (Fig. 10e), the A, B, and C ring of the two are found to have nearly identical conformations, but the differences in the D-ring are appreciable (Fig. 14). The most obvious difference is in the hydrogen bonding capabilities of the D-ring substituents. Whereas both agonist and antagonist can accept a hydrogen bond at O-20, only the agonist can also donate two hydrogen bonds.

## V. D-RING CONTROL OF ACTIVITY

The structural features that are required for binding to the progestin and estrogen receptors and the structural features that differentiate agonism from antagonism suggest that the A ring plays the primary role in binding, whereas the D ring plays the primary role in controlling activity. The possible means by which the steroid D ring might control activity include (1) inducing or stabilizing an essential conformational state in the receptor (allostery), (2) influencing the aggregation state of the receptor, or (3) participating in a direct interaction with DNA or chromatin (see Fig. 15).

In model (1), contact between the bound steroid and a distant part of the receptor (Fig. 15a) induces and/or stabilizes a change in the receptor conformation. If the appropriate D-ring substituent is missing, the steroid will bind, but the conformational change in the receptor will not occur and the

---

*Although the O-20 carbonyl of 18-deoxyaldosterone is a potential hydrogen bond acceptor, no hydrogen bonding involving this oxygen is observed in the solid state.

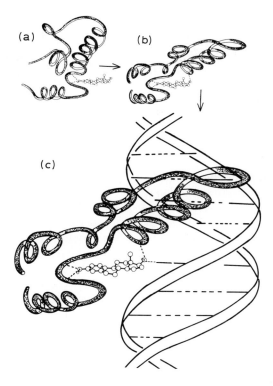

FIG. 15. Hypothesis: (a) Receptor binding involves tight contacts only to the steroid A ring. The receptor is in the "inert" conformation. (b) Substituents on the steroid D ring induce or stabilize an essential conformational state in the receptor (allostery). (c) The steroid D ring contacts a DNA base. This event is essential either for DNA-sequence recognition and/or the activation of transcription.

hormone will be more readily released. Such a mechanism would be compatible with the rapid off-rate of estrone that accounts for its weaker (than estradiol) binding to the estrogen receptor (Weichman and Notides, 1980).

Alternatively (2), the functional groups on the D ring might stabilize or destabilize the formation of different multimeric forms of the receptors. The nuclear processing steps essential for the expression of estrogenic activity, which are partially or completely impaired in estrogen antagonists (Horwitz and McGuire, 1978), could be the stabilization either of a conformational state (1) or of an aggregate state of the receptor (2) by the D ring. Tseng and Gurpide (1976) have found that only phenolic steroids possessing a 17β-hydroxy group compete with estradiol for nuclear binding.

Possibility (3) is intriguing, given our conclusion that the D ring is not bound tightly to the receptor. When the receptor–steroid complex interacts with DNA, the steroid D ring may be sufficiently exposed to contact the

DNA directly. A possible model for such an interaction is provided by the crystal complex of deoxycorticosterone and adenine (Weeks *et al.*, 1975), in which the carbonyl and hydroxyl substituents on the corticoid D ring form hydrogen bonds to the two nitrogens of adenine that would normally be involved in Watson–Crick base pairing (Fig. 16). Such contacts might be critically involved, either in DNA sequence recognition or in the activation of transcription by the steroid–receptor complex. An analogous mechanism has been proposed for the action of the catabolite gene-activator protein (CAP) and its cofactor AMP in *Escherichia coli* (Kline *et al.*, 1980; Ebright and Wong, 1981).

We presently favor the notion that the D ring has at least two roles: (1) stabilizing a specific conformational state in the receptor (allostery) and (2) participating in a direct steroid-DNA contact. We postulate a model whereby the D ring mediates both effects simultaneously (Fig. 15).

One implication of this model is worth mentioning. The similarity in shape between steroid structures, carcinogens, and base pairs has been the subject of speculation for over 20 years (Huggins and Yang, 1962; Hendry *et al.*, 1977). The binding of some carcinogens, their derivatives and metabolites to estrogen receptors (Schneider *et al.*, 1976; R. H. Ebright, unpublished data), the correlation between the presence of estrogen receptors and breast-tumor growth (King *et al.*, 1969; McGuire and Julian, 1971; Jensen *et al.*, 1971; Wittliff *et al.*, 1971), and our hypothesis that direct contact between the receptor-bound steroid and DNA occurs lend support to the following suggestion. One end of certain carcinogens might mimic the steroid A ring and thus bind to receptors. The receptor, activated by this binding, could enter the nucleus and carry the carcinogen to the specific site(s) on DNA involved in the steroid-regulated growth response. If the other end of the carcinogen (the end analogous to the steroid D ring) has

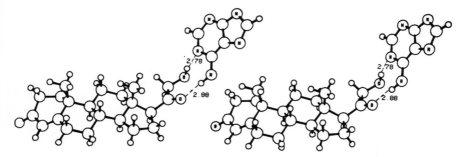

FIG. 16. X-ray crystal structure of a molecular complex between deoxycorticosterone and adenine. Note the hydrogen bonds between the steroid side chain and the two nitrogens of adenine that are responsible for Watson–Crick base pairing in DNA.

substituents that generate covalent bonding to the DNA, a mutation will be generated at these sites. In effect, the receptor might be "catalyzing" the formation of a covalent carcinogen-DNA adduct (i.e., premutational lesions) at a specific, regulatory site on DNA.

## VI. SUMMARY

Examination of the structures of compounds having high affinity for progestin and estrogen receptors strongly suggests that receptor binding is primarily the result of a tight association between the receptor and the steroidal A ring or the analogous ring on a nonsteroidal hormone analog. High-affinity binding to the progesterone receptor appears to be correlated to a complementary fit between amino acids of the receptor site and the inverted A-ring characteristic of certain steroids having 4,9-dien-3-one composition. Likewise, a phenolic ring similar to the A ring of estradiol apparently is sufficient to permit effective binding to the estrogen receptor. The data suggest that specific interactions between the D-ring region and the receptor play at best a minor role in receptor binding but are the most important factor in determining agonist versus antagonist behavior subsequent to binding.

Antagonists that compete for a steroid receptor site may be expected to have the A-ring composition and conformation necessary for receptor binding but to lack the D-ring conformational features and functional groups that induce or stabilize subsequent receptor functions. Antagonists might also be compounds with A-ring conformations appropriate for binding but other structural features that interfere with subsequent receptor functions essential to activity. The possible means by which D rings might control activity include (1) inducing or stabilizing a specific conformational state in the receptor (allostery), (2) influencing the aggregation state of the receptor, and/or (3) participating in a direct interaction with DNA or chromatin. It should be emphasized that these three mechanisms are not mutually exclusive.

## ACKNOWLEDGMENTS

Research supported in part by NIAMDD Grant No. AM-26546 and DDR Grant No. RR-05716. The organization and analysis of the data base associated with this investigation and several of the illustrations were carried out using the PROPHET system, a unique national computer resource sponsored by the NIH. The authors wish to express their appreciation to Q. Bright, G. Del Bel, C. DeVine, J. Gallmeyer, B. Giacchi, D. Hefner, K. McCormick, P. Strong, and M. Tugac for assistance in the organization and preparation of this manuscript.

# REFERENCES

Binart, N., Catelli, M. G., Geynet, C., Puri, V., Hähnel, R., Mester, J., Baulieu, E. E. (1979). *Biochem. Biophys. Res. Commun.* **91**, 812–818.

Borgna, J. L., and Rochefort, H. (1981). *J. Biol. Chem.* **256**, 859–868.

Brooks, S. C., Horn, L., Pack, B. A., Rozhin, J., Hansen, E., and Goldberg, R. (1980) *In* "Estrogens in the Environment" (J. A. McLachlan, ed.), pp. 147–167. Elsevier, New York.

Busetta, C., Courseille, C., Leroy, F., and Hospital, M. (1972). *Acta Crystallogr.* **B28**, 3293–3299.

Campsteyn, H., Dupont, L., and Dideberg, O. (1972). *Acta Crystallogr.* **B28**, 3032–3042.

Campsteyn, H., Dideberg, O., Dupont, L., and Lamotte, J. (1979). *Acta Crystallogr.* **B35**, 2971–2975.

Cooper, A., Gopalakrishna, E. M., and Norton, D. A. (1968). *Acta Crystallogr.* **B24**, 935–941.

Cooper, A., Kartha, G., Gopalakrishna, E. M., and Norton, D. A. (1969) *Acta Crystallogr.* **B25**, 2409–2411.

Courseille, C., Busetta, B., Precigoux, G., and Hospital, M. (1975). *Acta Crystallogr.* **B31**, 2290–2294.

Dideberg, O., Dupont, L., and Campsteyn, H. (1975). *Acta Crystallogr.* **B31**, 637–640.

Duax, W. L., and Norton, D. A. (1975). "Atlas of Steroid Structure," Vol. 1. Plenum, New York.

Duax, W. L., and Weeks, C. M. (1980). *In* "Estrogens in the Environment" (J. A. McLachlan, ed.), pp. 11–31. Elsevier, New York.

Duax, W. L., Weeks, C. M., and Rohrer, D. C. (1976). *In* "Topics in Stereochemistry" (E. L. Eliel and N. L. Allinger, eds.), Vol. 9, pp. 271–383. Wiley, New York.

Duax, W. L., Cody, V., Griffin, J. F., Rohrer, D. C., and Weeks, C. M. (1978a). *J. Toxicol. Environ. Health* **4**, 205–227.

Duax, W. L., Cody, V., Griffin, J., Hazel, J., and Weeks, C. M. (1978b). *J. Steroid Biochem.* **9**, 901–907.

Duax, W. L., Cody, V., and Hazel, J. (1978c). *Steroids* **30**, 471–480.

Duax, W. L., Weeks, C. M., and Strong, P. D. (1979). *Cryst. Struc. Commun.* **8**, 659–662.

Duax, W. L., Griffin, J. F., and Rohrer, D. C. (1981a). *J. Am. Chem. Soc.* **103**, 6705–6712.

Duax, W. L., Smith, G. D., Swenson, D. C., Strong, P. D., Weeks, C. M., Ananchenko, S. N., and Egorova, V. V. (1981b). *J. Steroid Biochem.* **14**, 1–7.

Duax, W. L., Griffin, J. F., Strong, P. D., Ulick, S., and Funder, J. W. (1982). *J. Am. Chem. Soc.* **104**, 7291–7293.

Duax, W. L., Griffin, J. F., Swenson, D. C., Strong, P. D., and Weisz, J. (1983a). *J. Steroid Biochem.* **18**, 263–271.

Duax, W. L., Fronckowiak, M. D., Griffin, J. F., and Rohrer, D. C. (1983b). *In* "Intramolecular Dynamics" (J. Jortner and B. Pullman, eds.), pp. 505–524. D. Reidel Publ., Dordrecht, The Netherlands.

Ebright, R. H., and Wong, J. R. (1981). *Proc. Natl. Acad. Sci. U.S.A.* **78**, 4011–4015.

Foresti Serantoni, E., Krajewski, A., Mongiorgi, R., Riva di Sanseverino, L., and Cameroni, R. (1975). *Cryst. Struct. Commun.* **4**, 189–192.

Griffin, J. F., Duax, W. L., and Weeks, C. M. (1983). "Atlas of Steroid Structure," Vol. 2. Plenum, New York (in press).

Hendry, L. B., Witham, F. H., and Chapman, O. L. (1977), *In* "Perspectives in Biology and Medicine" (R. L. Landau, ed.), Vol. 21, pp. 120–130. Univ. of Chicago Press, Chicago.

Hoffman, L. M. (1974). *In* "Recent Advances in Renal Physiology and Pharmacology" (L. G. Wesson and G. M. Fanelli, Jr., eds.), pp. 305–315. Univ. Park Press, Baltimore.

Horwitz, K. B., and McGuire, W. C. (1978). *J. Biol. Chem.* **253**, 8185–8191.

Huggins, C., and Yang, N. C. (1962). *Science* **137**, 257–262.

Jensen, E. V., and Jacobson, H. I. (1962). *In* "Recent Progress in Hormone Research" (R. O. Greep, ed.), pp. 387–414. Academic Press, New York.

Jensen, E. V., Block, G. E., Smith, S., Kyser, K., and DeSombre, E. R. (1971). *Nat. Cancer Inst. Monogr* **34**, 55–79.

Johnson, C. K. (1965). "*ORTEP,*" Report ORNL-3794. Oak Ridge National Laboratory, Tennessee.

Karmin, A., and Brown, E. A. (1972). *Steroids* **20**, 41–62.

Keasling, H. H., and Schueler, F. W. (1950). *J. Am. Pharm. Assoc.* **39**, 87–90.

King, R. J. B., and Mainwaring, W. I. P. (1974). "Steroid–Cell Interaction." Univ. Park Press, Baltimore.

King, R. J. B., Gordon, J., and Steggler, A. W. (1969). *Biochem. J.* **114**, 649–657.

Kline, E., Brown, C., Bankaitis, V., Montefiori, D., and Craig, K. (1980). *Proc. Natl. Acad. Sci. U.S.A.* **77**, 1768–1772.

Kontula, K., Janne, O., Vijko, R., de Jager, E., de Visser, J., and Zeelen, F. (1975). *Acta Endocrinol.* **78**, 574–592.

McGuire, W. L., and Julian, J. A. (1971) *Cancer Res.* **31**, 1440–1445.

Merriam, G. R., MacLusky, N. J., Picard, M. K., and Naftolin, F. (1980). *Steroids* **36**, 2589–2609.

Mickelson, K. E., and Westphal, U. (1980). *Biochemistry* **19**, 585–590.

Milgrom, E. (1981). *In* "Biochemical Actions of Hormones" (G. Litwack, ed.), Vol. 8, pp. 465–492. Academic Press, New York.

Mornon, J.-P., Delettre, J., Lepicard, G., Bally, R., Surcouf, E., and Bondot, P. (1977). *J. Steroid Biochem.* **8**, 51–62.

Mueller, G., and Kim, U.-H. (1978). *Endocrinology (Baltimore)* **102**, 1429–1435.

O'Malley, B. W., and Birnbaumer, L., eds. (1978). "Receptors and Hormone Action," Vol. 1. Academic Press, New York.

Pons, M., and Simons, S. (1981). *J. Org. Chem.* **46**, 3262–3264.

Precigoux, G., Busetta, B., Courseille, C., and Hospital M. (1975). *Acta Crystallogr.* **B31**, 1527–1532.

Raynaud, J. P., Ojasov, T., Bouton, M. M., and Philibert, D. (1979). *In* "Drug Design" (E. J. Ariens, ed.), Vol. 8, pp. 169–214. Academic Press, New York.

Raynaud, J. P., Philibert, D., and Azadian-Boulanger, G. (1973). *In* "Physiology and Genetics of Reproduction, Part A" (E. Coultinka and F. Fuchs, eds.), pp. 143–160. Plenum, New York.

Roberts, P. J., Pettersen, R. C., Sheldrick, G. M., Isaacs, N. W., and Kennard, O. (1973). *J. Chem. Soc. Perkins Trans.* 2 1978–1984.

Robertson, D. W., Katzenellenbogen, J. A., Long, D. J., Rorke, E. A., and Katzenellenbogen, B. S. (1982). *J. Steroid Biochem.* **16**, 1–13.

Schneider, S. L., Alks, V., Morreal, C. E., Sinka, D. K., and Dao, T. L. (1976). *J. Natl. Cancer Inst.* **57**, 1351–1354.

Segaloff, A., Gabbard, R. B., Flores, A., Borne, R. F., Baker, J. K., Duax, W. L., Strong, P. D., and Rohrer, D. C. (1980) *Steroids* **35**, 1335–1349.

Smith, H. E., Smith, R. G., Toft, D. O., Neergaard, J. R., Burrows, E. P., and O'Malley, B. W. (1974) *J. Biol. Chem.* **249**, 5924–5932.

Terenius, L. (1974) *Steroids* **23**, 909–918.

Tseng, L., and Gurpide, E. (1976) *J. Steroid Biochem.* **7**, 817–822.

Ulick, S., Marver, D., Adam, W. R., and Funder, J. W. (1979) *Endocrinology (Baltimore)* **104,** 1352–1356.

Weeks, C. M., Rohrer, D. C., and Duax, W. L. (1975). *Science* **190,** 1096–1097.

Weichman, B. M., and Notides, A. C. (1980). *Endocrinology (Baltimore)* **106,** 434–439.

Westphal, U., Stroupe, S. D., and Cheng, C.-L. (1977). *Ann. N.Y. Acad. Sci.* **286,** 10–28.

Westphal, U., Stroupe, S. D., Cheng, S.-L., and Harding, G. B. (1978). *J. Toxicol. Environ. Health* **4,** 229–247.

Wittliff, J. L., Hilf, R., Brooks, W. F., Savlov, E. D., Hall, T. C., and Orlando, R. A. (1971). *Cancer Res.* **32,** 1983–1992.

# CHAPTER 8

# Application of Immunochemical Techniques to the Analysis of Estrogen Receptor Structure and Function

## Geoffrey L. Greene

Ben May Laboratory for Cancer Research
The University of Chicago
Chicago, Illinois

BIOCHEMICAL ACTIONS OF HORMONES, VOL. XI

## I. INTRODUCTION

Undoubtedly the most significant conclusion to emerge from more than two decades of research on the mechanism of action of steroid hormones is that specific steroid-receptor proteins are involved in the regulation of gene expression in hormone-responsive tissues. Despite a wealth of descriptive data on the behavior of steroid–receptor complexes *in vivo* and *in vitro*, knowledge of the biochemical pathways involved is far from complete. However, a general hypothesis of steroid action has evolved, for all classes of steroid hormones, based largely on the use of radiolabeled hormones to identify the receptor proteins involved (Gorski *et al.*, 1965; Jensen *et al.*, 1968; Muldoon, 1980, Jensen *et al.*, 1982). According to this theory, free hormone enters a responsive cell through the plasma membrane and binds with high affinity to a specific receptor protein located in the cytoplasm. The steroid–receptor complex then undergoes a temperature- and steroid-dependent activation process to yield a nucleotropic complex that translocates to the nucleus, where it interacts with chromatin and in some way stimulates the production or accumulation of specific RNAs. The ultimate result is the production of specific intracellular and secreted proteins (Beato, 1980) that are involved in the growth and/or regulation of the target tissue and other tissues.

The processes involved in steroid uptake and binding to the appropriate receptor proteins, as well as virtually all of the intracellular interactions of steroid–receptor complexes, including activation, nuclear uptake, degradation, biosynthesis, and movement within target cells, remain obscure and controversial. In addition, knowledge of the composition, sequence, and physicochemical properties of all classes of steroid hormone receptors is very limited. There are several reasons for this lack of knowledge. First, purification of biologically active steroid receptors has been hampered by the low availability of these proteins, even in target tissues, as well as by difficulties encountered in the handling of receptor proteins. Second, it is not clear how the various forms of hormone–receptor complexes found in cell-free extracts of target tissues (Sherman *et al.*, 1978) are related to one another or which forms are biologically important. In addition, our ability to identify and locate the receptor proteins both *in vitro* and *in vivo* has, until recently, depended exclusively on the binding of a radiolabeled hormone to its receptor, a process that can be complicated by the presence of other binding proteins (Clark *et al.*, 1978; Mercer *et al.*, 1981). In cell-free extracts, steroid receptors can irreversibly lose their ability to bind steroid or can be modified in other ways as a consequence of their interaction with endogenous enzymes or with other poorly understood factors present in tissue or tumor extracts. Furthermore, receptor proteins occupied by endogenous steroid will not be detected either *in vivo* or *in vitro* unless an exchange assay is carried out, usually at elevated temperature. Radiolabeled steroids are also incapable of detecting receptor during early stages of receptor synthesis and during later stages of degradation and cannot distinguish between recycled or newly synthesized receptors. Finally, the labeled hormones currently available are not generally suitable for ultrastructural analysis of receptor interactions with specific components of the cytoplasm and/or nucleus of target cells. A more detailed knowledge of the mechanism of receptor-mediated hormone responses will require complete purification, characterization, and reconstitution of all important cellular components, including steroid-occupied and unoccupied receptor, chromatin acceptor sites, specific DNA-binding sites, resonsive genes, and other still unknown factors whose presence is required for complete response.

It is clear that a means of detecting, locating, and measuring receptor proteins that does not depend on the binding of a radiolabeled hormone would complement and extend our current understanding of receptor-mediated responses. Antibodies, and in particular monoclonal antibodies, are excellent candidates for alternative probes due to their potential specificity and high affinity for receptor proteins either in the presence or absence of steroid. In addition, antibodies can be readily immobilized to aid in the purification of receptors or they can be tagged with enzymes, electron-opaque substances, or radioisotopes to localize and/or quantify receptors in tissues, cultured cells, or cell-free extracts. Because of their potential sensitivity to three-dimensional changes in protein structure and, at the same time, their ability to recognize discrete regions of the polypeptide chain (less than six amino acids) (Kabat, 1956, 1960) as well as side-chain moieties, pure monoclonal antibodies offer the additional possibility of exploring the fine structure of receptor complexes, including the steroid-, chromatin-, and DNA-binding regions of these molecules.

For all of these reasons, we have prepared a series of polyclonal (Greene *et al.*, 1977, 1979, 1980b) and monoclonal (Greene and Jensen, 1981; Greene *et al.*, 1980a, 1980c) antibodies to calf uterine and human breast cancer estrogen receptors. As described in more detail below, these antibodies have proved to be useful and informative probes for receptor detection, purification, characterization, localization, and measurement in normal and neoplastic tissues and cultured cells. Several other laboratories have reported the preparation of polyclonal antibodies to steroid receptors, including estrogen (Al-Nuami *et al.*, 1979; Coffer *et al.*, 1980; Radanyi *et al.*, 1979; Raam *et al.*, 1981), progestin (Logeat *et al.*, 1981; Feil, 1983), and glucocorticoid (Govindan, 1979; Eisen, 1980) receptors. However, as of this writing there are only two other reports in the literature of monoclonal antibodies to steroid receptors: rat liver glucocorticoid receptor (Grandics *et al.*, 1982) and calf uterine estrogen receptor (Moncharmont *et al.*, 1982).

## II. PURIFICATION OF CALF AND HUMAN ESTROGEN RECEPTORS

An important step in the initial characterization of estrogen receptors and the preparation of specific antibodies was the partial purification of the receptor proteins. Although numerous purification schemes for various steroid receptors have been published, real progress has been achieved only in the past few years, primarily due to the preparation of suitable steroid-affinity adsorbents.

Estrogen receptors from low-salt extracts of calf uterus (Sica and Bresciani, 1979) and MCF-7 human breast cancer cells (Greene *et al.*, 1980c) have now been purified to near homogeneity in reasonable yields by chromatography through estradiol affinity adsorbents, usually in combination with heparin-Sepharose (Molinari *et al.*, 1977). Purification of progesterone receptors from chick oviduct, (Kuhn *et al.*, 1975; Puri *et al.*, 1982) rabbit uterus (Lamb *et al.*, 1982), and human uterus (Smith, 1981) by affinity chromatography, as well as by conventional methods, has also been reported. In addition, rat liver glucocorticoid receptor has been purified by chromatography through a steroid adsorbent followed by DNA cellulose (Govindan and Manz, 1980). A similar scheme has been used to purify androgen receptor from steer seminal vesicle (Chang *et al.*, 1982). Despite these successes, the composition, sequence, and function of steroid receptors remains largely a mystery due to a lack of sufficient amounts of purified receptors for detailed analysis and as a consequence of apparent receptor alterations that occur during handling and purification.

### A. PURIFICATION OF CALF UTERINE ESTROPHILINS

All of our initial immunizations were carried out with nuclear estradiol–receptor complex ($E^*R_n$) obtained from calf uteri after in vitro translocation of cytosolic receptor with [$^3$H]estradiol. Purification of this complex was achieved by a sequence of extraction in 400 mM KCl followed by ammonium sulfate precipitation, gel filtration through Sephadex G200, polyacrylamide-gel electrophoresis, and gel filtration through Sephacryl S200, as shown in Table I (Greene *et al.*, 1979). A 12,000-fold purification of receptor afforded a preparation of $E^*R_n$ that contained approximately 100% of the specific

TABLE I

PURIFICATION OF NUCLEAR ESTROPHILIN COMPLEX[a]

| Step | Protein (mg/kg tissue) | dpm/kg $\times 10^{-6}$ | S.A.[b] (dpm/mg $\times 10^{-3}$) | Yield (%) | Purification factor |
|------|----|----|----|----|----|
| Cytosol | 30,000 | 1,000 | 33 | 100 | 1 |
| Nuc. ext. | 1,500 | 475 | 317 | 47 | 10 |
| AS ppt. | 300 | 211 | 735 | 21 | 22 |
| G200 | 4 | 55 | 13,750 | 5 | 412 |
| PAGE | 0.34 | 40 | 117,000 | 4 | 3,510 |
| S200 | 0.025 | 10 | 400,000 | 1 | 12,000 |

[a]Reprinted with permission from Greene *et al.* (1979), *J. Steroid Biochem.* **11**, 333–341. Copyright 1979, Pergamon Press, Ltd.

[b]390,000 $\times 10^3$ dpm/mg is the theoretical specific activity for $M_r$ 68,000 and one E* per receptor.

radioactivity expected for pure steroid–receptor complex containing one molecule of [$^3$H]estradiol per protein molecule of $M_r$ 68,000. The overall yield was about 1%. Immunizations were carried out with estrophilin obtained after the polyacrylamide gel electrophoresis step (ca. 20–40% pure).

We have subsequently developed a two-step purification scheme for cytosolic estrophilin from calf uterus (unpublished results) that affords highly purified steroid–receptor complex (E*R$_c$) in good yield. This protocol, which is virtually identical to the protocol used to purify MCF-7 breast cancer cytosol estrophilin in our laboratory, now provides sufficient material for peptide mapping, amino acid composition and sequence, and immunochemical analysis of functional domains. A comparison of the structural and functional properties of calf uterine E*R$_c$ with those of MCF-7 human E*R$_c$ is in progress.

## B. PURIFICATION OF MCF-7 ESTROPHILIN

The use of affinity chromatography for the purification of steroid receptors has generally been limited by resistance of the bound receptor to elution under conditions compatible with its stability as well as by enzymatic or chemical cleavage of ester and amide groups in the spacer arms that link steroids to the supporting matrix. For estrogen receptors we (Greene *et al.*, 1980c), as well as others (Sica and Bresciani, 1979), solved the elution problem by including chaotropic salts such as sodium thiocyanate (Molinari *et al.*, 1977), with or without dimethylformamide (Musto *et al.*, 1977), in the eluting medium with estradiol to facilitate release of the receptor protein. The problem of adsorbent stability was solved in our work by using a thioether

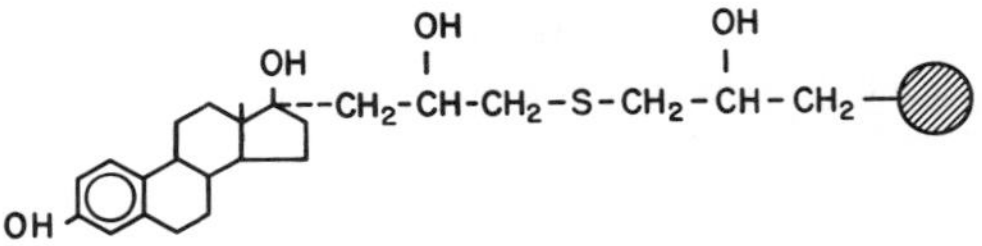

FIG. 1. Structure of estradiol affinity adsorbent. The shaded circle represents the Sepharose 6B matrix. [From Greene *et al.* (1980c).]

bridge to link estradiol to Sepharose 6B (Fig. 1). As a result, we have established a general purification protocol for estrogen receptor that is simple, reproducible, and gives a good yield of highly purified receptor protein as the steroid–receptor complex (E*R). The estradiol- and heparin-Sepharose columns used in this scheme both have high capacities for receptor, the former being 5–10 nmol of receptor per milliliter of adsorbent and the latter being about 1 nmol of E*R per milliliter of adsorbent. To obtain material suitable for immunization of animals, partial purification of MCF-7 cytosol estrophilin can be achieved by affinity chromatography alone, as shown in Table II. In this purification sequence, a 2-ml column of adsorbent retained 79% of the available receptor in 630 ml of MCF-7 cytosol. Elution with [$^3$H]estradiol in the presence of 10% dimethylformamide and 0.5 $M$ sodium thiocyanate, followed by removal of excess reagents by gel filtration, gave a 40% recovery of E*R$_c$ that was about 6% pure, based on the specific radioactivity expected for one molecule of E* bound to a 4 S protein of $M_r$ 65,000. The partially purified E*R$_c$ sedimented at about 4 S in salt-containing sucrose gradients and as a mixture of 4 S and 7 S components in low-salt gradients. It is possible to achieve more than a 1000-fold purification of estrophilin by steroid affinity chromatography alone if the column is washed extensively before elution of receptor with [$^3$H]estradiol.

Following the examples of Puca (Molinari *et al.*, 1977) and Bresciani (Sica and Bresciani, 1979), who used heparin-Sepharose to improve their purifica-

TABLE II
PURIFICATION OF MCF-7 ESTROGEN RECEPTOR[a]

| Stage | Protein (mg) | Total receptor[b] | | Yield (%) | Purity[c] (%) | Purification factor |
| | | nmol | Spec. act.[d] | | | |
| --- | --- | --- | --- | --- | --- | --- |
| Cytosol | 6212 | 7.26 | 1.2 | 100 | — | 1 |
| Affinity eluate | 3.2 | 2.87 | 897 | 40 | 6 | 767 |

[a]From Greene *et al.* (1980c).
[b]Determined by specific binding to Controlled-Pore glass beads.
[c]Assuming one E* bound to a 4–5 S protein of $M_r$ 65,000.
[d]In picomoles per milligram of protein.

TABLE III
PURIFICATION OF MCF-7 ESTROGEN RECEPTOR[a]

| Step | Protein (mg) | Total receptor[b] (nmol) | Spec. act. (pmol/mg) | Yield (%) | Purity[c] (%) | Purification factor |
|---|---|---|---|---|---|---|
| (1) Cytosol | 3979 | 5.61 | 1.41 | 100 | — | 1 |
| (2) Affinity eluate | N.D. | 4.58 | N.D. | 82 | — | — |
| (3) G25 eluate | 26.6 | 4.03 | 152 | 72 | 1 | 108 |
| (4) Heparin-sepharose eluate | 0.26 | 2.33 | 9058 | 42 | >59 | 6424 |

[a]From Greene (1983).
[b]Determined by specific binding to Controlled-Pore glass beads.
[c]Assuming one E* bound to a protein of $M_r$ 65,000 (determined by SDS-gel electrophoresis).

tion of calf uterine estrogen receptor, we modified our purification scheme to include chromatography of the partially purified $E^*R_c$ through a heparin-Sepharose column, as shown in Table III. To maximize the recovery of receptor, we omitted some of the washing reagents, such as 0.5 $M$ sodium thiocyanate, prior to elution of $E^*R_c$ from the steroid adsorbent. As a result, the overall recovery of receptor is typically 30–45%, and the purity ranges from 60% to greater than 90% when the affinity adsorbent is used in combination with heparin-Sepharose. We have isolated as much as 5 nmol (315 μg; $M_r$ 65,000) of receptor in a single experiment. Recent modifications of the protocol include omission of the gel filtration step prior to adsorption of the eluted $E^*R_c$ to heparin-Sepharose and replacement of the di-$n$-propyl thioether bridge in the steroid resin with a longer thioether bridge (unpublished results). Purifications of calf uterine and MCF-7 cytosol receptor are very reproducible with the modified protocol, affording relatively large quantities of highly purified estophilin.

Some of the properties of highly purified MCF-7 estrogen receptor are summarized in Table IV. Unlike the unpurified cytosol E*R, which sediments as an 8–9 S complex in low-salt gradients, and partially purified $E^*R_c$ (Table II), which sediments as a mixture of 4 S and 7–8 S complexes in the absence of salt, the purified receptor has lost its ability to aggregate and sediments as a 4.5 S–5.0 S complex in gradients containing either 10 m$M$ KCl or 400 m$M$ KCl. However, if purified $E^*R_c$ is mixed with receptor-depleted MCF-7 cytosol, a 7–8 S $E^*R_c$ complex is observed (unpublished results), indicating that the factors, or factor, responsible for the formation of 8 S receptor complex are removed during purification. An apparent molecular weight of 120,000 for purified $E^*R_c$, determined by high-performance liquid chromatography (HPLC) and sedimentation data in the presence of

TABLE IV
PROPERTIES OF PURIFIED MCF-7 ESTROGEN RECEPTOR[a]

|                              | Native[b] | Dissociated[c] |
|------------------------------|-----------|----------------|
| Sedimentation coefficient(s) | 4.5 S     | 4.5 S          |
| Stokes radius[d] (a)         | —         | 57.4 Å         |
| $M_r$ (s & a)                | —         | 120,000        |
| $M_r$ (SDS)                  | —         | 65,000         |
| No. hormone sites            | —         | 1              |

[a]From Greene (1982).
[b]Buffers containing 10 m$M$ KCl.
[c]Buffers containing 400 m$M$ KCl.
[d]Determined by gel exclusion high-pressure liquid chromatography.

0.4 $M$ KCl suggests the formation of a dimer under these conditions. When highly purified receptor was analyzed by SDS-gel electrophoresis under reducing conditions, one major band, $M_r$ 65,000, was observed when the gel was stained with silver (Merril *et al.*, 1981) or with Coomassie brilliant blue R-250 (Cleveland *et al.*, 1977) or when [125]I-labeled receptor was detected by autoradiography. It appears that specific radioactivity determinations, based on the Coomassie brilliant blue protein assay (Bearden, 1978), underestimate the purity of our preparations. It is interesting that, whereas the purified MCF-7 estrogen receptor migrates as a single band on SDS gels, purified calf uterine cytosol receptor migrates as two discrete bands, at $M_r$ 65,000 and $M_r$ 67,000. The two species derived from calf uterus appear to be intimately related to each other, as shown by peptide mapping with trypsin and *Staphylococcus aureus* V8 protease; no differences in peptide band patterns could be discerned on SDS gels. The nature of this basic difference between calf uterine estrophilin and MCF-7 receptor is not yet understood but could be related to fundamental differences in the source of each receptor (i.e., uterus versus mammary cancer cells), although Sica and Bresciani (1979) observed only a single polypeptide band ($M_r$ 70,000) on SDS gels for highly purified calf uterine cytosol E*R.

## III. PREPARATION AND CHARACTERIZATION OF POLYCLONAL ANTIBODIES

The availability in our laboratory of partially purified nuclear estradiol–receptor complex (E*$R_n$) from calf uterus led to the preparation of the first well-characterized antibodies to a steroid-receptor protein (Greene *et al.*, 1977). Rabbits, a goat, and rats (Greene *et al.*, 1979, 1980b) immunized with $E*R_n$ that was 10–20% pure (0.30–1.5 nmol of receptor per injection) produced antibodies that recognized all tested mammalian and nonmammalian estrogen receptors (Table V), including cytosol and nuclear estrophilin from reproductive tissues and tumors, as well as some antibodies that were species specific. Interaction of these antibodies with $E*R$ was detected and characterized by sucrose density gradient centrifugation, double antibody precipitation, gel filtration, and adsorption to protein A-Sepharose. In all cases these antibodies have been specific for estrogen receptors, showing no tendency to react with androgen or progesterone receptors, free estradiol, nonspecific binding components in human breast cancer cytosols, α-fetoprotein, or steroid-binding globulins. Similar cross-reacting antibodies have been produced by others in animals immunized with estrogen receptors from calf uterus (Rodanyi *et al.*, 1979), rat mammary tumor (Al-Nuami *et al.*, 1979), human myometrium (Coffer *et al.*, 1980), and human breast cancer (Raam *et al.*, 1981).

For virtually all of the experiments involving polyclonal antibodies, [$^3$H]estradiol ($E*$) has served as a marker for estrophilin, either before or after interaction of the receptor with antibody. Association of these antibodies with receptor does not cause the release of significant amounts of $E*$ from $E*R$ nor does it prevent the binding of hormone to uncomplexed receptor. However, goat antibody does cause a decrease in the affinity and the steroid-binding capacity of calf receptor (Greene *et al.*, 1979), probably

TABLE V

REACTIVITY CHARACTERISTICS OF DIFFERENT ANTIESTROPHILIN ANTIBODY PREPARATIONS[a]

| Antibody preparation | | | | Estrophilin source | | | | | |
|---|---|---|---|---|---|---|---|---|---|
| | | | | Uterus | | Human | | Oviduct | |
| | | Monoclonal | | | | Breast MCF-7 | | | |
| Source of immunogen | Host | Myeloma | Ig class | Calf | Rat | CA | Cell | Monkey | Hen |
| Calf uterus | Rabbit | | | + | + | + | + | + | + |
| (nuclear E*R) | Goat | | | + | + | + | + | + | + |
| | ACI rat | | | + | + | + | + | | |
| | Lewis rat | | | + | − | − | − | | |
| | Lewis rat | P3 | IgM | + | − | − | − | | |
| | Lewis rat | NSI | IgM | + | − | − | − | | |
| | Lewis rat | Sp2/0 | IgM | + | − | − | − | | |
| | Lewis rat | Sp2/0 | IgG2a | + | − | − | − | | |

[a]Reprinted by permission of the publisher from Jensen and Greene (1980), *in* "Functional Correlates of Hormone Receptors in Reproduction," by V. B. Mahesh and T. G. Muldoon (eds.), pp. 317–333. Copyright 1980 by Elsevier Science Publishing Co., Inc.

indicating the availability of a determinant on the uncomplexed receptor which, through its interaction with one or more of the goat antibodies, exerts this effect. In contrast, goat antibody has little or no effect on preformed E*R complexes, consistent with the hypothesis that this sensitive region is occluded or altered when the receptor is bound to steroid. Experiments are in progress to determine whether the goat antibody might be a good probe for detecting differencees between the binding of estrogens and anti-estrogens to unoccupied receptor; if different sites are involved or if the conformation of the antiestrogen–receptor complex is altered, this polyclonal antibody might be able to detect such changes. A similar study with rabbit antiestrophilin (Garcia et al., 1982) showed that this antibody decreased the association rate of tamoxifen and 5α-androstanediol with estrophilin from calf uterine nuclei but did not affect the binding of estradiol or monohydroxytamoxifen to receptor. Thus, this effect did not correlate with antiestrogenic activity but rather with ligand affinity for receptor.

Much of the useful information obtained thus far on the interaction of our polyclonal and monoclonal antibodies with estrophilins has been derived from sedimentation experiments in sucrose gradients. With [³H]estradiol serving as the marker for E*R complex, it is possible to observe the formation of discrete, nonprecipitating immune complexes, as indicated by shifts in the sedimentation rates of E*R or R in the presence of immunoglobulin from an immunized animal (i-Ig) but not from a control animal (n-Ig). As shown in Fig. 2, the interaction of excess rabbit i-Ig with the antigen, highly purified nuclear E*R from calf uterus, produces a shift in the E*R peak from 4.5 S to greater than 10 S in gradients containing 10 m$M$ KCl (low salt) or 400 m$M$ KCl (high salt). Crude nuclear E*R from calf uterus, which sediments at 5.2 S in high-salt gradients, reacts with rabbit i-Ig to give, in addition to the 10–12 S immune complex, a variable amount of a second immune complex that sediments at about 7–8 S (Greene et al., 1979). In contrast, the 4 S native cytosol form of estrophilin interacts with excess rabbit i-Ig to give a single immune complex at about 7.5–8 S in a salt-containing gradient, as seen in Fig. 3 for cytosol E*Rs from calf uterus and human breast cancer. Similar results have been obtained for all tested cytosol estrogen receptors. The formation of more rapidly sedimenting immune complexes (10–12 S) in the presence of our rabbit i-Ig appears to be a general phenomenon associated with nuclear E*R, heat-activated, or ammonium sulfate-precipitated cytosol E*R, and the 4.5 S calcium-stabilized cytosol receptor from calf and rat uterus (DeSombre et al., 1969).

We have observed similar patterns of interaction between goat antibody and cytosol or nuclear forms of estrophilin, except that all goat i-Ig·E*R complexes are less discrete and sediment beyond the 8 S region, indicating the formation of immune complexes that contain two or more antibodies

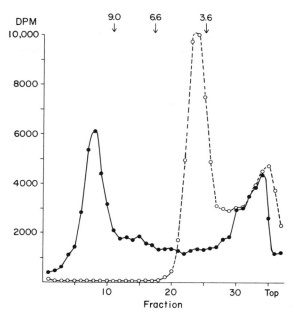

FIG. 2. Antibody-receptor interaction demonstrated by an increase in sedimentation rate of estradiol–receptor complex (E*R). Sedimentation profile for highly purified E*R complex from calf uterine nuclei, in 10–30% sucrose gradients containing 10 mM KCl, after incubation with immunoglobulin from an immunized (●) or control (○) rabbit. [Reprinted with permission from Greene *et al.* (1979), *J. Steroid Biochem.* **11**, 333–341. Copyright 1979, Pergamon Press, Ltd.]

bound to each E*R (Greene *et al.*, 1979). In addition, some of the goat antibodies are probably specific for calf E*R because smaller immune complexes are obtained when these antibodies interact with E*R from other species.

Of the polyclonal antiestrophilin antisera generated thus far in our laboratory, only one has been completely specific for the receptor used as the antigen. Immunoglobulin from a Lewis rat immunized with nuclear E*R from calf uterus recognizes only calf estrophilin, although the determinant recognized is present in cytosol as well as nuclear forms of calf estrogen receptor. All other animals, including several rats (ACI and Lewis strains), rabbits, and a goat, have produced antibodies that recognize estrophilins from all tested species and target tissues (Table V), regardless of the form (cytosol or nuclear extract) of estrogen receptor used as the antigen. In addition, immunizations have been as successful with denatured receptor as with intact estradiol–receptor complex.

Several major conclusions can be drawn from our studies on the interactions of these polyclonal antibodies with various estrophilins. First, there is

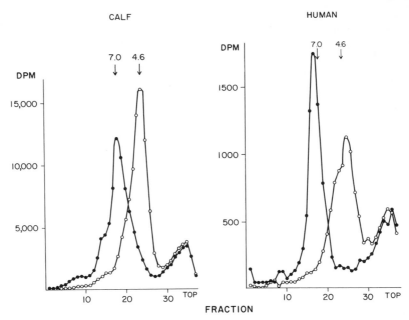

Fig. 3. Sedimentation profiles in 10–30% sucrose/400 m$M$ KCl gradients of calf uterine cytosol E*R and human breast cancer cytosol E*R in the presence of immunoglobulin from an immunized (●) or control (○) rabbit. [From Greene *et al.* (1977).]

obviously immunochemical similarity among estrogen receptors from mammalian and nonmammalian sources, indicating that one or more determinants, and thus amino acid sequences, have been conserved throughout the evolution of birds and mammals. In addition, we have some preliminary evidence that at least one of our polyclonal antibodies (from the Lewis rat immunized with MCF-7 cytosol E*R) can recognize nuclear E*R from *Xenopus* liver. Certainly the gross physical and chemical features of well-characterized estrogen receptors, such as those from calf uterus and from MCF-7 cells, are consistent with this observation (e.g., $M_r = 65,000–70,000$ for calf and human E*R). However, it is very likely that there is sequence heterogeneity, as shown by the different reactivity patterns of the goat antibody with estrophilins from various species and by the specificity of the one Lewis rat antibody for calf estrophilin. Despite the extensive cross-reactivity of several antibodies with various estrophilins these antibodies appear to be completely specific for the class of hormone receptor used as the antigen. In fact, all of the data published to date on the specificities of various steroid-receptor antibodies indicate that these antibodies are specific in each case for the class of hormone receptor used to generate them. Finally, the interaction of all of our polyclonal and monoclonal antibodies with cytosol and nuclear forms of estrophilin is consistent with the concept that nuclear receptor is derived from the cytosol, or native, receptor via a hormone-induced activation of the native receptor (Jensen *et al.*, 1968). For estrogen receptor, this activation process is usually accompanied by a change in the sedimentation rate of the E*R complex from 4 to 5 S in high-salt gradients (Jensen and DeSombre, 1973), a process that has been postulated to involve either dimerization of receptor (Notides *et al.*, 1975; Little *et al.*, 1975) or formation of a complex between receptor and another cytosol component (Yamamoto, 1974; Thampan and Clark, 1981). The greater increase in sedimentation rate accompanying the reaction of rabbit or goat i-Ig with nuclear or heat-activated E*R as compared with the cytosol complex (Figs. 2 and 3) suggests that more molecules of immunoglobulin can associate with activated receptor than with the native form. This observation is compatible with either explanation of receptor activation because a receptor dimer or a complex between receptor and another component might contain two or more determinants available to an antibody generated against the nuclear form of the receptor. With crude nuclear extracts, the formation with rabbit i-Ig of a 7.5 S immune complex as well as the 10–12 S complex may represent contamination of the nuclear extract with untransformed cytosol receptor. The exact nature and composition of the 5 S nuclear E*R has not yet been resolved. However, some of our monoclonal antibodies may be able to resolve this issue.

## IV. PREPARATION AND CHARACTERIZATION OF MONOCLONAL ANTIBODIES

Despite the fact that polyclonal antibodies generated in rabbits and a goat against estradiol–receptor complexes of calf uterus have proved useful for the study of receptor structure and function as well as for the purification and immunoassay of receptor, much of the work has been limited by the heterogeneity of antibodies present in animal sera; some of these antibodies recognize proteins other than estrophilin. To overcome these limitations, we have prepared monoclonal antibodies to calf uterine estrophilin and to MCF-7 human breast cancer estrogen receptor. As expected, the high affinity, monospecificity, and abundance of these monoclonal antibodies have permitted us to use them for the development of specific and sensitive immunoassays for human estrogen receptor, for the development of an immunocytochemical assay for primate and nonprimate estrophilin in several target tissues, for analysis of proteolytic fragments of receptor digests on sucrose density gradients as well as on nitrocellulose blots of SDS gels, for investigating sequence similarities and differences among various mammalian and nonmammalian estrophilins, and for establishing the distinction between estrogen receptors and other classes of steroid hormones. It is clear that monoclonal antibodies will prove to be powerful probes for investigating the structure, composition, and cellular interactions of all classes of steroid-hormone receptors.

## A. MONOCLONAL ANTIBODIES TO CALF UTERINE ESTROPHILINS

The first monoclonal antibodies to mammalian estrogen receptors were prepared in our laboratory by polyethylene glycol-mediated fusion of splenic lymphocytes from male Lewis rats, immunized with partially purified nuclear E*R from calf uterus (Table I), with mouse myeloma cells (P3-X63-Ag8, P3-NSI/l-Ag4-l, and Sp2/0-Agl4) (Greene *et al.*, 1980a). Approximately 9% of the resulting hybridoma cultures produced antibodies to the receptor protein, as determined by double antibody precipitation of crude nuclear E*R from calf uterus when E*R was incubated with hybridoma culture medium and goat antibody to Lewis rat Ig. Antiestrophilin-secreting hybrid lines were derived from all three mouse myeloma cell lines, although the P3 and NSI myelomas produced more viable hybrids than did the Sp2/0 myeloma. When cloned by limiting dilution, 56 cultures of hybridomas were obtained that secreted antiestrophilin. Ten of these clones, from all three myeloma lines, have been expanded and characterized; seven clones (from P3, NSI, and Sp2/0) secrete rat IgM and three (from Sp2/0) secrete rat IgG2a. By growing some of these clones as ascites tumors in athymic mice, we have been able to obtain as much as 30–40 mg of antibody at a time. The antibodies secreted by Sp2/0-derived hybridomas are particularly easy to purify by conventional techniques or by immunoadsorption because the hybrid cells synthesize only the immunoglobulin produced by lymphocytes from the immunized rat (Shulman et al., 1978). After repeated cloning, several of these hybridomas (Table V) have proved to be stable in long-term culture (at least several months) and when stored in liquid nitrogen (for 4 years).

Like the immunoglobulin (i-Ig) from the rat antiserum, all of the monoclonal rat IgG2a antibodies react with 4 S cytosol E*R (Fig. 4a) and 5 S nuclear E*R (Fig. 4b) of calf uterus to give 7–8 S immune complexes in salt-containing gradients. The monoclonal IgMs react with both forms of receptor (Fig. 4a, b) to give 12–13 S immune complexes (the IgM itself sediments at 12–13 S). In contrast to monoclonal IgG, which shows comparable affinity for

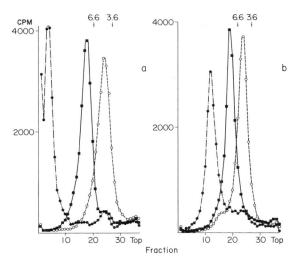

FIG. 4. Reaction of monoclonal IgG and IgM with calf uterine estrophilin. Sedimentation profiles in sucrose gradients containing 400 $mM$ KCl of E*R (0.6 pmol) from the following: (a) calf uterine cytosol (10–30% sucrose) and (b) calf uterine nuclei (10–50% sucrose), in the presence of Lewis rat n-Ig (○), 20 μg monoclonal i-IgG (■), or monoclonal i-IgM (●), 200 μg in (a) and 20 μg in (b). [From Greene *et al.* (1980a).]

cytosol and nuclear forms of calf E*R, the IgMs react preferentially with the nuclear form. The reasons for this distinction are not clear. All of the monoclonal antibodies produced against calf uterine estrophilin are specific for calf receptor, as are the antibodies present in the serum of the immunized rat. These antibodies react with occupied as well as unoccupied receptors and do not interfere with the ability of receptor to bind steroid, as determined by postlabeling immune complexes in sucrose gradients with E*.

By including [$^{35}$S]-methionine in the culture medium of hybridomas, we have prepared radiolabeled antibodies with specific activities in excess of 200 Ci/mmol. The advantage of this labeling method is that full immunochemical activity is retained and the purity of the secreted $^{35}$S-Ig is extremely high (>90%) with respect to labeled proteins. As shown in Fig. 5, interaction of a $^{35}$S-IgG (B72Spγ) with calf nuclear E*R can be recognized by the formation of an immune complex consisting of both $^{35}$S-IgG and E*R$_n$. When treated with an excess 5 S E*R$_n$ (Fig. 5a, open circles), all of the 7 S $^{35}$S-IgG (Fig. 5a, closed circles) is shifted to the 8–9 S region (Fig. 5b) along with that portion of the excess E*R$_n$ that reacted. As described below, these labeled antibodies make excellent probes for detecting intact receptor and receptor fragments on blots of SDS gels or in any situation where receptor is occupied

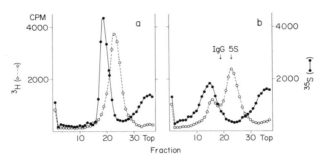

FIG. 5. Interaction between $^{35}$S-labeled monoclonal antiestrophilin (B72Spγ) and excess calf nuclear E*R. Sedimentation profiles in 10–30% sucrose gradients containing 400 m$M$ KCl of nuclear calf uterine E*R (○) and a limiting amount of monoclonal $^{35}$S-IgG (●): (a) in separate tubes and (b) after incubation together for 1 hr at 4°C. The arrows in (b) indicate the sedimentation positions of E*R$_n$ (5 S) and labeled IgG (7 S) corresponding to the peaks in (a). [From Greene *et al.* (1980a).]

with unlabeled steroid or otherwise unable to bind [$^3$H]estradiol. Labeled antibodies can be used for quantitative assays as well as qualitative analysis, thereby eliminating the need for labeled steroid in many systems.

## B. MONOCLONAL ANTIBODIES TO HUMAN ESTROPHILIN

Although the monoclonal antibodies prepared against calf estrophilin have proved useful for the characterization, assay, and purification of cytosol and nuclear forms of calf receptor, these antibodies are limited by their specificity for calf E*R and by their apparent recognition of only one region of the receptor molecule. All of the data accumulated thus far indicate that all 10 cloned hybridomas secrete antibodies (IgM or IgG) that recognize the same determinant or mutually exclusive determinants on the calf receptor. Because of our interest in being able to study estrogen receptors in other species, particularly in human reproductive tissues and breast cancer, we have directed our efforts for the past 3 years to preparing and characterizing monoclonal antibodies to human estrophilin.

With the successful partial purification of cytosol estrogen receptor obtained from MCF-7 human breast cancer cells we began, in 1979, to immunize male Lewis rats in order to generate monoclonal rat antibodies to human estrophilin. Steroid–receptor complex (E*R$_c$) eluted from our estradiol affinity adsorbent (about 5–10% pure) proved to be immunogenic in a male Lewis rat when injected by the method of Vaitukaitis *et al.* (1971). Fusion of splenic lymphocytes from this rat with mouse myeloma cells (P3-X68-Ag8 and Sp2/0-Agl4) yielded, after cloning by limiting dilution, three hybridoma cell lines, each of which secreted a unique idiotype of antibody that recognized a distinct region of the estrogen-receptor molecule (Table VI, D series). All three hybrids have now been stabilized by repeated cloning. The two P3-derived hybridomas (D58P3μ and D75P3γ) became stable only after they lost their ability to synthesize and secrete mouse myeloma heavy and light immunoglobulin chains. The spontaneous loss of myeloma immunoglobulin chains has been reported by others (Köhler and Milstein, 1976). Thus, all three hybridomas now secrete only rat Ig. These hybridomas have been in culture for almost 3 years and have been expanded repeatedly in athymic mice to produce, for D547Spγ and D75p3γ, a total of more than 100 mg of each antibody. Secreted antibodies are routinely purified by adsorption to Sepharose-conjugated goat antibody to rat IgG, or by chromatography on DEAE-cellulose for IgGs, or by filtration through Bio-Gel A-1.5m agarose for IgMs.

The characteristics of the antibodies present in Lewis rat antiserum and of the antibodies secreted by the three monoclonal hybridoma lines are summarized in Table VI. Whereas the rat antiserum cross-reacted with estrophilin from all sources tested, including hen oviduct and *Xenopus* liver, none of the isolated monoclonal antibodies recognized hen E*R. All three monoclonal antibodies recognized estrophilin from human breast cancer and from monkey uterus. When tested against calf and rat E*R, differences in cross-reactivity among the three monoclonal antibodies were observed. The

TABLE VI

CROSS-REACTIVITY OF MONOCLONAL ANTIBODIES TO HUMAN ESTROPHILIN

| | Receptor source | | | | | | |
|---|---|---|---|---|---|---|---|
| | Breast cancer | | Uterus | | | | Oviduct |
| Antibody[a] | MCF-7 | Human | Human | Monkey | Calf | Rat | Hen |
| Rat serum | + | + | + | + | + | + | + |
| D58P3μ | + | + | + | + | + | + | − |
| D75P3γ | + | + | + | + | − | − | − |
| D547Spγ | + | + | + | + | + | + | − |
| F88Spγ | + | | + | | + | + | + |
| F344Spμ | + | | + | | + | + | + |
| G5Spγ | + | | | | + | | − |
| G13Spγ | + | | | | | | |
| H222Spγ | + | + | + | | + | + | + |
| H226Spγ | + | + | + | | + | + | + |

[a]IgM antibodies indicated by μ and IgG by γ. P3 and Sp indicate hybridomas derived from P3-X63-Ag8 and Sp2/0-Ag14 mouse myeloma cells, respectively.

titer of the IgG from clone D547Spγ (Sp2/0) was considerably lower against calf and rat E*R than against MCF-7 E*R (Greene *et al.*, 1980c), whereas the IgM secreted by D58P3μ cross-reacts strongly with all tested mammalian estrophilins and the IgG secreted by D75P3γ appears to be virtually specific for primate receptor. Monoclonal IgGs from both D547Spγ and D75P3γ react with cytosol and nuclear E*Rs from primate sources to give 8 S immune complexes in salt-containing sucrose gradients (Figs. 6 and 7). Similar complexes are obtained with D547Spγ and E*Rs from nonprimate sources, such as calf and rat uterus. However, the Lewis rat antiserum reacts with primate E*Rs to give 10–12 S immune complexes (Fig. 6) and with estrophilins from nonprimate sources to give 8 S complexes, suggesting that there is at least one antibody in the rat serum that is primate specific. IgM secreted by D58P3μ forms 18–19 S immune with cytosol and nuclear E*Rs, in contrast to the 12–13 S complexes obtained with the calf-specific monoclonal antibodies. When any two of the D-series antibodies are mixed sequentially with MCF-7 cytosol E*R, a new immune complex containing E*R and each added antibody is obtained (Fig. 7), demonstrating that each antibody recognizes a unique and well-separated region of the human-receptor molecule. All three antibodies have been biosynthetically labeled with [$^{35}$S] methionine to produce functional immunochemical probes with high specific activities.

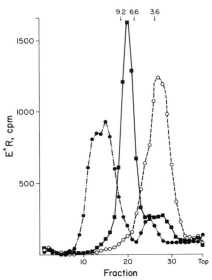

FIG. 6. Sedimentation profiles in 10–30% sucrose/400 mM KCl gradients of E*R (0.5 pmol) from human breast cancer cytosol in the presence of 25 μg of Lewis rat n-Ig (○), 25 μg of D547Spγ monoclonal IgG (■), or 10 μl of Lewis rat antiserum (●). [From Greene *et al.* (1980c).]

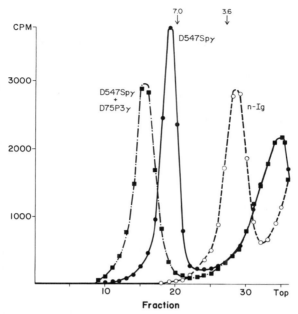

Fɪɢ. 7. Independent reactions of monoclonal antibodies with human estrophilin. Sedimentation profiles in 10–50% sucrose gradients containing 400 mM KCl of MCF-7 cell cytosol E*R (0.5 pmol) in the presence of 50 μg of Lewis rat n-Ig (○), 40 μg of D547Spγ monoclonal IgG (●), or 40 μg D547IgG followed by 50 μg D75Spγ IgG (■). [From Greene and Jensen (1982).]

The above results, taken with previous observations, show that in addition to the common antigenic determinant(s) recognized by rabbit, goat, and rat antiestrophilin, there is a determinant in mammalian receptor that is not present or available in crude preparations of hen E*R. Also, there are determinants characteristic of primate receptor that are either absent or modified in nonprimate estrophilins, such as those from calf and rat uterus. Finally, as mentioned previously, there is at least one determinant in calf receptor that is specific to that species. The availability of a library of antibodies with different specificities will undoubtedly facilitate the investigation of similarities and differences among estrogen receptor of different animal species.

The preparation of monoclonal rat antibodies to human estrogen receptor has been repeated twice by us and once by Larry Miller at Abbott Laboratories (Miller *et al.*, 1982) to produce a number of unique monoclonal antibodies that are being used in radiolabeled and unlabeled forms to detect, measure, and characterize mammalian estrogen receptors from several species and tissues. The properties of some of these antibodies are summarized in Table VI. Of particular significance in all of this work has been our ability to generate virtually unlimited amounts of pure, monospecific antibodies from relatively impure (5–10% of theoretical specific activity) preparations of receptor. Thus, the hybridization techniques developed by Köhler and Milstein (1975) are particularly applicable to the preparation of monoclonal antibodies to proteins, such as steroid receptors, whose lability and low concentration in target cells make them difficult to isolate in a highly purified form.

## V. APPLICATION OF IMMUNOCHEMICAL TECHNIQUES TO THE ANALYSIS OF RECEPTOR STRUCTURE AND FUNCTION

With the availability of radiolabeled and unlabeled forms of the monoclonal antibodies listed in Table VI, we have begun to study their application to the purification, cellular localization, and quantitative analysis of estrophilins in tissues and cultured cells from several species. These antibodies are also being used to facilitate cloning of the gene coding for estrogen receptor in MCF-7 cells and for mapping and characterizing the functional domains of the receptor molecule. Progress has been made in each of these areas of immunochemical analysis of receptor structure and function.

### A. Purification of Estrophilins by Immunoadsorption

One of the more important advantages of having highly specific antibodies that can recognize estrophilins from several sources is the use of such antibodies to purify various estrophilins by immunoadsorption. When coupled to Sepharose 4B, several antibodies have proved useful for the isolation of cytosol and nuclear forms of estrophilins from primate and nonprimate tissues and cultured cells. Two of the monoclonal antibodies specific for calf estrophilin, B36NSμ (IgM) and B72Spγ (IgG), have been used to purify cytosol and nuclear E*R from calf uterus. Immunoadsorbents prepared from either antibody, by covalent attachment of Ig to cyanogen bromide-activated Sepharose 4B (20 mg Ig per milliliter Sepharose), can bind more than 1 nmol of E*R per milliliter of adsorbent. However, elution of intact E*R has proved to be difficult due to the high avidity of these antibodies for receptor ($K_d \simeq 10^{-10}M$). The recovery of E*R has ranged from 25 to 50%, affording estrophilin that is >5% pure, based on the radioactivity expected for one molecule of E* bound to a 4–5 S protein of $M_r$ 65,000 (Greene and Jensen, 1981). Similar results were obtained when an immunoadsorbent prepared from D547Spγ IgG was used to partially purify cytosol E*R from calf uterus. The yield and purity of E*R were again about 25% and 5%, respectively.

However, when the same immunoadsorbent was used to isolate and purify MCF-7 cytosol estrophilin, it was not possible to elute receptor in a form capable of binding [$^3$H]estradiol. Our ability to dissociate intact calf E*R from the D547 antibody, which was prepared against MCF-7 human receptor, is undoubtedly due to the lower avidity of this antibody for nonprimate estrophilins (Greene *et al.*, 1980c). A modified version of the D547 immunoadsorbent, containing only 1 mg of IgG per milliliter of Sepharose 4B, has proved to be a particularly effective means of isolating and purifying MCF-7 cytosol estrophilin. The capacity of this column is greater than that of the earlier version (~2 nmol E*R per milliliter adsorbent), and nonspecific adsorption of proteins other than receptor is minimal. Although it is necessary, thus far, to elute occupied or unoccupied receptor under denaturing conditions (e.g., 1% SDS), we are able to obtain, in a single step, receptor that is virtually as pure as estrophilin that has been purified by chromatography on estradiol-Sepharose and heparin-Sepharose (unpublished results). The nearly quantitative yield of this purification method makes it a valuable source of receptor for peptide mapping and for determining the amino acid composition and sequence of estrophilin.

Immunoadsorbents prepared from highly cross-reactive antibodies, such as H222Spγ, should provide a general means of isolating estrophilins from mammalian or nonmammalian tissues containing relatively small amounts of receptor. For example, purification of estrogen receptor from rat uterus by conventional methods is impractical because of the difficulty in obtaining enough tissue to allow for extensive loss of receptor during purification. However, an immunoadsorbent prepared from D547Spγ or H222Spγ would be capable, in a single step, of providing sufficient amounts of highly purified rat uterine estrogen receptor for peptide mapping and/or analysis by SDS-gel electrophoresis and immunoblotting after elution with SDS. An added advantage is the ability of these adsorbents to bind either occupied or unoccupied receptor, as well as degraded or altered forms of estrogen receptors; this is particularly true for H222Spγ, which recognizes a stable and well-conserved determinant that is close to the steroid-binding site (Sobel, 1982). Finally, it is possible that such immunoadsorbents will facilitate the isolation of estrogen receptor molecules that are bound to important chromatin proteins, specific DNA sites, or perhaps other soluble proteins, factors, or RNAs that participate in the receptor-mediated response, thereby providing a means of identifying some of these moieties in cellular extracts. It is clear that the availability of immunoadsorbents that are capable of binding multiple forms of estrogen receptor from virtually any animal or tissue will greatly enhance our ability to compare and contrast estrophilins from all target tissues, regardless of source.

B. Quantitative Immunochemical Assay of Estrophilins

An important application of monoclonal antibodies to human estrophilin is the measurement of estrogen receptors in human breast cancers. Knowledge of the tumor content of estrophilin has been shown to be of significant clinical value as a guide to prognosis and therapy selection in the treatment of advanced breast cancer (DeSombre *et al.*, 1979). As shown in a clinical study at the University of Chicago (Jensen *et al.*, 1976), approximately two-thirds of patients whose cancers contain moderate to high levels of estrophilin respond to endocrine therapy. Current assays for estrogen receptor in breast cancer biopsies depend on the binding of radiolabeled estradiol to the receptor protein. Excess unbound hormone is separated from receptor-bound steroid by sucrose gradient ultracentrifugation, Dextran-coated charcoal, gel filtration, or adsorption of E*R to hydroxylapatite. All of these methods require fairly large amounts of tumor and are sensitive to changes in the ability of receptor to bind estradiol. In addition, receptor occupied by endogenous hormone can be detected only by an exchange assay, which frequently results in a loss of binding sites.

To overcome these limitations we have used two monoclonal rat antibodies (D547Spγ and D75p3γ) that bind to different regions of the estrogen receptor molecule to devise simple immunoradiometric (IRMA) and immunocolorimetric (ICMA) assays (Greene and Jensen, 1982). This work was done in collaboration with Chris Nolan at Abbott Laboratories. Simultaneous binding of the two monoclonal antibodies to MCF-7 E*R was demonstrated by the formation of a ternary–immune complex ($Ab_1 \cdot E^*R \cdot Ab_2$) that sediments at 11–13 S in salt-containing sucrose gradients (Fig. 7). As

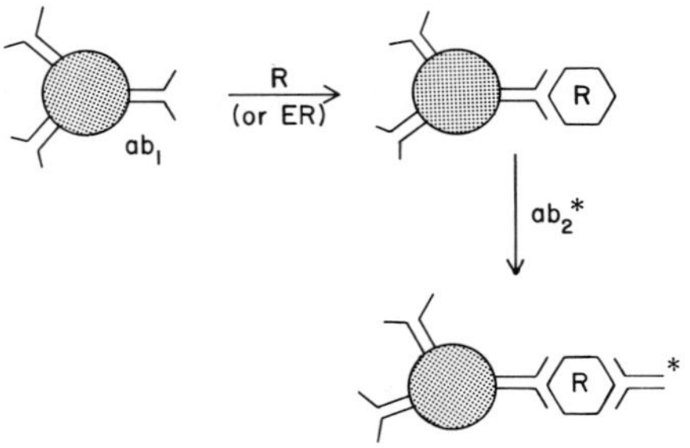

Fig. 8. System for the immunochemical measurement of estrogen receptors. A polystyrene bead, coated with one monoclonal antibody (D547Spγ), adsorbs unoccupied (R) or occupied (ER) receptor from tissue or tumor extract. Bound receptor adsorbs a second monoclonal antibody (D75P3γ) which has been labeled (*) either with $^{125}I$ for an immunoradiometric assay (IRMA) or with an enzyme such as horseradish peroxidase for an immunocolorimetric assay (ICMA). [From Greene and Jensen (1982).]

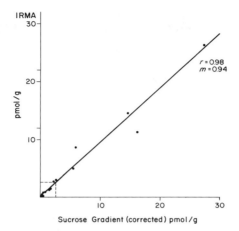

FIG. 9. The estrophilin contents of 18 human breast cancer cytosols as determined by the IRMA technique, compared with the results obtained by sucrose gradient ultracentrifugation. For the latter method, a subsaturating dose (0.5 nM) of [³H]estradiol was used and the results were corrected to total binding capacity expected for a saturating dose of steroid. The distinction between receptor-rich and receptor-poor tumors (dashed line) in postmenopausal patients occurs at a level of 2.5 pmol E*R per gram of tumor when excess E* is added to the cytosol. [From Greene and Jensen (1982).]

shown schematically in Fig. 8, polystyrene beads coated with D547SPγ IgG can adsorb either occupied (ER) or unoccupied (R) receptor present in a tumor or tissue extract. Radiolabeled (IRMA) or peroxidase conjugated (ICMA) D75P3γ is then used to measure the amount of receptor bound to the bead. When antibody-coated beads were incubated with different amounts of MCF-7 cytosol E*R, bound E*R was directly proportional to added E*R over a wide range of E*R concentrations, as determined both by direct measurement of [³H]estradiol on the beads and by measuring the amount of ¹²⁵I-labeled D75P3γ IgG bound after a second incubation with labeled antibody. When tumor cytosols from 18 human breast cancers were analyzed for receptor content by the IRMA method and the results were compared with estrophilin content determined by specific steroid binding on sucrose density gradients, the relative ranking of receptor levels was virtually the same for all 18 tumors (Fig. 9). This sandwich technique has since been modified to an immunocolorimetric assay at Abbott Laboratories and tested against an additional 64 breast cancer cytosols with equally good results. A commercial diagnostic kit that is simple, rapid, and does not depend on the binding of radioactive estradiol to receptor should be available soon.

An important conclusion can be drawn from Fig. 9 concerning the total amount of estrogen receptor present in the 18 breast cancer cytosols tested by the IRMA method. A comparison of the results for the IRMA and sucrose gradient techniques ($r = 0.98$; $m = 0.94$) indicates that there are no significant amounts of occupied receptor, or receptor that is unable to bind steroid, present in these cytosols. Although this study is hardly exhaustive, the data suggest that the amount of estrophilin determined by steroid-binding assays in breast cancer cytosols is very close to the total amount of immunoreactive receptor present.

## C. Immunocytochemical Localization of Estrophilins

Although the immunoradiometric, or immunocolorimetric, assay described above can provide useful quantitative information about estrophilin levels in breast cancers and other primate tissues, it is not possible to determine the intra- and intercellular distribution of receptors with this assay. Such information could be valuable both for determining the prognosis and therapy selection in breast cancers and for studying receptor dynamics in other estrogen-responsive tissues and cultured cells. Because many of the questions concerning the precise location of receptor within a target cell in the presence and absence of steroid remain unresolved, there is a definite need for methods that can detect and measure estrophilins at the light microscopic and electron microscopic levels in cells. In addition, our understanding of receptor regulation would be greatly enhanced if we could localize receptor during degradation as well as during synthesis and/or recycling. Also, questions about changes in receptor levels and distribution in reproductive tissues, and perhaps brain, during normal reproductive cycling might best be answered with immunocytochemical probes for the receptor molecules. Ultrastructural studies of target cells with receptor-specific immunochemical probes could reveal the presence and location of specific acceptor sites in the chromatin as well as DNA-binding sites in the nuclear matrix (Barrack and Coffey, 1980), if they exist. The same studies might also reveal specific binding sites for receptor in the cytoplasmic matrix, such as in microsomes (Little *et al.*, 1972) or other organelles or membranes (Pietras and Szego, 1979), as has been suggested in the literature. Immunocytochemical studies at the ultrastructural level might also provide insight into the intracellular interactions of estrogen antagonists, particularly if the effect of these antagonists is to direct receptors to different sites in the nucleus as has been suggested by Ruh and Baudendistel (1978) and Gardner *et al.* (1978). Finally, the nature of a second type of estradiol binder in the nucleus of target cells, designated "type II" sites (Eriksson *et al.*, 1978; Markaverich and Clark, 1979), whose levels correlate with growth even better than the classical type I sites, remains unresolved. It is not yet known whether these type II binders represent a modified form of receptor that might be recognized by receptor-specific antibodies or another protein unrelated to the type I receptor.

In order to answer some of these questions, we have used several of the monoclonal antibodies listed in Table VI to develop an immunocytochemical assay for estrophilins in tissue sections and in dispersed cells. In our laboratory we have used D547, D75, H222, and H226 IgGs to detect and localize estrophilin with an immunoperoxidase technique (Sternberger, 1974) in frozen, fixed sections of human breast tumors (King and Greene, 1983), human uterus, and other mammalian reproductive tissues as well as cultured MCF-7 cells. In this procedure, frozen sections (4–8 $\mu$m) are thaw mounted on uncoated glass slides, fixed in graded aqueous ethanols (35–100% ethanol), and incubated with one or more monoclonal rat antiestrophilin antibodies. Specifically-bound antibodies are visualized by the indirect immunoperoxidase method (Nadji, 1980), with goat antibody to Lewis rat IgG serving as a bridge between bound monoclonal antibodies and rat peroxidase–antiperoxidase complex (PAP); diaminobenzidine (DAB) serves as the chromogen.

As illustrated in Fig. 10A, specific nuclear localization of estrophilin is observed by the immunoperoxidase method in a tumor section cut from a receptor-rich human mammary infiltrating ductal carcinoma. No specific staining for receptor is observed in the receptor-poor infiltrating ductal carcinoma shown in Fig. 10C. Specific nuclear staining is abolished by addition of MCF-7 cytosol (20 pmol of estrophilin per ml), partially purified MCF-7 cytosol E*R (ca. 10% pure) (Fig. 10B), or receptor-depleted cytosol to which highly purified MCF-7 E*R (ca. 90% pure) has been added to the primary antibody (e.g., H226) prior to incubation of the antibody with the tissue section. The inclusion of receptor-depleted cytosol (receptor removed by adsorption to an estradiol affinity adsorbent) alone with the primary antibody does not reduce specific nuclear staining, indicating that only estrophilin competes for specific receptor sites in the tissue section. We have now analyzed frozen sections from more than 120 breast cancer biopsies by the indirect immunoperoxidase technique and correlated the intensity and distribution of specific staining for estrophilin in tumor cells with receptor levels determined by sucrose gradient analysis of tumor cytosols. Thus far, our ability to distinguish receptor-rich from receptor-poor tumors is very good (King and Greene, 1983); we have not failed to detect a receptor-rich tumor by this method. However, we have observed significant nuclear staining for estrophilin in a small number of tumors that would be classified as receptor-poor by conventional steroid-binding assays. A notable feature of these tumors is that specific staining is very heterogeneous, indicating the

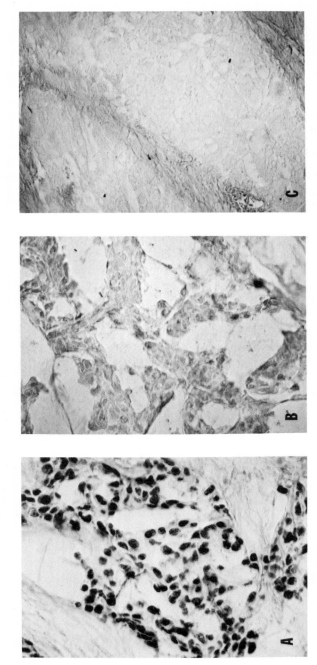

FIG. 10. Immunocytochemical localization of estrophilin in human breast cancers. Ethanol-fixed, frozen sections (8 μm) of receptor-rich (A,B) and receptor-poor (C) human mammary infiltrating ductal carcinomas were incubated with H226Spγ IgG (20 μg/ml) in the absence (A, C) or presence (B) of partially purified MCF-7 cytosol E*R (ca. 10% pure), followed by goat antibody to rat IgG and rat peroxidase–antiperoxidase complex (PAP). Bound antibodies were then visualized by treatment of the sections with diaminobenzidene. Estrogen receptor levels in these tumors were determined independently in fresh tumor cytosols by sucrose density gradient ultracentrifugation with [3H]estradiol.

possible presence of more than one population of tumor cells. Further clarification of these findings and their implications for prognosis and response to endocrine therapy in breast cancers will have to await correlation of our results with clinical response.

An issue that remains unresolved in our immunocytochemical studies is the intracellular location of estrogen receptor in responsive tissues in the presence and absence of estrogens. We have applied the immunoperoxidase technique to a variety of tissues and cells. They include the following: human breast cancer cells; normal breast tissue and uterus; rabbit ovary, uterus, pituitary, and liver before and after estradiol injection in immature, pseudopregnant, and ovariectomized animals; and cultured MCF-7 human breast cancer cells before and after treatment with estrogens and antiestrogens. Thus far, only nuclear staining has been observed in all receptor-containing tissues and cells studied, although all four of the above antibodies, each of which recognizes a unique determinant on the receptor molecule, bind both cytosol and nuclear forms of estrophilin with equally high avidity in tissue extracts. No nuclear staining is observed when control polyclonal rat IgG or monoclonal rat antibodies prepared against acetylcholine receptor or choline acetyltransferase are substituted for anti-ER antibodies. In addition, no specific nuclear staining is observed in nontarget tissues such as colon, pancreas, skeletal muscle, or receptor-negative breast cancers. In contrast, predominantly cytoplasmic staining has been observed when the same antibodies were used on formalin fixed, paraffin-embedded sections of human breast cancers, as reported by Mehrdad Nadji at the University of Miami (Jensen *et al.*, 1982). Shanti Raam (Raam *et al.*, 1982) has also reported specific cytoplasmic localization of estrophilin with polyclonal antiestrophilin in frozen, ethanol-fixed sections of human breast cancers and uterus, as well as in MCF-7 cells. The significance of these different staining patterns remains unresolved at this time. Our own data suggest that the majority of the estrogen receptor is always associated with the nucleus, although it is entirely possible that we are not detecting cytoplasmic receptor because determinants are unavailable to our antibodies due to receptor packaging or conformation in the cytoplasm. Experiments designed to resolve this important question are in progress.

## D. IMMUNOCHEMICAL MAPPING OF ESTROPHILIN

In ongoing studies to map the location of antigenic determinants on MCF-7 and calf estrophilins in relation to functional domains, the relative positions of nine unique determinants on the receptor have been determined by density gradient analysis of antibody-receptor interaction after

limited proteolysis of MCF-7 cytosol E*R with trypsin, chymotrypsin, mercuripapain or mercaptoethanol-activated papain (Sobel, 1982). As determined by ultracentrifugation in salt-containing (400 mM KCl) sucrose gradients, digestion with mercuripapain under controlled conditions degrades 4
S cytosol E*R from MCF-7 cells to a 3.3 S moiety, whereas chymotrypsin,
trypsin, and activated papain yield 2.6 S fragments. When these estradiol-
binding fragments were tested for reactivity with various antibodies, as
judged by the formation of a 7–8 S immune complex, it was found that
mercuripapain    treatment    eliminated    only    the    H226    determinant,
chymotrypsin eliminated D547 as well as H226, and trypsin and activated
papain eliminated H226, D547, and D75, whereas determinants for six other
antibodies were unaffected by these enzymatic digestions. For MCF-7 nuclear E*R the pattern was the same except that mercuripapain eliminated
the determinants for D75 and D547 as well as for H226. Assuming that
receptor is a single polypeptide chain and that the determinants are arranged in a linear fashion, the model shown in Fig. 11A is consistent with the
data. However, the tertiary structure of the molecule must be such that the
determinant for H226 is spatially proximal to the determinant for H222
because reaction of the intact receptor with one antibody prevents binding of

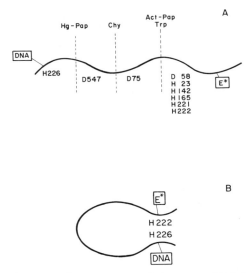

FIG. 11. (A) Map of antigenic determinants in relation to steroid-binding and DNA-binding
domains of the MCF-7 cytosol estrogen receptor. Dashed lines indicate sites of cleavage for
listed enzymes. Postulated recognition sites for 9 antibodies are shown. E*, estrogen-binding
region; DNA, DNA-binding region. (B) Postulated folding pattern for MCF-7 receptor to
account for mutual exclusion of H222Spγ and H226Spγ binding sites. [From Sobel (1982).]

the other antibody (Fig. 11B). From our studies on the immunochemical mapping of human estrogen receptor, it is clear that only one antibody, H226, appears to recognize a region of the receptor that is near the DNA-binding portion of the nuclear form of estrophilin and relatively distant from the steroid-binding domain (Fig. 11A). When tested for their ability to associate with $\varnothing$X174 double-stranded DNA in sucrose density gradients, none of the estradiol-binding fragments was able to recognize DNA, whereas the intact nuclear MCF-7 receptor co-sedimented with the DNA. However, preliminary results indicate that when nuclear E*R is cleaved with mercuripapain, a portion of the receptor molecule (without E*) retains its ability to bind to DNA, as shown by the formation of a ternary–immune complex consisting of $^{35}$S-H226 IgG, $\varnothing$X174 DNA, and mercuripapain-cleaved receptor. The immunochemical detection, purification, and analysis of such cleaved fragments as well as steroid-binding fragments should provide further insight into structure–function relationships for the receptor molecule.

## VI. SUMMARY

The foregoing studies demonstrate the feasibility and practicality of purifying estrogen receptors from at least two sources and preparing polyclonal or monoclonal antibodies to these proteins. Highly purified cytosol E*R can be obtained rapidly, reproducibly, and in good yield from calf uterus and from MCF-7 human breast cancer cells by a combination of steroid-affinity chromatography and selective adsorption to heparin-Sepharose. Purification of estrophilins by immunoadsorption also promises to be a valuable tool for obtaining unoccupied and steroid-occupied receptors for amino acid composition and sequence analysis.

For the preparation of polyclonal and monoclonal antibodies various animals, including several rabbits, a goat, and more than 10 rats, have been immunized with relatively small doses (0.3–1.5 nmol) of partially purified calf and human estrogen receptors (1–40% pure) to produce detectable titers of antiestrophilins at serum dilutions greater than 1:50,000, in some cases. We have performed four successful rat lymphocyte–mouse myeloma cell fusions to yield a number of stable rat–mouse hybridomas that secrete unique, and pure, monoclonal antibodies specific for estrogen receptors (Tables V and VI; B,D,F, and G Series). A separate fusion carried out at Abbott Laboratories (Miller *et al.*, 1982) produced several more monoclonal antibodies (Table VI; H series) that recognize additional regions of the receptor. Interaction of these antibodies with steroid-occupied and unoccupied forms of estrophilin from mammalian and nonmammalian sources has been studied extensively by sucrose density gradient ultracentrifugation, gel filtration, interaction with protein A-Sepharose, double antibody precipitation, immunoadsorption, immunoblotting, and immunocytochemistry techniques. Immune complexes can be detected and quantified by direct methods with radioactive tags for receptor ([$^3$H]estradiol or [$^{125}$I]estradiol), or for antibody ([$^{125}$I]- or [$^{35}$S]methionine), or with enzyme-conjugated antiestrophilin antibodies (immunocolorimetric assays). These complexes can also be detected and quantified by indirect immunoperoxidase and immunoradiometric methods with labeled antibodies that recognize the primary antiestrophilin antibody.

Although the monoclonal antibodies generated thus far appear to recognize a fairly extensive region of the estrogen-receptor molecule (Fig. 11), we have not obtained monoclonal antibodies that interfere with the binding of steroid to receptor or with the nonspecific binding of receptor to DNA. Thus, we are still missing probes for important and possibly extensive regions of the receptor. Efforts to obtain such potentially useful antibodies are in progress. These antibodies will be used in combination with existing antibodies to map and isolate functional domains of estrophilin after controlled digestion of intact receptor with various enzymes. As described earlier, unlabeled antibodies can be used to detect and characterize steroid-binding fragments on sucrose density gradients. In addition, radiolabeled antibodies (e.g., $^{35}$S-IgG) can be used to detect all immunoreactive receptor fragments on nitrocellulose blots of SDS gels (Towbin et al., 1979) after proteolysis (Cleveland et al., 1977). Interesting peptides will be isolated by immunoadsorption and sequenced. At least five of the available monoclonal antibodies recognize intact receptor on electrophoretic blots, although they differ in their ability to recognize receptor framents. Such studies will facilitate cross-species comparisons of estrogen receptors as well as a more detailed analysis of the composition of the receptor molecule in relation to its function.

Other ongoing and future applications of immunochemical techniques to studies on estrogen action that are being carried out in our own laboratory and in collaboration with other investigators include the following: cloning of the gene coding for estrogen receptor in MCF-7 cells; isolation and characterization of the native form of estrophilin (8–10 S) from tissue and cell extracts; detection and characterization of estrogen receptor in nuclear matrix preparations from chick livers; ultrastructural immunocytochemical localization of estrogen receptor in responsive tissues in the presence and absence of estrogens and antiestrogens, and isolation and characterization of estrophilins biosynthetically labeled in vitro or in culture with radioactive amino acids.

Although many questions about the structure and function of estrogen receptors and other steroid receptors remain unanswered, it is clear that the use of immunochemical techniques for the detection, measurement, purification, localization, and structural analysis of these proteins in responsive tissues and cultured cells will enhance our knowledge of the biochemical pathways involved in steroid hormone action. With their potential purity, specificity, and sensitivity, monoclonal antibodies are particularly attractive as independent probes for receptor proteins both *in vitro* and *in vivo*. These attributes are further enhanced by the ease with which such antibodies can be radiolabeled biosynthetically. As new monoclonal antibodies with different reactivity patterns toward various forms of steroid receptors and regions of the receptor molecules become available, we will be able to improve our understanding of the relation between structure, composition, and function of these proteins, an understanding based on information that cannot be obtained from steroid-binding studies alone. In addition, such antibodies may ultimately serve as valuable diagnostic, prognostic, and therapeutic reagents for various hormone-responsive diseases, such as human breast cancer and cancer of the prostate.

## ACKNOWLEDGMENTS

These investigations were supported by research grants from the American Cancer Society (BC-86), Abbott Laboratories, the National Cancer Institute (CA-02897), and by the Women's Board of the University of Chicago Cancer Research Foundation.

## REFERENCES

Al-Nuami, N., Davies, P., and Griffiths, K. (1979). *Cancer Treat. Rep.* **63**, 1147.
Barrack, E. R., Coffey, D. S. (1980). *J. Biol. Chem.* **255**, 7265–7275.
Bearden, J. C., Jr. (1978). *Biochim. Biophys. Acta* **533**, 525–529.
Beato, M., eds. (1980). "Steroid Induced Uterine Proteins." Elsevier, New York.
Chang, C. H., Rowley, D. R., Lobl, T. J., and Tindall, D. J. (1982). *Biochemistry* **21**, 4102–4109.
Clark, J. H., Hardin, J. W., Upchurch, S., Eriksson, H. (1978). *J. Biol. Chem.* **253**, 7630–7634.
Cleveland, D. W., Fischer, S. G., Kirschner, M. W., and Laemmli, U. K. (1977). *J. Biol. Chem.* **252**, 1102–1106.
Coffer, A. I., King, R. J. B., and Brockas, A. J. (1980). *Biochem. Int.* **1**, 126–132.
DeSombre, E. R., Carbone, P. P., Jensen, E. V., McGuire, W. L., Wells, S. A., Jr., Wittliff, J. L., and Lipsett, M. B. (1979). *N. Engl. J. Med.* **301**, 1011–1012.
DeSombre, E. R., Puca, G. A., and Jensen, E. V. (1969). *Proc. Natl. Acad. Sci. U. S. A.* **64**, 148–154.
Eisen, H. J. (1980). *Proc. Natl. Acad. Sci. U. S. A.* **77**, 3893–3897.
Eriksson, H., Upchurch, S., Hardin, J. W., Peck, E. J., Jr., and Clark, J. H. (1978). *Biochem. Biophys. Res. Commun.* **81**, 1–7.
Feil, P. D. (1983). *Endocrinology (Baltimore)* **112**, 396–398.

Garcia, M., Greene, G., Rochefort, H., and Jensen, E. V. (1982). *Endocrinology (Baltimore)* **110**, 1355–1361.

Gardner, R. M., Kirkland, J. I., and Stancel, G. M. (1978). *Endocrinology (Baltimore)* **103**, 1583–1589.

Gorski, G., Toft, D., Shyamala, S., Smith, D., and Notides, A. (1965). *Recent Prog. Horm. Res.* **24**, 45–80.

Govindan, M. V. (1979). *J. Steroid Biochem.* **11**, 323–332.

Govindan, M. V., and Manz, B. (1980). *Eur. J. Biochem.* **108**, 47–53.

Grandics, P., Gasser, D. L., and Litwack, G. (1982). *Endocrinology (Baltimore)* **111**, 1731–1733.

Greene, G. L. (1983). *In* "Gene Regulation by Steroid Hormones II" (A. K. Roy and J. H. Clark, eds.), pp. 191–200. Springer-Verlag, Berlin and New York.

Greene, G. L., and Jensen, E. V. (1981). *In* "Monoclonal Antibodies in Endocrine Research" (R. E. Fellows and G. S. Eisenbarth, eds.), pp. 143–155. Raven, New York.

Greene, G. L., and Jensen, E. V. (1982). *J. Steroid Biochem.* **16**, 353–359.

Greene, G. L., Closs, L. E., DeSombre, E. R., and Jensen, E. V. (1977). *Proc. Natl. Acad. Sci. U. S. A.* **74**, 3681–3685.

Greene, G. L., Closs, L. E., DeSombre, E. R., and Jensen, E. V. (1979). *J. Steroid Biochem.* **11**, 333–341.

Greene, G. L., Fitch, F. W., and Jensen, E. V. (1980a). *Proc. Natl. Acad. Sci. U. S. A.* **77**, 157–161.

Greene, G. L., Closs, L. E., DeSombre, E. R., and Jensen, E. V. (1980b). *J. Steroid Biochem.* **12**, 159–167.

Greene, G. L., Nolan, C., Engler, J. P., and Jensen, E. V. (1980c). *Proc. Natl. Acad. Sci. U. S. A.* **77**, 5115–5119.

Jensen, E. V., and DeSombre, E. R. (1973). *Science* **182**, 126–134.

Jensen, E. V., and Greene, G. L. (1980). *In* "Functional Correlates of Hormone Receptors in Reproduction" (V. B. Mahesh and T. G. Muldoon, eds.), pp. 317–333. Elsevier, New York.

Jensen, E. V., Suzuki, T., Kawashima, T., Stumpf, W. E., Jungblut, P. W., and DeSombre, E. R. (1968). *Proc. Natl. Acad. Sci. U. S. A.* **59**, 632–638.

Jensen, E. V., Smith, S., and DeSombre, E. R. (1976). *J. Steroid Biochem.* **7**, 911–917.

Jensen, E. V., Greene, G. L., Closs, L. E., DeSombre, E. R., and Nadji, M. (1982). *Recent Prog. Horm. Res.* **38**, 1–40.

Kabat, E. A. (1956). *J. Immunol.* **77**, 377–385.

Kabat, E. A. (1960). *J. Immunol.* **84**, 82–85.

King, W., and Greene, G. L. (1983). *Nature (London)* submitted.

Köhler, G., and Milstein, C. (1975). *Nature (London)* **256**, 495–497.

Köhler, G., and Milstein, C. (1976). *Eur. J. Immunol.* **6**, 511–519.

Kuhn, R. W., Schrader, W. T., Smith, R. G., and O'Malley, B. W. (1975). *J. Biol. Chem.* **250**, 4220–4228.

Lamb, D. J., Holmes, S. D., Smith, R. G., and Bullock, D. W. (1982). *Biochem. Biophys. Res. Commun.* **108**, 1131–1135.

Little, M., Rosenfeld, G. C., and Jungblut, P. W. (1972). *Hoppe-Seyler's Z. Physiol. Chem.* **353**, 231–242.

Little, M., Szendro, P., Teran, C., Hughs, A., and Jungblut, P. W. (1975). *J. Steroid Biochem.* **6**, 493–500.

Logeat, F., Vu Hai, M. T., and Milgrom, E. (1981). *Proc. Natl. Acad. Sci. U. S. A.* **78**, 1426–1430.

Markaverich, B. M., and Clark, J. H. (1979). *Endocrinology (Baltimore)* **105**, 1458–1462.

Mercer, W. D., Edwards, D. P., Chamness, G. C., and McGuire, W. L. (1981). *Cancer Res.* **41**, 4644–4652.

Merril, C. R., Goldman, D., Sedman, S. A., and Ebert, M. H. (1981). *Science* **211**, 1437–1438.

Miller, L. S., Tribby, I. I. E., Miles, M. R., Tomita, J. T., and Nolan, C. (1982). *Fed. Proc., Fed. Am. Proc. Exp. Biol.*, **41**, Abstract 1459.

Molinari, A. M., Medici, N., Moncharmont, B., and Puca, G. A. (1977). *Proc. Natl. Acad. Sci. U. S. A.* **74**, 4886–4890.

Moncharmont, B., Su, Jui-Lan, and Parikh, I. (1982). *Biochemistry* **21**, 6916–6921.

Muldoon, T. G. (1980). *Endocrinol. Rev.* **1**, 339–364.

Musto, N. A., Gunsalus, G. L., Miljkovic, M., and Bardin, C. W. (1977). *Endocr. Res. Commun.* **4**, 147–157.

Nadji, M. (1980). *Acta Cytol.* **24**, 442–447.

Notides, A., Hamilton, D. E., and Auer, H. E. (1975). *J. Biol. Chem.* **250**, 3945–3950.

Pietras, R. J., and Szego, C. M. (1979). *J. Steroid Biochem.* **11**, 1471–1483.

Puri, R. K., Grandics, P., Dougherty, J. J., and Toft, D. O. (1982). *J. Biol. Chem.* **257**, 10831–10837.

Raam, S., Nemeth, E., Tamura, H., O'Brian, D. S., and Cohen, J. L. (1982). *Eur. J. Cancer Clin. Oncol.* **18**, 1–12.

Raam, S., Peters, L., Rafkind, I., Putnam, E., Longcope, C., and Cohen, J. L. (1981). *Molec. Immunol.* **18**, 143–156.

Radanyi, C., Redeuilh, G., Eigenmann, E., Lebeau, M. C., Massol, N., Secco, C., Baulieu, E. E., and Richard-Foy, H. (1979). *C. R. Acad. Sci. Paris, Series D.* **288**, 255–258.

Ruh, T. S., and Baudendistel, L. J. (1978). *Endocrinology (Baltimore)* **102**, 1838–1846.

Sherman, M. R., Pickering, L. A., Rollwagen, F. M., and Miller, L. K. (1978). *Fed. Proc., Fed. Am. Proc. Exp. Biol.* **37**, 167–173.

Shulman, M., Wilde, C. D., and Köhler, G. (1978). *Nature (London)* **276**, 269–270.

Sica, V., and Bresciani, F. (1979). *Biochemistry* **18**, 2369–2378.

Smith, R. G., d'Istra, M., and Van, N. T. (1981). *Biochemistry* **20**, 5557–5565.

Sobel, N. (1982). Ph.D. thesis, Univ. of Chicago, Chicago, Illinois.

Sternberger, L. A. (1974). "Immunocytochemistry." Prentice-Hall, Englewood Cliffs, New Jersey.

Thampan, T. N. R. V., and Clark, J. H. (1981). *Nature (London)* **290**, 152–154.

Towbin, H., Staehelin, T., and Gorden, J. (1979). *Proc. Natl. Acad. Sci. U. S. A.* **76**, 4350–4354.

Vaitukaitis, J., Robbins, J. B., Nieschlag, E., and Ross, G. T. (1971). *J. Clin. Endocrinol. Metab.* **33**, 988–991.

Yamamoto, K. R. (1974). *J. Biol. Chem.* **249**, 7068–7075.

# CHAPTER 9

# Role of the Estrogen Receptor in Estrogen-Responsive Mammalian Cells

*Henri Rochefort and Bruce Westley*

Unité d'Endocrinologie Cellulaire et Moléculaire
U 148 INSERM
Montpellier, France

BIOCHEMICAL ACTIONS OF HORMONES, VOL. XI
Copyright © 1984 by Academic Press, Inc.
All rights of reproduction in any form reserved.
ISBN 0-12-452811-2

# I. INTRODUCTION

The presence of specific estrogen-binding proteins (generally termed receptors or estrophilins*) in estrogen target tissues, the translocation of the estrogen–receptor complex into the cell nucleus, and the subsequent stimulation of RNA and protein synthesis were first described 20 years ago (Jensen and Jacobson, 1962). These findings led to the formulation of a model of estrogen action (Mueller *et al.*, 1961; Jensen *et al.*, 1972; Baulieu *et al.*, 1971), which still appears to be valid and which provides the conceptual framework for most current research on the mechanism of action of all steroids and related hormones. According to this model, estrogen enters the estrogen-responsive cell and binds noncovalently but with high affinity to estrogen-receptor proteins located in the cytosol (operationally defined as the 100,000 g supernatant of a cell homogenate). This binding induces a change in the receptor (termed activation) that results in the translocation of the estrogen–receptor complex into the nucleus and/or its retention in chromatin. The initiation of responses to estrogens are contingent on the retention of the estrogen–receptor complex in the nucleus (Gorski and Gannon, 1976).

The demonstration in a variety of experimental systems (but mostly in birds and amphibia) that the synthesis of specific proteins is increased by estradiol via an increased level of the mRNA coding for these proteins led to the concept that the estrogen–receptor complex might act by stimulating the transcription of estrogen-responsive genes by interacting with nearby regulatory DNA sequences. The events that occur after the binding of the steroid to the receptor, which result in the nuclear translocation of the estrogen–receptor complex and the induction of new mRNA molecules, are still obscure.

In addition to their effects on the biosynthesis of specific proteins, estrogens increase cell proliferation and stimulate general cellular metabolism. This pleiotropic effect (Tomkins, 1975) is poorly understood and, as it may also be triggered by other hormones and growth factors, it cannot be considered as a specific response to estrogens.

Although it is widely accepted that the estrogen receptor is directly involved in mediating the effects of estrogens, most of the evidence is somewhat indirect and circumstantial (for reviews see Jensen *et al.*, 1972; O'Malley and Means, 1974). The most convincing arguments are as follows:

---

*In this chapter, estrogen receptor is defined as the estrogen-binding protein (or estrophilin) found in the cytosol of target tissue saturated with physiological concentrations of hormones and translocated into the nucleus, even though the role of these binding proteins in estrogen action has not been directly demonstrated.

1. There is no example of a cell type that responds to estrogen but does not contain estrogen receptors, and conversely, most cells that do not respond to estrogen contain little or no estrogen receptor.
2. The affinities of various estrogens for the estrogen receptor are generally correlated with both their ability to translocate the receptor to the nucleus and their ability to elicit an estrogenic response.
3. The proportion of the estrogen receptors that become occupied *in vivo* can be varied by administering different doses of estrogen, and the magnitude of the response is related to the degree of occupation of the receptor.

In this chapter, we present some of the work that was undertaken in our laboratory to clarify the biological significance of the estrogen receptor and its interactions with DNA. In Section II, we describe experiments in which the affinities of the estrogen receptor for estrogens and androgens were correlated with the ability of these ligands to translocate the estrogen receptor into the cell nucleus and elicit estrogen-specific responses. These experiments provide evidence that in the mammalian systems we have studied most of the ligands, including androgens, that interact with the estrogen receptor are able to elicit estrogenic responses and therefore suggest that the receptor rather than the ligand determines the specificity of the response.

Antiestrogens inhibit the effects of estrogens and are therefore potentially powerful tools for dissecting the mechanism of estrogen action. The nonsteroidal antiestrogens, nafoxidine, tamoxifen, and Ci628, competitively inhibit the binding of estrogen to the estrogen receptor. In Section III, various properties of estrogen– and antiestrogen–receptor complexes are compared in an attempt to define the steps or modifications to the estrogen receptor that occur after the binding of the hormone and are required for the full activation induced by estrogens.

Estrogen receptors bind DNA *in vitro*. This interaction has been widely interpreted as a property of the receptor that is required for its biological action, even though the interaction of the receptor and DNA has not been demonstrated *in vivo*. In Section IV, the binding of various forms of the estrogen receptor to DNA are compared and the biological significance of this binding discussed.

The experiments described in this chapter were performed using several different estrogen-responsive systems. Most of the studies on the estrogen receptor were performed using rat, lamb, or calf uteri because of the availability and high receptor content of this tissue and the extensive literature on its estrogen receptor. The response of the uterus to estrogen is complex, the synthesis of certain proteins such as the induced protein (IP) increases shortly after estradiol administration and this is followed by an increase in the weight of the uterus (for more detailed review see Gorski and Gannon, 1976; Katzenellenbogen, 1980). Other experiments were performed on MCF-7 cells. This cell line was established from the pleural effusion of a patient with metastatic breast cancer and contains high concentrations of estrogen receptor. In this sytem, estrogen increases cell division, the level of progesterone receptor, and the production of a 52,000-dalton glycoprotein (52K protein) in the culture medium (Westley and Rochefort, 1980).

## II. THE SPECIFICITY OF ESTROGEN ACTION IN MAMMALS IS DETERMINED BY THE ESTROGEN RECEPTOR

The precise role of the receptor is unknown; its function, for instance, could be primarily to transport the steroid into the nucleus. Alternatively, the steroid might induce the transport of the receptor onto specific sites in the chromatin. In the first instance, the response would be specific for the steroid while in the second it would be specific for the receptor. In this section, we describe experiments that justify the concept that the estrogen-receptor protein determines the biological effects of estrogens.

### A. BINDING OF ANDROGENS TO THE ESTROGEN RECEPTOR

Figure 1 shows binding curves of 2 androgens 5α-androstane, 3β, 17β-diol (Adiol, Fig. 1a), and 5 androstene-3β 17β-diol (5 Adiol, Fig. 1c) in cytosol prepared from rat uteri. The dissociation constant for the binding was 16.6 nM for Adiol and 6.5 nM for 5 Adiol (Fig. 1b and 1d). That this relatively high-affinity binding was to the estrogen receptor and not the androgen receptor was shown by competition experiments in which the binding of [³H]Adiol was measured in the presence of a series of unlabeled steroids (Fig. 2). The binding was competed very efficiently by estrogens and the antiestrogen tamoxifen and less efficiently by androgens such as Adiol and 5α-dihydrotestosterone (DHT). Compared to estradiol, however, these androgens dissociated rapidly from the estrogen receptor, and as we have noted for other low-affinity ligands, notably the antiestrogen tamoxifen, the binding constant was modified by antibodies raised against the estrogen receptor (Garcia *et al.*, 1982).

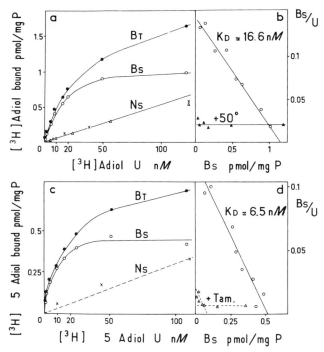

FIG. 1. Binding of ³H-labeled androgens to uterine-estrogen receptor. Rat uterine cytosol was incubated with increasing concentrations of [³H]5α Androstane, 3β, β17 diol (Adiol) (a and b) or 5 Androstene, 3β, 17β diol (5 Adiol) (c and d) either alone or in the presence of a 100-fold excess of nonradioactive steroid. The concentration of the total bound ³H-labeled hormone ($B_T$) was determined by dextran-coated charcoal assay. The unbound concentration (U) represents the difference between total and bound steroids. The specifically bound ³H-labeled steroid (Bs) was obtained by subtracting the nonspecific binding (NS) from the total binding. The specific bindings determined in a and c and after heating of the same cytosol at 50°C for 45 minutes (+50°C, b) or after competition by 1 μM tamoxifen (Tam, d) were plotted in b and d according to Scatchard. [From Garcia and Rochefort (1979).]

## B. Nuclear Translocation of the Estrogen Receptor by Androgens

Before it had been established that androgens interact with the estrogen receptor, we demonstrated that micromolar concentrations of androgens (DHT and testosterone) translocate the estrogen receptor into the nucleus of rat uteri *in vitro* (Rochefort *et al.*, 1972). The estrogen-receptor sites were

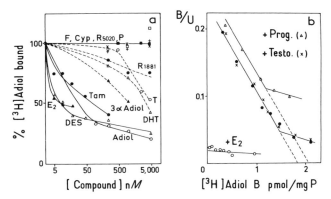

FɪG. 2. Binding stereospecificity of [³H]Adiol to the uterine-estrogen receptor. Calf-uterine cytosol was incubated for 4 hours at 2°C with the hormones. The bound [³H]Adiol was then determined by DCC adsorption. (a) Competition experiments. The cytosol was incubated with 50 nM [³H]Adiol and increasing concentrations of the following competitors: E₂ (▲), DES (△), Adiol (○), tamoxifen (Tam: ●). DHT (△— —△), testosterone (T; ○— —○), 5α-androstane-3α, 17β-diol (3 α Adiol: ▲— —▲), R1881 (●— —●), cortisol (F; x), cyproterone acetate (Cyp: ■), R5020 (+), and progesterone (P; □). Results are expressed as the percentage of the binding in control samples without competitor and are plotted against the log of the concentration of competitor by Scatchard plot. (b) Varying concentrations of [³H]Adiol alone (●) or together with 50 nM E₂ (○). Testosterone (x), or progesterone (△) were incubated with calf-uterine cytosol, and the [³H]Adiol binding was measured as in Fig. 1. Values were plotted according to Scatchard. In this cytosol, the number of specific binding sites for [³H]E₂, [³H]testosterone, and [³H]R5020 were 1.98, 0.08, and 2.08 pmol/mg protein, respectively, as determined separately by Scatchard plots. [From Garcia and Rochefort (1979).]

quantified by binding of [³H]estradiol at 0–2°C and as this did not appear to involve the exchange of androgens, there was little evidence from this early study to suggest that androgens bind to the estrogen receptor. We now understand that this was because both DHT and testosterone are very easily displaced by estradiol at 0–2°C since they dissociate very rapidly from the estrogen receptor (Rochefort and Garcia, 1976; Garcia and Rochefort, 1978).

We then demonstrated that DHT translocates both the rat uterine androgen (at microgram doses) and estrogen receptor (at milligram doses) into the nucleus *in vivo*. Injection of microgram amounts of DHT had no effect on uterine growth or on the incorporation of [³H]leucine into protein. In contrast, milligram doses of DHT increased both [³H]leucine incorporation and uterine weight. In addition, there was a correlation between the degree of stimulation of leucine incorporation and the amount of estrogen receptor translocated to the nucleus by DHT (Fig. 3) (Garcia and Rochefort, 1977).

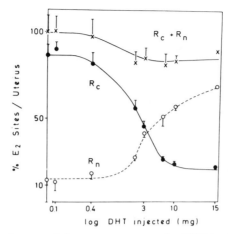

FIG. 3. Nuclear translocation of the estrogen receptor by DHT *in vivo*. Immature rats received one single subcutaneous injection of DHT or the vehicle only. The cytosol and KCl particulate extracts of uteri were prepared 3 hours later. The cytosol ($R_c$) and nuclear ($R_n$) estradiol receptor were subsequently labeled *in vitro* by exchange and finally measured by dextran-coated charcoal assay. Each determination was made in duplicate from five to ten uteri. Results of three to five experiments are represented as the mean ± 1 SEM. The effect of increasing doses of DHT is represented. x shows the sum of the sites in the nucleus and cytosol. [From Rochefort and Garcia (1976).]

## C. ESTROGEN-SPECIFIC EFFECTS OF ANDROGENS

Several proteins such as the IP, the progesterone receptor, and the 52K protein are considered to be specifically regulated by estrogens because they are not induced by other classes of steroids such as progestins, glucocorticoids, and physiological doses of androgens. In contrast, the effect of estradiol on leucine incorporation and uterine growth are pleiotropic responses, which may also be triggered by other mitogens. It was therefore important to study the induction of specific proteins to define the receptor responsible for mediating the effects of high doses of androgens. It was first shown that in the uterus the IP was also stimulated by high doses of DHT both *in vitro* (Ruh *et al.*, 1975) and *in vivo* by using a double labeling technique (Garcia and Rochefort, 1977) or by labeling with [35S]methionine (Rochefort *et al.*, 1980a). In contrast, the IP was not regulated by physiological concentrations of androgens, which translocate only the androgen receptor into the nucleus. These results were subsequently extended to other estrogen-specific responses. In DMBA mammary tumors, the levels of progesterone receptor were increased by high doses of DHT (Garcia and Rochefort, 1978; M. Garcia, 1983). In MCF-7 human breast cancer cells, two estrogen-responsive proteins, the progesterone receptor and the 52K protein, have been studied, Zava and McGuire (1978) showed that high concentrations of DHT increased the level of the progesterone receptor. We have shown that while DHT was inactive at physiological concentrations that exclusively occupy and activate the androgen receptor it induced the 52K glycoprotein at pharmacological concentrations (Westley and Rochefort, 1980). This induction was blocked by the antiestrogens tamoxifen and 4-hydroxytamoxifen (Fig. 4). We also tested the effects of adrenal androgens such as 5α-androstene 3β, 17β-diol (Adiol) and 5α-androstane 3β, 17β-diol (5 Adiol), which have a much higher affinity for the estrogen receptor (Fig. 1). These androgens induced the 52K protein at near physiological concentrations (Fig. 5). For all estrogen-agonists studied, we found that their ability to induce the 52K protein was proportional to their affinity for the estrogen receptor (Adams *et al.*, 1981; Fig. 5).

In all these experiments, the possibilities that the androgen is metabolized to or is contaminated by estrogens have been excluded. For instance, if the DHT had been contaminated by estrogens, then the observed binding would have been of high affinity and the steroid bound to the receptor would not have exchanged with [³H]estradiol so easily at 0–2°C. The direct interaction of labeled androgens with the estrogen receptor (Garcia and Rochefort, 1979) and experiments with antibodies raised against the estrogen receptor (Garcia *et al.*, 1982) also argue against this possibility.

The progesterone receptor is also able to bind androgens at high concentrations and might therefore be responsible for eliciting the estrogenic effects of high doses of androgens. However, the progesterone receptor is not translocated to the nucleus by androgens (Rochefort and Garcia, 1976), and progesterone is clearly unable to trigger estrogen-specific responses such as the accumulation of the IP, the progesterone receptor, or the 52K protein. We therefore conclude that the progesterone receptor could not be responsible for the observed estrogenic effects of androgens.

These results show that, at least in mammals, estrogen-induced proteins are specifically regulated by ligands able to activate the estrogen receptor, such as estrogens and some androgens. The informational molecule that interacts with the chromatin appears therefore to be the protein rather than the hormone, the function of the steroid being primarily to trigger and maintain the receptor in an activated state. These results also suggest that the receptor interacts specifically and directly with nuclear components.

In mammals, therefore, progesterone and androgen receptors appear to be unable to trigger estrogen-specific responses. This is in contrast to birds, where both progesterone and estrogen induce ovalbumin and conalbumin

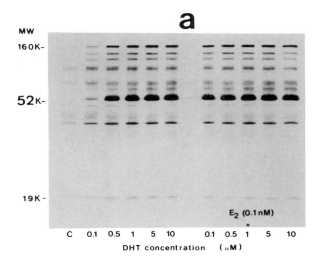

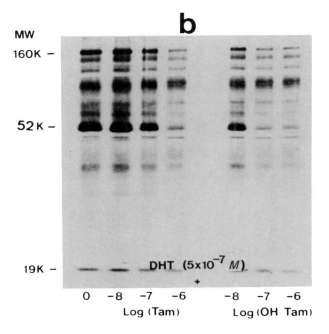

FIG. 4. Estrogenic effect of DHT on secreted proteins in MCF-7 human breast cancer cells. (a) The MCF-7 cells were cultured for 2 days with increasing concentrations of DHT without or with 0.1 nM estradiol. The proteins were then labeled by [$^{35}$S]methionine analyzed by SDS-polyacrylamide-gel electrophoresis and revealed by fluorography.

(b) Same protocol as (a) but the cells were treated by 0.5 μM DHT and indicated concentrations of tamoxifen (Tam) or monohydroxytamoxifen (OH-Tam). [From Rochefort *et al.* (1980).]

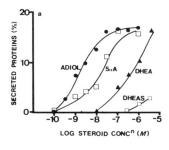
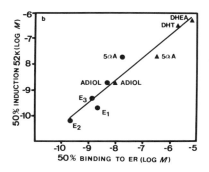

FIG. 5. Induction of 52K protein in MCF-7 cells by adrenal androgens. (a) Dose–response curves for the synthesis of 52K protein in MCF-7 cells. Ordinate, percentage of 52K protein in the secreted proteins, minus that in the control lacking steroid hormone. Dehydroepiandrosterone (DHEA), DHEA sulfate (DHEAS); androstane-3β,17β-diol (5αA); 5 androstenediol (Adiol). (b) Correlation between the concentration required for half-maximum induction of the 52K protein and the $K_D$ or $K_i$ for binding to ER. $K_D$ values were obtained by Scatchard plot. The $K_i$ values were obtained by competition with 17β-[$^3$H]estradiol. Estradiol ($E_2$); estrone ($E_1$); estriol ($E_3$). [From Adams *et al.* (1981).]

synthesis in the oviduct (McKnight, 1978). This suggests that the interaction of steroid receptors with chromatin in mammals may be more specific than in lower vertebrates.

## III. USE OF NONSTEROIDAL ANTIESTROGENS TO STUDY THE MECHANISM OF ESTROGEN ACTION

Nonsteroidal antiestrogens antagonize specifically the effects of estrogens *in vivo*, although they may also show estrogenic activity when administered alone. These drugs, which are metabolized *in vivo*, interact with the estrogen receptor with quite different characteristics from some of their metabolites (Capony and Rochefort, 1978; Borgna and Rochefort, 1980). To use antiestrogens as tools for understanding estrogen action, it is therefore important to define conditions under which they are either full estrogen antagonists or partial agonists and also to ensure that the compound used is actually responsible for the antagonist activity.

### A. PROBLEMS AND CHOICE OF THE EXPERIMENTAL SYSTEM

In humans, synthetic nonsteroidal antiestrogens are extensively used to treat postmenopausal breast cancer since they prevent the growth of some estrogen-receptor positive tumors. Because the antitumoral effect of tamoxifen is probably not exclusively due to its antiestrogenic activity and as the mechanism of the regulation of cell proliferation is more complex than that of gene expression, the effects of tamoxifen on cell proliferation are not considered in this chapter. In this section, we discuss systems in which these drugs have been demonstrated to inhibit well-defined estrogen-specific responses.

The degree of both the antagonistic and the agonistic effects of antiestrogens varies with the species, the tissue, the timing of administration, and the response being studied. For instance, in the chicken, tamoxifen is only an estrogen antagonist and does not induce ovalbumin or conalbumin synthesis. In the rat it increases the weight of the uterus but when administered continuously with estradiol, it antagonizes the uterotrophic effects of estradiol.

The arguments presented in Sections I and II suggest that the estrogen receptor mediates the effects of estrogens, and it is generally believed that antiestrogens also exert their effects by interacting with the estrogen receptor. It would therefore be predicted that the complex formed between the estrogen receptor and an estrogen should have different physicochemical properties from that formed with an antiestrogen in order to account for the different biological activities of the two types of complex. The elucidation of these differences should help to define an important step(s) in the mechanism of action of both estrogens and antiestrogens.

Our general approach has therefore been to compare the interactions of the estrogen receptor with antiestrogens in systems where antiestrogens are partial or full antagonists. The MCF-7 human breast cancer cell line has been used as the system of choice. In these cells, the biological activity of ligands can be established since they are metabolized less than *in vivo*, and any metabolism that does occur can be easily monitored. Moreover, several estrogen-regulated proteins can be studied. The effects of tamoxifen in MCF-7 cells depends on the response being studied. Tamoxifen acts as a partial estrogen agonist in that it induces the progesterone receptor (Horwitz and McGuire, 1978), whereas it is a full estrogen antagonist for the induction of the 52K glycoprotein by estradiol (Westley and Rochefort, 1980).

It has been proposed that the rate of dissociation of a ligand–receptor complex may be used to differentiate steroid agonists from antagonists and, indeed, many antiestrogens such as tamoxifen, Ci628, and nafoxidine, have a lower affinity than estradiol for the estrogen receptor and dissociate from it more rapidly. However, the observations that androgens are able to trigger estrogenic responses (see Section II) and that recently identified metabolites of the antiestrogens tamoxifen (Borgna and Rochefort, 1981) and Ci628 (Katzenellenbogen *et al.*, 1981) have a high affinity for the estrogen receptor but are potent antiestrogens argue against this simple view (Rochefort *et al.*,

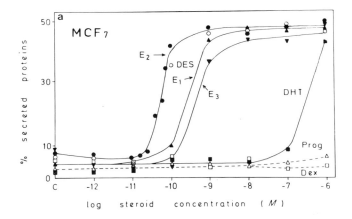

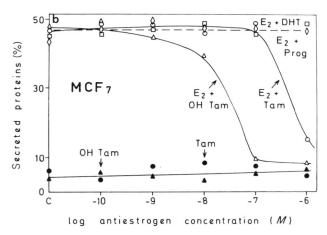

FIG. 6. (a) Induction of the 52K protein by various hormones. Withdrawn MCF-7 cells were cultured for 48 hours in medium containing charcoal-treated serum plus various concentrations of estradiol (●), diethylstilbestrol (○), estrone (▲), estriol (▼), 5α-dihydrotestosterone (■), progesterone (△), or dexamethasone (□). The cells were then labeled with [35S]methionine, the secreted proteins were analyzed on SDS polyacrylamide gels, and the percentage of [35S]methionine in the secreted proteins, which was due to the 52K protein, was estimated by scanning of the fluorographs. (b) Effect of antiestrogens. Withdrawn MCF-7 cells were cultured for 48 hours in medium containing charcoal-treated serum plus various concentrations of tamoxifen (●) or hydroxytamoxifen (▲) alone or charcoal-treated serum containing estradiol (0.1 nM) plus various concentrations of tamoxifen (○), hydroxytamoxifen (△), progesterone (◇), or 5α-dihydrotestosterone (□). The cells were then treated as described in (a). [Reprinted with permission from Westley and Rochefort (1980). Copyright 1980 by M.I.T. Press.]

1979). To circumvent the problems inherent in the use of antiestrogens that dissociate rapidly from the estrogen receptor, we have used 4-hydroxy-tamoxifen (OH-Tam), a metabolite of tamoxifen. [$^3$H]OH-Tam binds to an 8S cytosol receptor with the same affinity as estradiol (Borgna and Rochefort, 1980), and polyclonal antibodies raised against the calf uterine estradiol receptor have the same affinity for estradiol and OH-Tam receptor complexes (Garcia and Rochefort, 1979). Using the induction of the 52K glycoprotein in MCF-7 cells as a response, 4-hydroxytamoxifen (OH-Tam) is about 20-fold more active as an antiestrogen than tamoxifen (Fig. 6) and shows little, if any, estrogenic activity. In addition, MCF-7 cells do not interconvert tamoxifen and OH-Tam.

### B. DIFFERENCES IN ESTROGEN RECEPTOR ACTIVATION BY ESTROGENS AND ANTIESTROGENS

It was established 10 years ago (Rochefort *et al.*, 1972; Clark *et al.*, 1973) that antiestrogens are able to translocate the estrogen receptor into the nucleus in the rat uterus, and this was subsequently shown for the chicken oviduct (Sutherland *et al.*, 1977). The translocated estrogen-receptor– antiestrogen complex is only partly active since antiestrogens stimulate the synthesis of some (progesterone receptor) but not all (52K protein) estrogen-induced proteins (Fig. 6) in MCF-7 cells. The activation of the receptor, which is classically defined as the biochemical process that allows the receptor to be located in the nucleus (Jensen *et al.*, 1974; Milgrom, 1981), is not therefore synonymous with the process that transforms the receptor into a form having a full biological activity.

To try to discriminate between the partially activated receptor, which translocates to the nucleus but has little biological activity, and a fully activated receptor, we have compared the ability of estradiol and OH-Tam to activate the cytosol estrogen receptor in a cell-free system. Two types of ligand-induced changes of the estrogen receptor may be defined: those that are triggered by both agonists and antagonists and that may be responsible for nuclear translocation and those that are triggered only by agonists. The second category may be involved in complete activation of the estrogen receptor leading to its biological activity.

### 1. Changes in the Receptor Induced by Both Estrogens and Antiestrogens

It has been shown that the estrogen-receptor activation can be inhibited *in vitro* by molybdate (Mauck *et al.*, 1982). The estrogen receptor was therefore incubated with [$^3$H]estradiol or [$^3$H]OH-Tam in the presence or absence of molybdate. Incubation of [³H]OH-Tam with the rat uterus estrogen receptor at 25°C induced the 4–5 S transformation that is detected by sedimentation through sucrose gradients containing KCl (Rochefort *et al.*, 1983).

As the nuclear translocation of the estrogen receptor may be a consequence of its increased binding to DNA, we have also tested the ability of the OH-Tam–estrogen–receptor complex to bind to DNA. A high concentration of calf thymus DNA displaced the peak of [³H]OH-Tam–estrogen–receptor complex during centrifugation through sucrose gradients, showing that all of the complexes could bind to DNA (Borgna and Rochefort, 1980). Molybdate prevented the binding of the OH-Tam–estrogen–receptor complex to DNA. The observation that OH-Tam can induce both the 4–5 S transformation and the binding of the estrogen receptor to DNA suggest that neither are criteria for the full activation of the estrogen receptor.

## 2. Changes in the Receptor Induced by Estrogens but Not Antiestrogens

The experiments described above show that the OH-Tam–estrogen–receptor complex has many features in common with the estradiol–receptor complex. More recently, however, we have identified three criteria by which they two types of complexes may be distinguished.

*a. Interaction of the Estrogen Receptor with Monoclonal Antibodies.* The B36 monoclonal antibody, which was raised against the nuclear calf uterus receptor, clearly discriminates between the cytosol and nuclear estrogen receptor (Greene *et al.*, 1980). It has a lower affinity for the molybdate-stabilized estrogen receptor than for the heat-activated estrogen receptor of calf uterine cytosol (Borgna *et al.*, submitted). We have recently shown that the B36 antibody discriminates between the estrogen receptor bound to estradiol or OH-Tam. For instance, the molybdate-stabilized estrogen receptor interacted more strongly with the B36 antibody when complexed with OH-Tam than with estradiol (Borgna *et al.*, submitted).

*b. Rate of Dissociation after Estrogen Receptor Activation.* The dissociation rates of estradiol and OH-Tam– estrogen–receptor complexes formed at 0°C vary somewhat, depending on the source of the estrogen receptor (Table I). For instance, the dissociation rates of the calf uterine estradiol and OH-Tam–estrogen–receptor complexes were similar. In contrast, the lamb uterine OH-Tam–estrogen–receptor complex dissociated threefold faster, and the chick oviduct OH-Tam–estrogen–receptor complex dissociated threefold slower than the estradiol–estrogen–receptor complexes prepared from the same tissues. The rate of dissociation of estradiol–estrogen–receptor complexes decreases after warming (Shyamala and Leonard, 1980). This decrease is one of the criteria that has been proposed to define the activation of the receptor *in vitro*. Indeed, this decreased dissociation rate is blocked by molybdate and the nuclear estradiol– estrogen–receptor complex dissociates more slowly than the cytosol complex (deBoer and Notides, 1981). As the estrogen– and antiestrogen– estrogen–receptor complexes could not be distinguished by their rate of dissociation, the effect of warming on the dissociation rate was measured for

TABLE I

EFFECT OF MOLYBDATE ON THE DISSOCIATION RATE $(K^-)$ OF DIFFERENT ESTROGENS AND ANTIESTROGENS FROM THE ESTROGEN RECEPTOR[a]

| A. Species specificity $(K^-$ in $10^{-4}$ sec$^{-1})$[b] | | | | | | |
|---|---|---|---|---|---|---|
| | Calf | Lamb | Rat | Mouse | Chicken | MCF-7 |
| Temperature (C) | 20° | 20° | 20° | 20° | 15° | 20° |
| $E_2$ Control | 0.47 | 0.14 | 0.64 | 1.27 | 0.68 | 0.51 |
| $E_2$ + Molybdate | 1.10 | 0.28 | 2.40 | 4.01 | 1.75 | 1.04 |
| Increase % | 135 | 100 | 275 | 215 | 155 | 105 |
| OHT Control | | | | | | |
| OHT + Molybdate | 0.56 | 0.47 | 0.69 | 0.88 | 0.20 | 1.92 |
| Increase (%) | 0 ± 10 | id | id | id | id | id |

| B. Ligand specificity $(K^-$ in $10^{-4}$ sec$^{-1})$[c] | | | |
|---|---|---|---|
| | Temperature | Control | + Molybdate | Increase (%) |
| $E_2$ | 20° | 0.14 | 0.28 | 100 |
| $E_1$ | 20° | 6.60 | 11.91 | 80 |
| $E_3$ | 20° | 0.31 | 0.68 | 120 |
| 5 Adiol | 0° | 0.63 | 1.13 | 80 |
| OHT | 20° | 0.47 | 0.47 | ≈0 |
| T | 0° | 2.30 | 2.30 | ≈0 |
| Ci 628 | 0° | 0.85 | 0.85 | ≈0 |

[a]Reprinted by permission from Rochefort and Borgna (1981), *Nature (London)* **292**, 257–259. Copyright © 1981 Macmillan Journals Ltd.

[b]Species specificity. The dissociation rate constants of $E_2$ and OH-Tam from the cytosol-estrogen receptor of calf, lamb, rat and mouse uterus, of chicken oviduct, and of the MCF-7 human breast cancer cell line have been determined at 20°C or 15°C (chicken), following heat activation in the presence or absence of 10 mM sodium molybdate as described in Fig. 7. The $K^-$ values calculated after correction for nonspecific binding and their percentage increase due to molybdate are presented. For OH-Tam studies, the difference between the two linear regressions drawn through the points obtained with and without molybdate was nil or less than 10%.

[c]Ligand specificity. The $K^-$ from the cytosol-estrogen receptor of lamb uterus has been determined at 20°C or 0°C, as described in Fig. 2, for the following estrogens (estradiol = $E_2$; estrone = $E_1$; estriol = $E_3$; and androsta-5-ene 3 β, 17 β-diol = 5 Adiol) and antiestrogens (CI 628; tamoxifen = T, and 4-hydroxy-tamoxifen = OH-Tam).

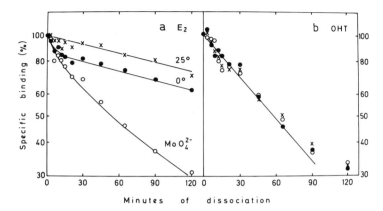

FIG. 7. Dissociation rate of estradiol (a) and 4-hydroxytamoxifen (b) from the estrogen receptor before and after heat activation. Lamb uterine cytosol prepared in the presence (○) or
absence (●, x) of 10 mM Mo $O_4^{2-}$ was incubated for 2 hours with 5 nM [$^3$H]estradiol or [$^3$H]4-
hydroxy-*trans*-tamoxifen. One part of the cytosol without Mo $O_4^{2-}$ was activated by a 30-
minute treatment at 25°C, the other part was maintained at 0°C, the dissociation rate was then
determined at 25°C, following the addition of 1μM unlabeled $E_2$ at time 0. The specific binding
to the estrogen receptor was determined by charcoal assay, the nonspecific binding was evalu-
ated in a parallel experiment performed with 1 μM unlabeled $E_2$. The complexes were stable
during the course of the assay. x (25°C), preactivated receptor; ● (0°C), nonpreactivated
receptor; ○ (Mo $O_4^{2-}$), molybdate-treated estrogen receptor. [Reprinted by permission from
Rochefort and Borgna (1981), *Nature (London)* **292**, 257–259. Copyright © 1981 Macmillan
Journals Ltd.]

both complexes. Because incubation at 0°C leads to a gradual decrease in the
rate of dissociation (Fig. 7a), the dissociation rate of the warmed complex was
compared to that of a complex incubated at 0°C in the presence of molybdate
(Fig. 7a). The estradiol– estrogen–receptor complexes prepared from different tissues always dissociated slower after warming at 25°C than after incubation at 0°C in the presence of molybdate. In contrast, the dissociation rate of
the OH-Tam– estrogen–receptor complexes, whether warmed at 25°C or
incubated at 0°C with molybdate, were always the same (Fig. 7b). These
results implied that by this *in vitro* criterion of activation, the estrogen
receptor could be transformed by estradiol but not OH-Tam.

These results were then extended to other slow and fast dissociating estrogen– and antiestrogen–receptor complexes (Table I). All the estrogen
agonists tested (estradiol, estrone, estriol, and androsta-5-ene-3β 17β diol)
activated the receptor, even though the absolute rate of dissociation of the
different complexes varied more than tenfold. None of the three estrogen
antagonists tested (4-hydroxytamoxifen, tamoxifen, Ci628) activated the estrogen receptor by this criterion (Rochefort and Borgna, 1981).

More recently (Rochefort *et al.*, 1983), we have shown that the difference is a consequence of the formation of the ligand–estrogen–receptor complex and not an indirect effect of the ligands on other factors present in the cytosol. A cytosol containing preformed [$^3$H]OH-Tam–estrogen–receptor complexes was mixed at 2°C with a cytosol containing nonradioactive estradiol, and conversely a cytosol containing preformed [$^3$H]estradiol–estrogen–receptor complexes was mixed with cytosol containing nonradioactive OH-Tam. The addition of the nonradioactive ligand had no effect on the dissociation rate of the radioactive ligand. These mixing experiments therefore show that it is the nature of the ligand interacting directly with the estrogen receptor that is responsible for the modification of the properties of the estrogen receptor. This suggests that one criterion for the activation of the estrogen receptor is an increased stability of the ligand–estrogen–receptor complex as reflected by a decrease in the dissociation rate. An estrogen thus appears to have a higher affinity for the activated estrogen receptor while the affinity of an antiestrogen remains constant after estrogen-receptor activation. These results are consistent with our previous findings that when tamoxifen and estrogen are incubated together with calf uterine estrogen receptor, the competition by tamoxifen for the binding of estradiol to the estrogen receptor decreases as the time of incubation increases. We now believe that the decrease in the efficiency with which tamoxifen competes for estradiol (indicating that the binding was not at equilibrium) (Rochefort and Capony, 1977) was partly due to the different dissociation rate of the two ligands and partly to the gradual transformation of the estrogen receptor into a form having a higher affinity for estrogens.

## C. Affinity for DNA

Another criterion for the activation of the estrogen receptor is its binding to DNA *in vitro*. As discussed in Section III,B,1, DNA may bind all of the OH-Tam–estrogen–receptor complexes if a high enough concentration of DNA is used. More recently, the apparent affinities of the binding of estradiol and OH-Tam–estrogen–receptor complexes to DNA adsorbed to cellulose have been measured. The OH-Tam–estrogen–receptor complex had a lower affinity for DNA than did the estradiol–estrogen–receptor complex, although the amount of receptor retained on the DNA at the highest concentration of DNA-cellulose was the same (Evans *et al.*, 1982). This difference was confirmed by evaluating the binding of the estradiol and OH-Tam–estrogen–receptor complexes to DNA using sucrose density gradient centrifugation to separate the free and DNA-bound complexes.

The results, taken together, strongly suggest that estradiol activates while

OH-Tam only partially activates the estrogen receptor. The apparent affinity of ligands for the estrogen receptor and their ability to transform the 4 S form of the estrogen receptor into a 5 S form do not discriminate between a fully activated and a partially activated or inactive estrogen receptor. By contrast, the hormone- and DNA-binding sites and an antigenic domain of the estrogen receptor would appear to be differently modified during the process of activation by estrogen and by antiestrogen. These results would be consistent with a model in which the activated complex formed between the receptor and agonists has a higher affinity both for DNA and for the agonists and that these two properties are required for the initiation of estrogenic effects in the cell nucleus.

## IV. BIOLOGICAL SIGNIFICANCE OF THE INTERACTION OF THE ESTROGEN RECEPTOR WITH DNA

As noted in Section I, the model for the mechanism of estrogen action in which the estradiol–receptor complex regulates the transcription of estrogen-responsive genes has been the dominant model of steroid hormone action for many years. This model requires that the estrogen–receptor complex interacts with chromatin. One possibility is that, as for the cyclic AMP receptor in procaryotes, the estrogen receptor interacts directly with DNA. The only results obtained so far on the interaction of the estrogen receptor with DNA have been obtained *in vitro* and concern the interaction with nonspecific DNA sequences. They, therefore, cannot explain the specific effect of estrogens on the induction of a limited number of proteins.

Recently, in other systems, mouse mammary tumor virus and chick oviduct, the glucocorticoid (Payvar *et al.*, 1981) and progesterone (Mulvihill *et al.*, 1982) receptors, respectively, have been demonstrated to interact with a higher affinity with certain DNA sequences, some of which are located in the 5' region of the regulated genes and may be involved in their regulation. Such data are not yet available for the estrogen receptor. In contrast, the characteristics of the low-affinity binding of the estrogen receptor to nonspecific DNA are well known (Yamamoto and Alberts, 1976; Rochefort *et al.*, 1980b). This interaction has been characterized by several techniques such as retention on DNA cellulose and ultracentrifugation in sucrose or metrizamide gradients. The interaction is reversible, is of low affinity, and is neither sequence nor species specific. The estrogen receptor does, however, interact more strongly with double-stranded DNA than with single-stranded DNA or other polyanions and the interaction is inhibited by intercalating drugs, indicating that a double helical structure appears to be required for binding (André *et al.*, 1976).

The interaction of the estrogen receptor with nonspecific DNA sequences is of interest for several reasons. First, it is an easy test that has been used to measure the activation of the receptor *in vitro*. Second, it is possibly involved in or responsible for the translocation of the receptor into the nucleus. Indeed, the amount of receptor that is translocated does not appear to be limited by the number of receptor-binding sites in the nucleus (acceptor sites), and this is compatible with the high proportion of the DNA that is accessible in chromatin. Third, a comparison of the affinity of this interaction *in vitro* with the biological activity of estrogens *in vivo* might explain some cases of estrogen unresponsiveness and thereby provide evidence for the biological significance of this estrogen–receptor–DNA interaction. Fourth, it could be used to map the domains of the receptor that are involved in the binding to chromatin. It is well known, for instance, that after proteolysis with trypsin or a $Ca^{2+}$-activated protease, the 8 S receptor is irreversibly transformed into 4 S proteolyzed forms that are unable to interact with DNA (André and Rochefort, 1973; Sherman *et al.*, 1978).

In this section, we summarize the results of experiments that were performed in an attempt to assess the biological significance of this estrogen–receptor–DNA interaction.

### A. COMPARISON OF CYTOSOLIC AND NUCLEAR FORMS OF THE ESTROGEN RECEPTOR AND THEIR BINDING TO DNA

To determine which, if any, of the different forms of the estrogen receptor that have been identified *in vitro* might be biologically active *in vivo*, the size and DNA-binding ability of the nuclear lamb uterine receptor was compared with different forms of the cytosol receptor (André *et al.*, 1978). The nuclear receptor was prepared from lamb endometrial nuclei after translocation of the estrogen receptor by incubation of uteri at 37°C in the presence of [$^3$H]estradiol. The receptor was extracted in low-salt conditions by extensive micrococcal nuclease digestion. The predominant form of the micrococcal nuclease extracted receptor sedimented at 6 S, i.e., somewhat slower than the 8 S cytoplasmic receptor but faster than the 4 S forms of the cytoplasmic receptor produced either by the action of trypsin or a $Ca^{2+}$-activated protease. When the different forms of the receptor were analyzed by gel filtration, ion exchange chromatography and their densities were measured on metrizamide gradients, the 8 S cytosol receptor always behaved similarly to the receptor extracted from nuclei by micrococcal nu-

TABLE II

COMPARISON BETWEEN THE "MICROCOCCAL" NUCLEAR RECEPTOR AND THE DIFFERENT FORMS OF THE CYTOSOL ESTROGEN RECEPTOR[a,b]

| Form of receptor | S value | Stokes radius (nm) | Calculated MW | DEAE cellulose KCl conc. required for elution (M) | Density[c] in metrizamide gradients (g/cc) | Binding to calf thymus (DNA) |
|---|---|---|---|---|---|---|
| Nuclear | | | | | | |
| Micrococcal nuclease extracted RE[d] | 6 | 5.2 | 130,000 | 0.23, 0.30 | 1.239 | + |
| Cytosol | | | | | | |
| 8 S "native" | 8 | 5.3 | 170,000 | 0.23, 0.30 | 1.238 | + |
| 4 S trypsinized | 4 | ND | ND | ND | 1.20 | − |
| 4 S Ca²⁺-activated protease | 4.5 | 2.9 | 55,000 | 0.10 | 1.275 | − |

[a] These results were obtained with nonpurified nuclear receptor from lamb endometrium. The molecular weights were calculated from the S value, and the Stokes radius according to the method of Siegel and Monty.

[b] Reprinted with permission from André et al. (1978). Copyright 1982 American Chemical Society.

[c] Results from Baskevitch and Rochefort (1981).

[d] RE = estrogen receptor.

clease but differently from the 4 S forms of the cytosol receptor produced by partial proteolysis (Table II).

The interaction of these different forms of receptors with DNA was then determined by the ability of calf thymus DNA to displace the peaks of receptor during velocity sedimentation on sucrose gradients. The 8 S cytosol receptor and the nuclease-extracted nuclear receptor bound to DNA, whereas the 4 S forms of the cytosol receptor did not.

These results clearly show that the receptor that is extracted from nuclei by micrococcal nuclease digestion is similar by several criteria to the 8 S cytosol receptor and retains an ability to bind DNA. The reason for the difference in the rates of sedimentation but not the stokes radius of these two forms is unknown but might reflect different degrees of asymmetry or different interactions with other molecules during the two isolation procedures. The observation that the nuclear receptor is still able to bind DNA *in vitro* is consistent with the concept that the receptor interacts with DNA *in vivo*. The observation that the 4 S form of the cytosol receptor that is formed by the $Ca^{2+}$-activated protease does not bind to DNA and is different by most criteria from the micrococcal nuclease-extracted nuclear receptor suggests that nuclear translocation is unlikely to occur as a result of proteolysis by the $Ca^{2+}$-activated protease. It remains conceivable, however, that this protease might be involved in the inactivation and processing of the estrogen receptor. It is also possible that a different type of partial proteolysis of the estrogen receptor would favor rather than prevent the binding of the estrogen receptor to DNA.

## B. BIOLOGICAL ACTIVITY OF THE ESTROGEN RECEPTOR IS CORRELATED WITH ITS DNA-BINDING AFFINITY

The comparison of the responsiveness of various tissues to estrogen with the ability of their estrogen receptors to bind DNA may provide evidence for the biological significance of the estrogen-receptor–DNA interaction. For example, the characterization of the interaction of DNA with the glucocorticoid receptors from mutant glucocorticoid-resistant lymphoma cell lines has shown that receptors from unresponsive cells may have either a higher (nt$^i$) or lower (nt$^-$) affinity for DNA (Higgins and Gehring, 1978). In this section, we have attempted to correlate the low-affinity binding of the estrogen receptor for DNA *in vitro* with the biological activity of estrogen receptors in several systems that do not respond to estrogens.

Table III summarizes examples in which the affinity of the estrogen receptor for DNA is modified either naturally or artificially. Agents such as molybdate and pyridoxal phosphate, which block the binding of receptors to DNA,

TABLE III
VARIATIONS IN THE AFFINITY OF THE ESTROGEN RECEPTOR FOR DNA[a]

| Component affected | No affinity | Decreased affinity | Increased affinity |
|---|---|---|---|
| (A) Cytosol receptor | Partial proteolysis ($Ca^{2+}$, trypsin) Molybdate[b] | Antiestrogens (OH Tamoxifen) | Estrogen unresponsive mammary tumors ($C_3H$, $R_3$) |
| (B) DNA | Pyridoxal $PO_4^{2+}$[c] Intercalating drugs (Ethidium bromide, ellipticine) | | BUdR Substitution |

[a]The *in vitro* interaction of RE to DNA can be prevented or modulated by modifications of the cytosol receptor (A) or of DNA (B). Results from our laboratory are described in the text.
[b]Results from Mauck *et al.* (1982).
[c]Results from Cake *et al.* (1978).

have been used mostly *in vitro* and we have not studied their mechanism of action. The OH-Tam–estrogen–receptor complex is biologically inactive in certain systems and appears to have a lower affinity for nonspecific DNA than the estradiol–estrogen–receptor complex (see Section III). We discuss below the estrogen-receptor–DNA interaction in estrogen-unresponsive cells containing estrogen receptor.

## 1. Estrogen-Unresponsive Mammary Tumors

Approximately 50% of human mammary tumors that contain estrogen receptors do not respond to estrogen. $C_3H$ mouse mammary tumors provide a model for this class of human mammary tumors. Estrogens do not affect the growth of these tumors or their levels of progesterone receptor (Baskevitch and Rochefort, 1983). These tumors, however, contain estrogen receptors that translocate into the nucleus *in vivo* after injection of estrogen (Vignon and Rochefort, 1978). The ability of the cytosol-estrogen receptor to bind to calf thymus DNA has recently been characterized (Baskevitch *et al.*, 1983). The apparent affinity of the estrogen receptor for DNA was two- to threefold higher than that of the uterine receptor of the same $C_3H$ mice or of rats. Although the reason for the increased affinity of this receptor for DNA is unknown, experiments in which cytosol from tumors and uteri are mixed might provide evidence for a cytosol protease present in the $C_3H$ mammary tumors that increases the *in vitro* affinity of the estrogen receptor for DNA (Baskevitch and Rochefort, submitted).

## 2. Inhibition of Estrogen Responsiveness Following the Incorporation of Bromodeoxyuridine into Cellular DNA

When MCF-7 cells are grown in the presence of 5 μg/ml of 5-bromodeox-yuridine (BudR), the induction of the 52K glycoprotein and the progesterone receptor by estradiol is inhibited (Garcia *et al.*, 1981). Other proteins that are not regulated by estradiol are not affected. This antiestrogenic effect appears to depend on the incorporation of BudR into DNA since it requires a lag of 24 hours and because both ARA-C (a DNA synthesis inhibitor) and thymidine (which competes with BudR for incorporation into DNA) inhibit the effect. This effect of BudR is an example of an inhibition of steroid hormone action that is probably located at the DNA level. Although the basis for this inhibition is unknown, it is tempting to speculate that the incorporation of BudR into DNA interferes with the normal interaction of the receptor with DNA. This interference could occur either at low-affinity sites or at the higher-affinity sites, which may exist close to estrogen-regulated genes. The *in vitro* affinity of estrogen receptors for BudR-substituted DNA is higher than for normal DNA (Kallos *et al.*, 1978), and estrogen receptors are extracted less efficiently by salt from the nuclei of cells grown in the presence of BudR (P. P. Baskevitch, unpublished data; Rochefort *et al.*, 1980; Kallos *et al.*, 1980).

These observations are consistent with the concept that the increased affinity of the receptor for BudR-substituted DNA causes the unresponsiveness to estrogen. Thus, whereas in the case of 4-hydroxytamoxifen, the inactivity of the 4-hydroxytamoxifen–receptor complex is correlated with a lower affinity for DNA; in the case of the $C_3H$ mammary tumor and MCF-7 cells grown in the presence of BudR, the unresponsiveness is correlated with an increased affinity of the estrogen–receptor complex for DNA. These findings suggest some analogy to the results obtained with mutant lymphoma cell lines that do not respond to glucocorticoids. The receptors of these mutants have either a higher (nt$^i$ phenotype) or lower (nt$^-$ phenotype) affinity for DNA. Clearly one explanation of these data is that both an increased and a decreased affinity of the steroid–receptor complex for DNA decreases its biological activity. Interpreted in the light of the model of steroid action presented in the introduction, in both cases the steroid–receptor complexes are inhibited from interacting with the higher-affinity sites that are postulated to lie close to hormonally responsive genes.

A model has been proposed in which steroid–receptor complexes reach higher-affinity DNA sites by translocation from low-affinity nonspecific sites (Palmiter *et al.*, 1978). In the case of an nt$^i$ phenotype where the receptor binds with a higher affinity to DNA, the receptor would be retained on nonspecific sequences and unable to reach the higher-affinity sites. In the case of an nt⁻ phenotype, the lowered affinity of the estrogen receptor for nonspecific DNA sequences might also prevent the receptor reaching the higher-affinity sites.

## V. CONCLUDING REMARKS

The data presented in this chapter strongly support the hypothesis that the estrogen receptor (Jensen and Jacobson, 1962; Jensen *et al.*, 1972) located in estrogen-target tissue mediates estrogen action. They also indicate that the nuclear translocation of estrogen receptor is not synonymous with the activation that is responsible for its biological action. The availability of different systems in which nuclear translocation does occur but in which the translocated receptors are inactive might allow other criteria of receptor activation, which are related to the biological response, to be defined.

It is interesting to note that even though the mammalian estrogen receptor was the first steroid receptor to be described, much less is known about its mechanism of action at the molecular level than for the glucocorticoid and the progesterone receptors.

It is anticipated that the understanding of estrogen action at the molecular level will soon be improved as purified estrogen receptors and cloned estrogen-regulated genes become available. These components would allow the binding of the receptor to putative regulatory sequences within and close to the hormonally regulated genes to be studied and may allow the development of *in vitro* systems in which transcription is regulated by the steroid–receptor complex.

Estrogen-responsive systems in mammals continue to have several potential advantages over other systems. First, estrogen-responsive cell lines are available that should allow genetic studies to be performed. Second, the existence of systems that have become unresponsive to estrogens, either spontaneously (e.g., estrogen-receptor positive, hormone-independent mammary tumors) or as a result of treatment with compounds such as BudR or antiestrogens might allow important steps in the mechanism of estrogen action to be defined by comparision with estrogen-responsive systems. Third, monoclonal antibodies against the estrogen receptor are now available and should allow the different functional domains of various forms of the estrogen receptor to be mapped (see Chapter 8, this volume).

Finally, estrogen-responsive cell lines also provide excellent systems with which to study the mechanism of the hormonal regulation of cell proliferation. The relationship between the modulation of gene expression and the regulation of cell proliferation by estrogens can now be studied in cell culture at the molecular level and might, in the near future, result in important progress in the understanding of steroid hormone action.

## ACKNOWLEDGMENTS

This chapter is based on the original work performed by our colleagues whose names appear in the cited publications. This work was supported by the "Institut National de la Santé et de la Recherche Médicale," the "Centre National de la Recherche Scientifique," the "Association pour le Développement de la Recherche sur le Cancer," and the University of Montpellier. We thank Edith Barrie for her skillful preparation of manuscript.

## REFERENCES

Adams, J., Garcia, M., and Rochefort, H. (1981). *Cancer Res.* **41**, 4720–4726.
André, J., and Rochefort, H. (1973). *FEBS LETT.* **32**, 330–334.
André, J., Pfeiffer, A., and Rochefort, H. (1976). *Biochemistry* **15**, 2964–2969.
André, J., Raynaud, A., and Rochefort, H. (1978). *Biochemistry* **17**, 3619–3626.
Baskevitch, P. P., and Rochefort, H. (1981). *Mol. Cell Endocrinol.* **22**, 195–210.
Baskevitch, P. P., and Rochefort, H. (1983). *In* "Drug and Hormone Resistance in Neoplasia" (N. Bruchovsky and J. H. Goldie, eds.), Vol. I. CRC Press (Uniscience), in press.
Baskevitch, P. P., and Rochefort, H. (1984). Submitted.
Baskevitch, P. P., Vignon, F., Bousquet, C., and Rochefort, H. (1983). *Cancer Res.* **43**, 2290–2297.
Baulieu, E. E., Alberga, A., Jung, I., Lebeau, M. C., Mercier-Bodard, C., Milgrom, E., Raynaud, J. P., Raynaud-Jammet, C., Rochefort, H., Truong, H., and Robel, P. (1971). *Recent Prog. Horm. Res.* **27**, 351–419.
Borgna, J. L., and Rochefort, H. (1980). *Mol. Cell. Endocrinol* **20**, 71–85.
Borgna, J. L., and Rochefort, H. (1981). *J. Biol. Chem.* **256**, 859–868.
Borgna, J. L., Fauque, J., and Rochefort, H. (1984). Submitted.
Cake, M. H., DiSorbo, D. M., Litwack, G. (1978). *J. Biol. Chem.* **253**, 4886–4891.
Capony, F., and Rochefort, H. (1978). *Mol. Cell. Endocrinol.* **11**, 181–198.
Clark, J. H., Anderson, J. N., and Peck, E. J. (1973). *Steroids* **22**, 707–718.
deBoer, W., and Notides, A. C. (1981). *Biochemistry* **20**, 1285–1289.
Evans, E., Baskevitch, P. P., and Rochefort, H. (1982). *Eur. J. Biochem.* **128**, 185–191.
Garcia, M. (1983). Ph.D. thesis, USTL, University of Montpellier, France.
Garcia, M., and Rochefort, H. (1977). *Steroids* **29**, 111–126.
Garcia, M., and Rochefort, H. (1978). *Cancer Res.* **38**, 3922–3929.
Garcia, M., and Rochefort, H. (1979). *Endocrinology (Baltimore)* **104**, 1797–1804.
Garcia, M., Westley, B., and Rochefort, H. (1981). *Eur. J. Biochem.* **116**, 297–301.
Garcia, M., Greene, G., Rochefort, H., and Jensen, E. V. (1982) *Endocrinology (Baltimore)* **110**, 1355–1361.
Greene, G., Fitch, G. W., and Jensen, E. V. (1980). *Proc. Natl Acad. Sci. U.S.A.* **77**, 157–161.
Gorski, J., and Gannon, F. (1976). *Annu. Rev. Physiol.* **38**, 425–450.
Higgins, S. J., and Gehring, U. (1978). *In* "Advances in Cancer Research," Vol. 28, pp. 313–397. Academic Press, New York.

Horwitz, K. B., and McGuire, W. L. (1978). *Endocrinology (Baltimore)* **103**, 1742–1751.
Jensen, E. V., and Jacobson, H. I. (1962). *Recent Prog. Horm. Res.* **18**, 387–414.
Jensen, E. V., Mohla, S., Gorell, T., Tanaka, S., and DeSombre, E. R. (1972). *J. Steroid Biochem.* **3**, 445–458.
Jensen, E. V., Mohla, S., Gorell, T., and DeSombre, E. R. (1974). *In* "Vitamins and Hormones," Vol. 32, pp. 89–127. Academic Press, New York.
Kallos, J., Fasy, T. M., Hollander, V. P., and Bick, M. D. (1978). *Proc. Natl. Acad. Sci. U.S.A.* **75**, 4896–4900.
Kallos, J., Hollander, V. P., Baskevitch, P. P., and Rochefort, H. (1980). *Ann. N.Y. Acad. Sci.* **346**, 415–418.
Katzenellenbogen, B. S. (1980). *Annu. Rev. Physiol.* **42**, 17–35.
Katzenellenbogen, B. S., Pavlik, E. J., Robertson, D. W. and Katzenellenbogen, J. A. (1981). *J. Biol. Chem.* **256**, 2908–2915.
McKnight, G. S. (1978). *Cell* **14**, 400–413.
Mauck, L. A., Day, R. N., and Notides, A. C. (1982) *Biochemistry* **21**, 1788–1793.2
Milgrom, E. (1981). *In* "Biochemical Actions of Hormones" (G. Litwack, ed.), Vol. VIII, pp. 465–491. Academic Press, New York.
Mueller, G. C., Gorski, J., and Aizawa, Y. (1961). *Proc. Natl. Acad. Sci. U.S.A.* **47**, 164–167.
Mulvihill, E. R., LePennec, J. P., and Chambon, P. (1982). *Cell* **28**, 621–632.
O'Malley, B. W., and Means, A. R. (1974). *Science* **183**, 610–620
Palmiter, R. D., Mulvihill, E. R., McKnight, G. S., and Senear, A. W. (1978). *Cold Spring Harbor Symp. Quant. Biol.* **42**, 639–647.
Payvar, F., Wrange, O., Carlstedt-Duke, J., Okret, S., Gustafsson, J. A., and Yamamoto, K. R. (1981). *Proc. Natl. Acad. Sci. U.S.A.* **78**, 6628–6632.
Rochefort, H., and Garcia, M. (1976). *Steroids* **28**, 549–560.
Rochefort, H., and Capony, F. (1977). *Biochem. Biophys. Res. Commun.* **75**, 277–285.
Rochefort, H., and Borgna, J. L. (1981). *Nature (London)* **292**, 257–259.
Rochefort, H., Lignon, F., and Capony, F. (1972). *Biochem. Biophys. Res. Commun.* **47**, 662–670.
Rochefort, H., Garcia, M., and Borgna, J. L. (1979). *Biochem. Biophys. Res. Commun.* **88**, 351–357.
Rochefort, H., Garcia, M., Vignon, F., and Westley, B. (1980a). *In* "Steroid Induced Uterine Proteins" (M. Beato, ed.), pp. 171–182. Elsevier, New York.
Rochefort, H., André, J., Baskevitch, P. P., Kallos, J., Vignon, F., and Westley, B. (1980b). *J. Steroid Biochem.* **12**, 135–142.
Rochefort, H., Borgna, J. L., and Evans, E. (1983). *J. Steroid Biochem.*, **19**, 64–74.
Ruh, T. S., Wassilak, S. G., and Ruh, M. F. (1975). *Steroids* **25**, 257–273.
Sherman, M. R., Pickering, L. A., Hollwagen, F. M., and Miller, L. K. (1978). *Fed. Proc.* **37**, 167–173.
Shyamala, G., and Leonard, L. (1980). *J. Biol. Chem.* **255**, 6028–6031.
Sutherland, R. L., Mester, J., Baulieu, E. E. (1977). *Nature (London)* **267**, 434–435.
Tomkins, G. M. (1975). *Science* **189**, 760–763.
Vignon, F., and Rochefort, H. (1978). *Cancer Res.* **38**, 1808–1814.
Westley, B., and Rochefort, H. (1980). *Cell* **20**, 352–362.
Yamamoto, K. R., and Alberts, B. M. (1976). *Annu. Rev. Biochem.* **45**, 721–746.
Zava, D. T., and McGuire, W. L. (1978). *Science* **199**, 787–788.

# CHAPTER 10

# Catechol Estrogens*

*Eytan R. Barnea, Neil J. MacLusky, and Frederick Naftolin*

Department of Obstetrics and Gynecology
Yale University School of Medicine
New Haven, Connecticut

*The following abbreviations are used throughout this chapter: HPLC, high-performance liquid chromatography; 4-MeO-$E_1$, 4-methoxyestrone, 1,3,5(10)-estratriene-3,4-diol-17-one-4-methyl ether; 2-MeO-$E_1$, 2-methoxyestrone, 1,3,5(10)-estratriene-2,3-diol,17-one-2-methyl ether; 4-MeO-$E_2$, 4-methoxyestradiol, 1,3,5(10)-estratriene-3,4,17$\beta$-triol-4-methyl ether; 2-MeO-$E_2$, 2-methoxyestradiol, 1,3,5(10)-estratriene-2,3,17$\beta$-triol-2-methyl ether; 4-OH-$E_1$, 4-hydroxyestrone, 1,3,5(10)-estratriene-3,4-diol-17-one; 2-OH-$E_1$, 2-hydroxyestrone, 1,3,5(10)-estratriene-2,3-diol-17-one; 4-OH-$E_2$, 4-hydroxyestradiol, 1,3,5(10)-estratriene-3,4,17$\beta$-triol; 2-OH-$E_2$, 2-hydroxyestradiol, 1,3,5(10)-estratriene-2,3,17$\beta$-triol; $E_1$, estrone, 1,3,5(10)-estratriene-3-ol-17-one; $E_2$, estradiol, 1,3,5(10)-estratriene-3-17$\beta$-diol; $E_3$, estriol, 1,3,5(10)-estratriene-3,16$\alpha$,17$\beta$-triol; $EE_2$, 17$\alpha$-ethinylestradiol, 1,3,5(10)-estratriene-17$\alpha$-ethinyl-3,17$\beta$-diol; CE, catechol estrogens; MeCE, methoxy derivatives of catechol estrogens.

BIOCHEMICAL ACTIONS OF HORMONES, VOL. XI

# I. INTRODUCTION

The catechol estrogens (CEs) are formed by A-ring hydroxylation of the circulating hormonal estrogens at positions 2 or 4. In man, CE formation represents a major route of estrogen metabolism, rivaling 16α-hydroxylation in quantitative importance (Fishman, 1963). The biologic role of CEs, however, is not at all clear.

A-ring hydroxylation has long been considered to be a potential pathway of estrogen metabolism. As early as 1940, Westerfeld proposed that CE formation might represent one of the ways in which estrogens are broken down. It was almost 20 years later, however, before the first direct evidence for in vivo CE formation was obtained when Krachy and Gallagher (1957) and Engel et al. (1957) demonstrated for the first time that [$^{14}$C]estradiol is converted to 2-methoxyestrogens (MeCE) in postmenopausal women. The route of formation of these compounds was postulated to involve initial CE formation and subsequent methylation of the CEs by catechol-o-methyl transferase (COMT). Confirmation of this hypothesis was provided by Fishman (1963), who isolated radioactive 2-OH-E$_1$ from human urine after the intravenous infusion of labeled E$_2$.

Initially, CEs were considered to be nothing more than estrogen degradation products. This view was supported by studies on the pharmacologic properties of CEs, which suggested that they were relatively weak estrogen agonists. During the late 1960s and early 1970s, however, a number of reports appeared that challenged the assumption that CEs were biologically inactive. First, Breuer, Knuppen, and their co-workers (Breuer et al., 1968; Knuppen et al., 1969) reported that CEs are excellent competitors for COMT, raising the possibility that they might form a direct biochemical link between the metabolism of estrogens and catecholamine neurotransmitter systems. Later reports demonstrated that 2-hydroxyestrogens can bind to hypothalamic and pituitary estrogen receptors (Davies et al., 1975); they also can influence gonadotrophin release (Naftolin *et al.*, 1975a). Since then, considerable progress has been made toward elucidating the biosynthesis, metabolism, and actions of CEs in humans as well as in experimental animals. The purpose of this chapter is to review the current status of our understanding of the biologic importance of CEs. First, the pathways involved in CE formation and metabolism will be discussed, together with information on the concentrations of CEs in tissues and biologic fluids in health and disease. Subsequently, the pharmacologic effects of CEs will be reviewed within the context of their mechanism of action. Finally, we will assess the evidence for a specific role for CE biosynthesis in the mechanism of estrogen action.

## A. Estrogen Formation, Mechanism of Action, and Metabolism: An Overview

Androgens are converted to estrogens by an enzyme complex that is commonly referred to as aromatase. In women, the major site of estrogen synthesis is the ovary, while peripheral aromatization accounts for an additional 30% of overall estrogen production. During pregnancy, these sources are augmented by the placenta. In addition, in some tissues there may be low levels of estrogen biosynthesis which, although contributing little to overall estrogen production, may exert powerful local estrogenic effects. Examples of this are provided by the brain (Naftolin *et al.*, 1975b; MacLusky and Naftolin, 1981) and the levator ani muscle (Bardin and Catterall, 1981), both of which are responsive to estrogens synthesized locally from circulating androgens.

The accepted model for the mechanism of estrogen action involves an initial binding reaction between the steroid and the cytoplasmic receptor sites, which is followed by translocation of the estrogen–receptor complexes to the cell nucleus. Within the nucleus, the receptor complexes bind to the chromatin, initiating changes in RNA and protein synthesis that are ultimately responsible for the overall estrogenic response (Jensen and DeSombre, 1973; Gorski and Gannon, 1977).

There are three main pathways of estrogen metabolism. In many tissues $E_2$ is converted to $E_1$ through a reversible reaction catalyzed by estradiol-17$\beta$ dehydrogenase. $E_1$ itself can be hydroxylated either on the D ring at position 16, resulting in the formation of 16$\alpha$ or 16$\beta$ $E_1$ which can then be reduced to give $E_3$ and epiestrol, or alternatively on the A ring to give the CEs. The extent and direction of estrogen metabolism along each of these pathways has a considerable impact on the biologic activity of the hormone. Thus, in the endometrium estradiol-17$\beta$ dehydrogenase activity

Fɪɢ. 1. Pathways of estrogen synthesis and metabolism. I (androgens), II (estrogens), III (2- and 4-hydroxyestrogens = CE), IV (methoxy-CE = MeCE). (X) denotes either (= O) or (OH).

may regulate the activity of circulating $E_2$ by converting it to the less-potent estrogen, $E_1$ (Gurpide, 1978). As we shall see shortly, the biologic activities of the CEs and the 16-hydroxylated estrogens are different; hence, the partitioning of estrogen metabolism between the A ring and 16-hydroxylation pathways may be an important factor in determining the nature and extent of the response to circulating estrogens (Martucci and Fishman, 1977, 1979).

## B. Chemical Synthesis of Catechol Estrogens

Chemically, the CEs are extremely unstable compounds that readily undergo autoxidation, especially at neutral or alkaline pH. This property hampered early attempts to synthesize and purify CEs. However, with the introduction of "reducing chromatography," under the protection of ascorbic acid (Gelbke and Knuppen, 1972), and the advent of high-performance liquid chromatography techniques (Williams and Goldzeiher, 1979; Aten *et al.*, 1982; MacLusky *et al.*, 1982), the problems of chromatographically separating CEs from other estrogens have largely been resolved.

The first chemical synthesis of a CE was reported by Niederl and Vogel (1949). They reported the preparation of 2-OH-$E_1$ by nitration of $E_1$, reduction to the *o*-aminophenol followed by formation and thermal decomposition of the diazonium salt. The yield obtained by this procedure was, however, very low. Later, Loudon and Scott (1953), Fishman *et al.* (1960), Coombs (1960), Knuppen *et al.* (1961), and Rao and Axelrod (1960) all developed methods to improve the yields of 2-OH-E$_1$, but these procedures were all relatively laborious. A direct oxidation method that was faster, while still giving good 2-hydroxyestrogen yields, was reported by Yoshizawa *et al.* (1972). Methods for 4-hydroxyestrogen synthesis were reported by Gold and Schwenk (1958), Hecker and Walk (1960), and Fishman *et al.* (1960). As with the early procedures for 2-hydroxyestrogen synthesis, these methods were fairly lengthy and arduous.

Perhaps the most convenient and simple methodology for large-scale synthesis of 2- and 4-hydroxyestrogens was introduced by Stubenrauch and Knuppen (1976). This procedure entails an initial nitration reaction and subsequent separation of the resulting 2- and 4-nitro compounds. These are reduced to the corresponding aminoestrogens, oxidized to the 2,3- or 3,4-quinones and finally reduced to 2- and 4-hydroxyestrogens. Overall yields are high, of the order of 30–40% for each of the 2- and 4-hydroxylated products.

For the preparation of high specific activity labeled CEs, somewhat different procedures are required to deal with the extremely small masses of starting labeled monophenolic estrogen and catechol product. A simple method for the high yield synthesis of labeled 2-hydroxyestrogens was described by Jellinck and Brown (1971), using mushroom tyrosinase under carefully defined conditions to limit the extent of further metabolism. A convenient small-scale procedure that generates both the 2- and the 4-hydroxyestrogens was reported by Gelbke *et al.* (1973). Room temperature incubation of monophenolic estrogens with potassium nitrosodisulfonate (Fremy's Salt) in acetone-water-acetic acid solution generated the 2- and 4-hydroxyestrogens in one step, with yields of approximately 12% and 7%, respectively.

## C. Measurement of 2- and 4-Hydroxylase Activities *in Vitro*

The task of devising a method for the specific and sensitive assay of 2- and 4-hydroxylase activities in biologic materials has proven to be extremely difficult. Although several authors have developed assay techniques, controversy still rages over the question of which of these techniques, if any, most accurately reflects *in vivo* 2- and 4-hydroxylase activity. The first method for 2-hydroxylase determinations was reported by Fishman and Norton (1975). It employed as an index of enzyme activity the quantity of $^3H_2O$ formed during incubation of the tissue samples with [2-$^3$H]monophenolic estrogen.

Subsequently, the same approach was extended to 4-hydroxylation, using [4-$^3$H]E$_2$ as substrate (Jellinck, 1980; Fishman and Norton, 1983). This method has considerable advantages in terms of speed and simplicity over the other methods available. Moreover, since it measures substrate utilization rather than product formation, it obviates the problems inherent in trying to measure the labile catechol products of the A-ring hydroxylation reactions. However, these advantages are at least partially offset by the fact that $^3$H release from [2-$^3$H]E$_2$ or [4-$^3$H]E$_2$ may occur through reactions *other* than specific enzyme-catalyzed 2- or 4-hydroxylation—for example, through chemical hydroxylation (Fishman and Norton, 1983) or through the action of peroxidase (Jellinck, 1980).

The other methods for assay of estrogen hydroxylase activity all depend on isolation of the CE products. Ball *et al.* (1978a,b) studied the hydroxylation of [$^3$H]E$_2$ in tissue homogenates by chromatographically separating the entire range of CEs produced, as well as the products of further CE metabolism. Although providing valuable information regarding the various routes of estrogen metabolism, such methods are too arduous to provide a useful, routine hydroxylase assay because of the extensive nature of further CE metabolism. Thus, other authors have attempted to devise a procedure that will "trap" the CEs produced by A-ring hydroxylation in an easily measured form. The first of these methods, devised from a similar procedure for assay of catecholamines, made use of the ability of COMT to methylate CEs and thereby to convert them to relatively stable methoxy derivatives. Utilizing a tritium-labeled S-adenosyl methionine (SAM) methyl donor, the methoxy products of the reaction can be measured by simple organic solvent extraction and scintillation counting (Merriam *et al.*, 1976; Paul *et al.*, 1977a; Barbieri *et al.*, 1978; Hoffman *et al.*, 1979a). Recently, Hersey and co-workers (1981a) have reported a more direct procedure, in which the CE products of [$^3$H]E$_2$ metabolism are prevented from undergoing significant further metabolism by adding ascorbic acid and a large excess of unlabeled CEs, as well as carrying out the reaction at 30°C instead of physiologic temperatures. The radiolabeled CEs are then separated from [$^3$H]E$_2$ by chromatography on neutral alumina.

There is currently no consensus as to which of these assay methods provides the more reliable estimates of A-ring estrogen hydroxylase activity. Each method appears to have advantages as well as drawbacks. The COMT-coupled method has been widely used in a variety of tissues (Paul *et al.*, 1977a; Barbieri *et al.* 1978; Hoffman *et al.*, 1979a). It remains uncertain, however, whether this method is truly stoichiometric in trapping *all* of the CEs produced in the system as methoxyestrogens. The tritium release method obviates this problem by measuring substrate utilization rather than product formation; but, as the recent studies of Hersey *et al.* (1981b) and Fishman and Norton (1983) indicate, there is a component of the tritium release reactions from both $[2\text{-}^3\text{H}]\text{E}_2$ and $[4\text{-}^3\text{H}]\text{E}_2$ that represents non-enzymic, nonspecific processes. Overshadowing all of the methods developed to date is the problem of clearly distinguishing between enzymic and nonenzymic CE formation. The C-2 and C-4 positions in the steroidal estrogens are susceptible to electrophilic attack from such species as singlet oxygen, superoxide radical, hydroxyl radical, and peroxides. These can be generated under *in vitro* incubation conditions by photolytic activation, interaction of oxygen with $\text{Fe}^{2+}$ ion or lipid peroxidation. Thus, unfortunately, the very conditions that are optimal for the formation and isolation of CEs in tissue homogenates or subcellular fractions may provide an excellent basis for nonspecific 2- or 4-hydroxylation (for discussion, see Fishman and Norton, 1983).

These problems make it necessary to treat the available data on measurements of 2- and 4-hydroxylase activity with a degree of circumspection. However, there are sufficient points of agreement between the results obtained by different workers, with different methodologies, to allow some general conclusions to be drawn. The majority of studies indicate that 2-hydroxylase is probably a microsomal enzyme (Ball and Knuppen, 1980; Fishman and Norton, 1983); the sole exception to this generalization is the recent report of Hersey *et al.* (1981a,b) that the majority of 2-hydroxylase activity in frozen rabbit hypothalami is found in the cytosol fraction. Studies on the properties of the liver 2- and 4-hydroxylase enzymes suggest that they both require NADPH and oxygen for activity and in all probability are cytochrome *P*-450 dependent (Hecker and Marks, 1965; Paul *et al.*, 1977; Ball and Knuppen, 1980). The brain microsomal 2-hydroxylase appears to be similar but not identical to the liver enzyme. Its $K_m$ for hydroxylation of $\text{E}_2$ is higher than that for the liver (93 $\mu M$ versus 11 $\mu M$, Hoffman *et al.*, 1979a); and recent work by Fishman and Norton (1983) indicates that the brain enzyme, unlike the liver, may have a preference for NADH rather than NADPH as cofactor.

The distribution of 2- and 4-hydroxylase activity within the body has been extensively studied. There is general agreement that the most active organs with respect to CE biosynthesis are the liver and the brain. How active the brain is in relation to the liver, however, remains a subject of some controversy. The first demonstration of 2-hydroxylase in the rat brain, by Fishman and Norton (1975) using the tritium release method, suggest that per unit weight of tissue 2-hydroxylase activity in the hypothalamus *exceeded* that in the liver by about 3:1. Subsequent studies using product isolation and COMP-coupled methodologies have generally given much lower estimates of brain 2-hydroxylase activity, ranging from about 40- to 100-fold lower than those in the liver (Paul *et al.*, 1977a; Ball *et al.*, 1978b; Barbieri *et al.*, 1978; Hoffman *et al.*, 1979a).

Within the central nervous system, the highest 2-hydroxylase activities appear to be present in the diencephalon. Thus, in the rat brain the hypothalamus has the highest content of 2-hydroxylase, with lower activities in other brain structures (Fishman and Norton, 1975; Paul et al., 1977; Barbieri et al., 1978). In the human fetus, 2-hydroxylase activity is distributed rather more evenly, extending through the hypothalamus, limbic brain, parietal cortex, and pituitary (Fishman et al., 1976; Ball et al., 1978b).

A variety of other tissues have also been shown to have at least some capacity for 2-hydroxylation, including kidney, testis, ovary, adrenal, lung, heart muscle, and placenta (Barbieri et al., 1978; Hoffman et al., 1979a; Smith and Axelrod, 1969; Milewich and Axelrod, 1971; Barnea and Naftolin, 1983). An interesting recent development is the report of Hoffman et al. (1979b) that some human breast cancer specimens contain increased 2-hydroxylase activities as well as elevated COMT levels, suggesting that one of the consequences of the neoplastic transformation in these tissues may be a change in the pattern of estrogen metabolism. These observations echo the earlier reports from Acevedo and his co-workers of 2-hydroxylation in hypertrophic and carcinomatous human prostate (Acevedo and Goldzieher, 1965) and in pheochromocytoma tissue (Acevedo and Beering, 1965).

There is some indication that 2-hydroxylase activity is under gonadal steroid control. Male rat liver contains a higher 2-hydroxylase activity than is the case in females (Barbieri et al., 1978). This sex difference is a function of testosterone in the male, with castration reducing and testosterone replacement restoring rates of hepatic 2-hydroxylation (Hoffman et al., 1979a). During the estrous cycle, Fishman et al. (1980b) have reported cyclic changes in hypothalamic 2-hydroxylase, with highest activities being present between proestrus and estrus, falling to a nadir at metestrus.

Drug treatments can also have marked effects on CE formation. Liver 2-hydroxylase activity is increased by spermidine and 3,4-benz(a)pyrene but unaffected by phenobarbital (Jellinck and Perry, 1967; Conney, 1967). Recent studies by Fishman and his collaborators (1980b) using the tritium-release assay have shown that 2-hydroxylase activity in the male rat brain is decreased by morphine treatment and increased after administration of the narcotic antagonist, naloxone. These interesting results raise the possibility that endogenous opioid peptides may modulate brain 2-hydroxylase activity.

### D. Metabolism of Catechol Estrogens

CEs are rapidly and extensively metabolized. Quantitatively, the predominant route of metabolism is via COMT-catalyzed methylation. This reaction exhibits a degree of specificity with respect to which of the catechol hydroxyls are methylated. Thus, in absolute terms the excretion of 2-methoxyestrogens exceeds that of the 3-methyl 2-hydroxyestrogens by at least 2:1

(Knuppen *et al.*, 1970; Femino *et al.*, 1974). In the case of the 4-hydroxyestrogens, methylation occurs almost exclusively on the 4 position (Ball *et al.*, 1971).

COMT is widely distributed throughout the body (Axelrod and Tomchick, 1958). Expressed per milligram of protein, highest COMT activity is found in the liver, closely followed by the placenta (Gugler *et al.*, 1970; Barnea *et al.*, 1983). However, red blood cells are a very important additional source of COMT activity and are probably responsible for a considerable fraction of total CE methylation (Bates *et al.*, 1977; Merriam *et al.*, 1980a). CEs represent the best known natural substrates for COMT, with $K_m$s for interaction, with this approximately at least 10- to 40-fold lower than those for the catecholamines themselves (Ball *et al.*, 1972b; Merriam, *et al.*, 1980c; Barnea *et al.*, 1983). This has important consequences not only for the metabolism of CEs but also for the relationship between estrogens and the catecholamine system. The high affinity of CEs for COMT makes them excellent competitive inhibitors of catecholamine methylation; indeed, there is evidence to suggest that elevated CE concentrations may significantly prolong the half-life of catecholamines in the circulation (Ball and Knuppen, 1980) (see Section III,E).

The CEs and methoxyestrogens both readily form water-soluble conjugates. In common with the monophenolic estrogens, they can be conjugated to sulfates or glucuronides. The CEs themselves appear to be preferentially conjugated to glucuronide, while in the case of the methoxyestrogens the sulfates predominate over glucoronides by about 5:1 (Ball, 1976; Ball *et al.*, 1977). Unlike the monophenolic estrogens, CEs and methoxyestrogens can also form thioether conjugates with glutathione (Kuss, 1967; Jellinck and Elce, 1969) while the CEs alone can form covalent thioether linkages with proteins (Hoppen *et al.*, 1974). The quantitative importance of thioether formation in the metabolism of CEs remains somewhat uncertain: although 2-hydroxyestrogen-glutathione conjugates have been demonstrated in the rat, *in vitro* as well as *in vivo*, a similar metabolic pathway has not so far been identified in man (Ball and Knuppen, 1980). Nevertheless, the capacity of CEs to form thioethers with proteins is of considerable theoretical importance as a possible mechanism for estrogen-induced cellular damage (Kappus *et al.*, 1973; Bolt and Kappus, 1974; Tsibris, 1979).

### E. Infusion Studies in Man: Formation and Clearance of Catechol Estrogens *In Vivo*

Continuing on from the pioneering reports of Krachy and Gallagher (1957), Engel *et al.* (1957), and Fishman *et al.* (1960), there have been numerous studies of the biosynthesis and clearance of CEs in man. These studies emphasize the importance of CEs as major, and in some circumstances even the predominant, metabolites of estrogens. In addition, they show that CEs are extremely rapidly metabolized and cleared from the circulation.

The general pattern of $E_2$ metabolism in man is well illustrated by the results of an elegant series of studies performed in Fishman's laboratory (Fishman et al., 1966, 1969, 1970). Following the oral administration of radiolabeled $E_2$, a proportion (40%) undergoes rapid conjugation and is not subsequently metabolized at either the 2- or 16-position. Of the circulating, nonconjugated $E_2$, the great majority undergoes oxidation to $E_1$. The $E_1$ thus formed serves as a substrate for extensive further metabolism. Approximately two-thirds of the circulating estrogens are excreted in the urine. Close to 30% of the urinary metabolites represent 2-substituted compounds, while about 15% represent 16-hydroxylated or 16-keto estrogens (predominantly $E_3$). The fate of the remaining 30–40% of circulating $E_2$ that is not excreted in the urine remains a mystery. Only around 5% of the total estrogen metabolites pass into the feces, since the majority of estrogens excreted in bile are reabsorbed through the enterohepatic circulation. It seems likely from $[16\alpha\text{-}^3H]E_2$ tracer studies that essentially all of the "missing" metabolites are substituted at the 16-position. They probably do not represent A-ring cleaved- or protein-conjugated metabolites formed as a result of 2-hydroxylation, since only about 30% of the "missing" fraction can be accounted for by metabolism at C-2 (Fishman et al., 1970).

Although CEs are rapidly methylated in the bloodstream, the methoxyestrogens are not necessarily just metabolic end products. Demethylation of methoxyestrogens was first demonstrated by Yoshizawa and Fishman (1970). These authors administered the $[2\text{-},3\text{-}^{14}CH_3]$monomethyl ethers and the $[2,3\text{-}^{14}CH_3]$dimethyl ether of 2-OH-$[6,7\text{-}^3H]E_2$ to two men and one woman. Their results indicated that some demethylation of the dimethyl ether occurred, yielding urinary 2-hydroxyestrogens. Surprisingly, however, no demethylation of the monomethyl ethers was observed. In contrast, Ball and his co-workers observed substantial (about 30%) demethylation of 2-MeO-$E_1$ after oral administration to men (Ball et al., 1977; Ball and Knuppen, 1980). These results indicate that demethylation of methoxyestrogens may occur to some extent in vivo. The physiologic significance of this reaction remains uncertain, but it may provide a route for pharmacologically increasing circulating CE levels (Ball and Knuppen, 1980).

As indicated earlier, the metabolic clearance rates (MCRs) of CEs are extremely rapid. Table I summarizes the MCR values for $E_2$ and a variety of CEs and methoxyestrogens, calculated from the results of $[^3H]$estrogen infusions in man. Estimates of MCR for the 2-hydroxyestrogens range from 13,000–90,000 1/day, more than 10-fold higher than for $E_2$ itself. The 4-hydroxyestrogens are cleared at slightly lower rates (about 16,000–19,000

TABLE I

Metabolic Indices of Primary Estrogens, CE and MeCE, Assembled from Various Publications[a]

| Compound | MCR 1/day | $K_m$ rat liver COMT $(\mu M)$[b] | $K_m$ human liver COMT $(\mu M)$[c] | Relative binding affinity for TEBG ([³H]testosterone-1)[d] |
|---|---|---|---|---|
| $E_2$ | 1350 (Tagatz and Gurpide, 1973) | N.D. | N.D. | 0.32 ± 0.09 |
| 4-OH-$E_2$ | 16,500 ± 1,500 (Pfeiffer *et al.*, 1982a) | 13.6 ± 5.6 | — | — |
| 2-OH-$E_2$ | 13,000 (Kono *et al.*, 1980) | 8.6 ± 2.7 | 15 | 0.070 ± 0.006 |
| 2-MeOH-$E_2$ | — | N.D. | N.D. | 2 ± 0.4 |
| $E_2$ | 2,500 (Tagatz and Gurpide, 1973) | N.D. | N.D. | — |
| 4-OH-$E_1$ | 19,000 ± 10,000 (Pfeiffer *et al.*, 1982a) | 10.1 ± 2.9 | 20 | — |
| 2-OH-$E_1$ | 51,000 ± 6,000 (Merriam *et al.*, 1980a) | 12 ± 3.4 | 20 | — |
| | 89,600 ± 15,700 (Longcope *et al.*, 1982) | | | |
| 2-MeOH-$E_1$ | [2,040 ± 240] (Longcope *et al.*, 1982) | N.D. | N.D. | — |
| $E_3$ | — | N.D. | — | — |
| 2-OH-$E_3$ | — | 11.2 ± 51 | 25 | — |

[a]The value for 2-MeO-$E_1$ represents an estimate derived from studies of the fate of injected 2-OH-$E_1$ and is therefore given in brackets. N.D. = no detectable competition for COMT-catalyzed methylation.

[b]Rat liver $K_m$ values from Merriam *et al.* (1980a).

[c]Human liver $K_m$ values from Ball *et al.* (1972a).

[d]Relative binding affinities for TEBG are from Dunn *et al.* (1980).

1/day) than the 2-hydroxyestrogens. These rapid clearance rates probably reflect methylation of the CEs by COMT, as well as rapid conjugation of the CEs and their methoxy metabolites (Merriam *et al.*, 1980a; Longcope *et al.*, 1982). The difference between the MCR values of the 2- and 4-hydroxyestrogens is consistent with the notion that COMT methylation plays an important role in the metabolism of these steroids, since there is an approximately 2-fold difference between the 2- and 4-hydroxy compounds in their $K_m$ for interaction with COMT.

Very little work has been done so far on the MCRs of CEs in experimental animals. The available information suggests that the situation in rats is probably similar to that in man. Thus, Kono *et al.* (1981) found that the plasma MCR of 2-OH-$E_1$ in male rats was approximately 50,000 ml/hour, more than 100 times that of $E_2$ in the rat (Tapper *et al.*, 1972).

## F. Catechol Estrogen Concentrations in Body Fluids

### 1. Blood

Measurements of circulating CEs are consistent with the hypothesis that these unconjugated CEs do not accumulate in the bloodstream. The first assay for measuring CEs in biological fluids, a radioimmunoassay, was developed by Yoshizawa and Fishman (1971). The antibody used was directed against 2-OH-$E_1$ and had only marginal cross-reactivity with the majority of other estrogens, except for 2-OH-$E_2$ (18% cross-reactivity compared to 2-OH-$E_1$). With this radioimmunoassay and unchromatographed extracts of human plasma, estimates of unconjugated circulating 2-OH-$E_1$ concentrations ranging from 28–39 pg/ml in young men and 108–295 pg/ml in young women to 1.2–3.6 ng/ml in late pregnancy were obtained (Yoshizawa and Fishman, 1971). Subsequently, other authors also developed radioimmunoassay procedures for the 2-hydroxyestrogens (Ball *et al.*, 1978a; Cecchini *et al.*, 1980). These procedures gave results that were qualitatively similar to those of Yoshizawa and Fishman (1971), but somewhat lower in absolute magnitude (Ball *et al.* 1978a: men, 45–65 pg/ml; cycling women 50–95 pg/ml; late pregnancy, 105–220 pg/ml). Finally, Kono *et al.* (1980) Merriam, and their collaborators refined the procedure of Ball *et al.* (1978a) by introducing a Sephadex LH-20 chromatography step to separate 2-OH-$E_1$ and 2-OH-$E_2$ prior to assay. With this methodology, the levels of 2-hydroxyestrogens measured in nonpregnant human plasma were reduced still further, although the results for pregnancy samples were in excellent agreement with those of Ball *et al.* (1978a) and Cecchini *et al.* (1980) (<15 pg/ml in young men and normally cycling women; pregnancy, 1st trimester, 10–34 pg/ml; 2nd trimester, 43–65 pg/ml; 3rd trimester, 67–284 pg/ml; Kono *et al.*, 1980; Merriam *et al.*, 1980a).

It is not possible at present to determine which of these disparate estimates of circulating 2-OH-$E_1$ concentrations are correct. However, a reasonable interpretation of the data is that unchromatographed plasma extracts may contain substances other than 2-OH-$E_1$ that cross-react to a limited extent with the 2-OH-$E_1$ antibody. If this interpretation is valid, then the lower estimates obtained by Kono, Merriam, and their collaborators (1980) would seem most likely to be correct.

Estimates of total organic solvent extractable CEs and methoxyestrogens in plasma do not necessarily provide an accurate picture of the availability of the steroids to the tissues for two reasons. First, as with the monophenolic estrogens, it is necessary also to consider the contribution from blood steroid-binding proteins. In man, the majority of the circulating testosterone and estradiol is bound to testosterone and estradiol-binding globulin (TEBG). The recent work of Dunn *et al.* (1980) has shown that 2-OH-$E_2$ and 2-MeO-$E_2$ do bind to TEBG: indeed, the affinity of 2-MeO-$E_2$ for this protein is extraordinarily high, exceeding that for either $E_2$ or testosterone (Table I; Fig. 2). Second, as one might predict from a knowledge of CE metabolism, the great majority of circulating CEs appear to be present in conjugated form. Thus, Ball and his co-workers found that in plasma samples from normal cycling women, radioimmunoassay measurements of 2-OH-$E_1$ after hydrolysis of steroid conjugates exceeded those obtained on fresh plasma extracts by at least 20:1 (Ball *et al.*, 1978b; Ball and Knuppen, 1980).

## 2. Other Body Fluids

The excretion of CEs and methoxyestrogens in urine has been studied extensively over the last 20 years. Endogenous 2-MeO-$E_1$ was first identified by Loke and Marrian (1958) in extracts of enzymatically hydrolyzed late pregnancy urine. These findings were later confirmed by Frandsen (1959), who also identified 2-MeO-$E_2$ in pregnancy urine. Quantification of nonmethylated CEs in human urine did not occur until more than a decade later, when chromatographic methods suitable for separation of the labile catechols became available. With the advent of this newer methodology, however, Gelbke and his collaborators were able to show that the concentration of 2-OH-$E_1$ in late pregnancy urine are within the same range as those of 2-MeO-$E_1$ (Gelbke and Knuppen, 1973; Gelbke *et al.*, 1973b).

Quantitatively, 2-OH-$E_1$ and its 2-methylated derivative represent the major 2-substituted estrogens in human pregnancy urine. They are not, however, the only urinary products of CE metabolism: studies in a number of laboratories have demonstrated the existence in urine of the entire range of 2-hydroxyestrogens and 2-methoxyestrogens (2-OH-$E_1$, 2-OH-$E_2$, 2-OH-$E_3$; 2-MeO-$E_1$, 2-MeO-$E_2$, 2-MeO-$E_3$) (Gelbke *et al.*, 1975; Gelbke and Knuppen, 1973; Cohen *et al.*, 1978).

The urinary excretion rates for 2-MeO-$E_1$ and 2-OH-$E_1$ in the menstrual cycle are at least one order of magnitude lower than those found during pregnancy (see Table II). The increase in excretion of both steroids in pregnancy commences within the first trimester (nonpregnant, periovulatory women: 2-OH-$E_1$, 41 µg/day; 2-MeO-$E_1$, 23 µg/day. Pregnant, first trimester 2-OH-$E_1$, 370 µg/day; 2-MeO-$E_1$, 141 µg/day) and continues to a maximum during the third trimester (*Emons et al.*, 1979; Ball *et al.*, 1979).

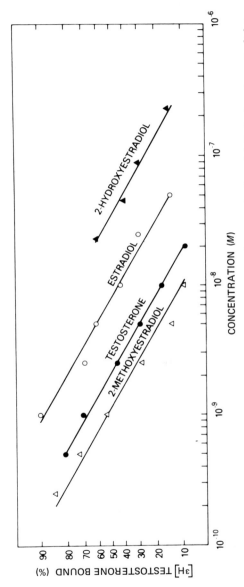

FIG. 2. Displacement of [3H]testosterone from human testosterone and estrogen-binding globulin by 2-methoxyestradiol, testosterone, estradiol, and 2-hydroxyestradiol. [From Dunn *et al.* (1981).]

TABLE II
URINARY EXCRETION OF 2-OH-E$_1$ AND 2-MeO-E$_1$ IN WOMEN ($\mu$g/24 hour)[a]

| Pregnancy | | Menstrual cycle | | |
|---|---|---|---|---|
| 2-OH-E$_1$ | 2-MeO-E$_1$ | 2-OH-E$_1$ | 2-MeO-E$_1$ | References |
| | 110 | | 1.9–2.9 | Adlercreutz *et al.*, 1968, 1974 |
| | | 10–60 | | Ball *et al.*, 1975 |
| 190–2000 | 60–1150 | 21 ± 12 | 15.4 ± 6.9 | Ball *et al.*, 1979 |
| 110–2100 | | 14.5–50 | | Chattoraj *et al.*, 1978 |
| 100–300 | 200–1000 | | | Cohen *et al.*, 1978 |
| 110–2100 | | | | Gelbke *et al.*, 1975 |
| | 100–350 | | | Gelbke and Knuppen, 1976 |
| | 25–1000 | | | Hobkirk and Nilsen, 1963 |
| | 200–300 | | | Scheike *et al.*, 1973 |
| | 50–240 | | | Wotiz and Chattoraj, 1964 |

[a]Adapted from Ball and Knuppen (1980).

The other biologic fluids in which 2-hydroxyestrogens and 2-methoxy-estrogens have been detected are bile and amniotic fluid. During pregnancy, Adlercreutz *et al.* (1973) found a steady increase in the biliary excretion of 2-MeO-E$_1$ between the 10th and 32nd weeks of gestation. The same group also detected free and conjugated 2-MeO-E$_1$ in amniotic fluid and reported the presence of 1.2 ± 0.8 ng/ml of 2-MeO-E$_1$ in pools of umbilical cord plasma.

## G. CATECHOL ESTROGEN CONCENTRATIONS IN TISSUES

Studies on CE levels in tissues have yielded contradictory results. Early measurements by Merriam *et al.*, (1976) and Paul and Axelrod (1977) obtained using a radioenzymatic (COMT-based) method suggested that the concentrations of free 2-hydroxyestrogens in brain and liver were extremely high (4–30 ng/g tissue). Later workers have been unable to confirm these observations. Ball and Knuppen (1980) used the same radioenzymatic procedure but incorporated extensive purification steps to separate authentic 2-OH-E$_1$ from other catechols present in the tissues. Under these conditions, estimates of brain 2-OH-E$_1$ content were far lower than those of Merriam *et al.* (1976) and Paul *et al.* (1977), of the order of 0.4–0.8 ng/g. Using radioimmunoassay, Fishman and Martucci (1979) obtained even lower estimated (<6 pg/g tissue) of free 2-OH-E$_1$ in rat brain. As with measurements of circulating 2-hydroxyestrogen concentrations, it seems reasonable to suppose that the disparities in values for tissue CE levels are a function of interference in the assays from other tissue components and hence that the lower estimates are more likely to be correct.

## II. PATHOPHYSIOLOGY OF CATECHOL ESTROGEN METABOLISM

In addition to the changes of CE production associated with different reproductive states, there are a variety of pathophysiologic conditions that are known to result in alterations in CE biosynthesis and metabolism.

### A. THYROID DYSFUNCTION

It has long been known that thyroid hormones influence estrogen metabolism. Fishman *et al.* (1963) demonstrated that hyperthyroid patients or normal subjects administered thyroxine have low urinary excretion of $E_3$ and high excretions of 2-MeO-$E_1$ or 2-OH-$E_1$. In contrast, hypothyroid patients were found to have decreased $E_2$ hydroxylation and increased 16α-hydroxylation. The authors concluded that C-2 and 16α-hydroxylation, but not 2-OH-$E_1$ methylation, are influenced by thyroid hormone.

In hamster liver, Keith (1977) found that thyroid hormone was able to stimulate formation of 2-OH-$E_2$ from $E_2$. Hoffman *et al.* (1979), however, were unable to confirm an effect of thyroid hormone on 2-hydroxylase activity in rat liver microsomes. These authors reported that hypo- and hyperthyroidism in rats *both* reduced liver 2-hydroxylase activity. The reason for these disparities remains uncertain, but they may at least in part reflect species differences in the effects of thyroid status.

### B. LIVER DISEASE

Alterations in the rates of estrogen A-ring or D-ring hydroxylation have been associated with liver disease. Zumoff *et al.* (1968) reported that patients with cirrhosis of the liver exhibit a fivefold decrease in the rate of 2-hydroxylation accompanied by a substantial increase in 16α-OH-$E_1$ and $E_3$ production, compared to normal subjects. This was ascribed to cholestasis and damage to the liver microsomal fraction containing the 2-hydroxylase enzyme (Hellman *et al.*, 1970; Zumoff *et al.*, 1970). More recently, Kreek *et al.* (1982) studied A-ring and D-ring hydroxylation rates in patients with a variety of other liver disorders. In patients with lupoid hepatitis and alcoholic cirrhosis, 2-hydroxylation was markedly decreased. As expected, this change was accompanied by an increase in $16\alpha$-hydroxylation. In contrast, patients with chronic active hepatitis without fibrosis showed no change in estrogen metabolism.

The consequences of the marked shift in estrogen metabolism from 2-hydroxylation to 16-hydroxylation can be quite dramatic. As indicated by Fishman and Martucci, $16\alpha$-OH-$E_1$ is a potent estrogen with a low-binding affinity for testosterone-estradiol-binding globulin. Thus, increased $16\alpha$-hydroxylation and decreased 2-hydroxylation of $E_1$ can lead to a generalized hyperestrogenization (Fishman and Martucci, 1980).

## C. Effects of Body Composition

Fluctuations in body weight, and in particular in body fat, have a profound effect on estrogen metabolism. Thus, in obese subjects, there is an increase in the production of 16-hydroxylated estrogens and a decrease in 2-hydroxylation. In contrast, patients with anorexia nervosa have relatively high rates of 2-hydroxylation (Fishman *et al.*, 1975).

## D. Catechol Estrogens and Breast Cancer

There is now a considerable body of evidence to suggest that breast cancer may be accompanied by changes in estrogen metabolism. Although some early studies suggested that overall estrogen metabolism was similar in normal subjects and patients with breast cancer (Crowley *et al.*, 1965; Scheike *et al.*, 1973), other workers have found a definite trend toward increased D-ring hydroxylation. Zumoff *et al.* (1966) reported that in men with breast cancer there was a diminution of $E_1$, 2-OH-$E_1$, and 2-MeO-$E_1$ formation and a marked increase in $E_3$ production compared to healthy controls. Similarly, Hellman *et al.* (1971) found a slight decrease in 2-OH-$E_1$ and significant increase in $E_3$ excretion in a group of postmenopausal women with breast cancer. A decrease in the rate of $16\alpha$-hydroxylation and concomitant increase in 2-OH-$E_1$ formation in women with breast cancer was reported by Fishman and Hellman (1976) after calusterone ($7\beta,17\alpha$-dimethyl testosterone) administration.

## E. Abnormal Pregnancy

Very little is known of the concentrations of CEs in body fluids in abnormal pregnancies. Although it is well established that the urinary concentrations of other estrogen metabolites such as $E_3$ and estetrol may change in some pathophysiologic conditions of pregnancy, there have been very few studies of the effects of these conditions on CE metabolism. Adlercreutz and his co-workers (Adlercreutz and Luukainen, 1970; Adlercreutz *et al.*, 1974) found that urinary 2-MeO-$E_1$ excretion was elevated in twin pregnancy (300 μg/24 hours versus 110 μg/24 hours in normal pregnancy) but reduced in pregnancy with anencephalic fetus 50 μg/24 hours). Recurrent jaundice in pregnancy slightly increased the excretion of 2-MeO-$E_1$ to 200 μg/24 hours.

These observations are difficult to interpret in the absence of parallel 2-hydroxyestrogen measurements, since it remains unclear whether the changes in 2-MeO-$E_1$ excretion reflect altered 2-hydroxylation or a shift in the ratio of methoxyestrogens to free CEs in the urine. Whatever the mechanism of the pathologic changes, however, the possibility must still be considered of altered CE metabolism leading to adverse biologic effects. In this context, it is of interest that recent studies in our laboratory (Barnea *et al.* 1983) have demonstrated significantly lower term placental COMT activities in severely hypertensive women than in normal mothers.

## III. PHARMACOLOGIC EFFECTS OF CATECHOL ESTROGEN ADMINISTRATION

### A. Effects on the Female Reproductive Tract

The estrogenic potencies of 2-OH-$E_1$ and 3-methyl 2-OH-$E_1$ were first tested by Niederl and Vogel (1949). Both compounds were found to have no significant estrogenic effects in rat. Similar results were obtained by Gordon *et al.* (1964). In 1978, however, Wotiz *et al.* reported that high doses of 2-OH-$E_1$ administered frequently (50 μg every 3 hours for 21 hours) could elicit a uterotrophic response. Martucci and Fishman (1977, 1979) examined the uterotrophic potencies of a number of rigorously purified CEs, administered either as subcutaneous paraffin pellets or as subcutaneous infusions from Alzet osmotic pumps. The results of these experiments revealed a striking difference between the 2- and 4-hydroxyestrogens: although 4-OH-$E_1$, 4-MeO-$E_1$, and 4-MeO-$E_2$ all induced marked uterine growth, the 2-hydroxyestrogens under the same conditions were relatively weak uterotrophic agents. Thus, 2-OH-$E_2$ induced a uterine response only at high doses, while 2-OH-$E_1$, 2-MeO-$E_1$, and 2-MeO-$E_2$ all were completely inactive. Moreover, there was no evidence of antagonistic effects of the 2-hydroxysteroids: simultaneous administration of 2-OH-$E_1$ and produced the same results as alone (Martucci and Fishman, 1977). The essential features of

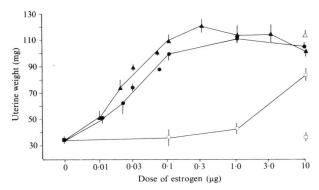

Fig. 3. Uterine weight (means±SEM) response to estradiol (▲), 4-hydroxyestradiol (●), and 2-hydroxyestradiol (○) given for 3 days to 23 day-old Sprague-Dawley rats (4–6 per group). The effects of 10 μg estrone (△) and 2-hydroxyestrone (□) are also shown. [From Franks et al. (1982a).]

these observations have since been confirmed by a number of authors, in both immature and ovariectomized adult female rats (Kanojia, 1977; Jellinck and Newcombe, 1980; Ball and Knuppen, 1980; Kono et al., 1981; Franks et al., 1982a).

In addition to the above-mentioned studies with uterine weight as an end point, there have been a number of studies of the effects of CEs on specific uterine biochemical "markers" of estrogen action. Interestingly, the results of these studies have not always followed the same pattern as overall uterotrophic responses. For example, as early as 1955, Mueller showed that 2-OH-$E_2$ was more effective than monophenolic estrogens ($E_1$, $E_2$, and $E_3$) in stimulating the uptake of formate ion by rat uterine strips. More recently, Kelly and Abel (1980, 1981) have demonstrated that CEs stimulate prostaglandin production from rat and human uterus, with potencies equal to or greater than those of $E_2$. Likewise, Tsibris et al. have reported that 2- and 4-hydroxyestrogens are more potent inhibitors of human cervical guaiacol peroxidase activity than either $E_1$ or $E_2$ (Tsibris et al., 1982).

At least part of the variability in response of the uterus to CEs can be ascribed to metabolic factors. As we have already seen, CEs are metabolized very rapidly in vivo and thus must be administered at high doses in order to simply reach the tissues in biologically effective concentrations. These metabolic factors are of considerably less importance under in vitro conditions or in vivo when the steroids are delivered directly to their site of action. The impact of metabolism on the actions of CEs is perhaps best illustrated by the results of recent studies by Franks et al. (1982a) and Hersey et al. (1982a) on the synthesis of the so-called "Induced Protein" in the immature rat uterus.

Synthesis of this protein is under estrogenic control and in general correlates well with the extent of uterine cell nuclear receptor translocation (Hersey *et al.*, 1982a). In the intact animal, there are large differences between the doses of $E_2$, 4-OH-$E_2$, 2-OH-$E_2$, and 2-OH-$E_1$ required to induce similar levels of cell nuclear-receptor binding (Jellinck and Newcombe, 1980; Mac-Lusky *et al.*, 1981; Kirchhoff *et al.*, 1981). Under *in vitro* incubation conditions, however, all four of these steroids are capable of stimulating induced protein synthesis (Franks *et al.*, 1982a; Hersey *et al.*, 1982a), and only relatively small differences are observed between the steroids with respect to their abilities to induce nuclear estrogen receptor translocation (Hersey *et al.*, 1982a).

## B. Effects of Catechol Estrogens on Brain and Pituitary Function

### 1. Gonadotrophin Release

The effects of CEs on the regulation of gonadotrophic secretion are many and varied. In common with the monophenolic estrogens, CEs can produce both positive and negative feedback effects on pituitary gonadotrophin release. In addition, however, they also appear to be capable of eliciting some responses that are qualitatively different from those produced by monophenolic estrogens under the same experimental conditions.

The first report of a CE effect on gonadotrophin secretion, by Naftolin *et al.* (1975a), indicated that the subcutaneous administration of 2-OH-$E_1$ to prepubertal male rats results in a severalfold increase in circulating LH concentrations. This was exactly the opposite of the negative feedback response that would be expected in this animal model in response to $E_1$ or $E_2$ injections and raised, for the first time, the possibility that 2-hydroxyestrogens might act as endogenous estrogen antagonists (Naftolin *et al.*, 1975a). 2-Hydroxyestrogen-induced increases in LH were also reported by Morishita *et al.* (1976), using 2-OH-$E_2$ in prepubertal male rats, by Gethmann and Knuppen (1976) in ovariectomized estradiol-primed female rats and by Martucci and Fishman (1979) in ovariectomized females administered 2-OH-$E_1$ by continuous infusion. In contrast, Rodriguez-Sierra and Blake (1980, 1982a) were unable to demonstrate any effect of 2-OH-$E_1$ on LH release after administration of 2-OH-$E_1$ or 2-OH-$E_2$ to prepubertal male or female rats. This apparent disparity probably reflects the complexity of the effects of the 2-hydroxyestrogens on gonadotrophin release, rather than any real discrepancy in the results. The facilitatory effects of 2-OH-$E_1$ on LH levels in prepubertal rats are acutely sensitive to both the time at which blood samples are withdrawn and the dose of steroid used. Thus, at doses of 50–100 μg/per rat, a facilitatory effect may be observed, while even slightly higher doses may elicit the opposite response of inhibition of LH release. In addition, there is a possibility that some of the above-mentioned studies may have been affected by impurities in the early commercial supplies of 2-hydroxyestrogens (for discussion, see MacLusky *et al.*, 1981).

In man, a similar pattern of mixed inhibition and facilitation of gonado-trophin release by 2-hydroxyestrogens has been observed. Adashi *et al.* (1981) and Schinfeld *et al.* (1980a) administered 2-OH-E$_1$ to hypogonadal women; in the former study by intravenous injection, in the latter by 4-hour continuous infusion. The only significant effects (an initial LH rise, followed by suppression of LH levels) were observed with the continuous infusions when the subjects were primed with estrogens prior to the 2-OH-E$_1$ treatment. In men, Merriam *et al.* (1981) reported that very high (3–6 mg/day) intravenous doses of 2-OH-E$_1$ are required to suppress LH and FSH secretion; while 2-OH-E$_2$ was found to inhibit LH secretion at much lower dose levels (200–800 μg/day).

The effects of the 4-hydroxyestrogens on gonadotrophin release are unlike those of their 2-hydroxy isomers and in general seem to resemble those of the parent monophenolic steroids. Thus, Martucci and Fishman (1979) found that 4-OH-E$_1$ administered continuously from osmotic pumps suppressed circulating LH levels in ovariectomized rats. Confirmation of the potency of 4-hydroxyestrogens as inhibitors of LH release was obtained by Franks *et al.* (1981) and Emons *et al.* (1981a), who found that 4-OH-E$_2$ treatments decreased circulating LH concentrations in adult male and ovariectomized female rats, respectively. With respect to positive feedback effects, Franks *et al.* (1980) reported that 4-OH-E$_2$ is as potent as E$_2$ with respect to the advancement of pregnant mare's serum gonadotrophin-induced ovulation in prepubertal female rats. Similarly, Ball *et al.* (1981) found that injections of 4-OH-E$_2$ benzoate into ovariectomized female rats elicited a phasic pattern of LH release similar to that induced by E$_2$.

Whether the effects of CEs on gonadotrophin release are mediated through actions on the hypothalamus, the pituitary, or both remains uncertain. However, *in vitro* studies have clearly demonstrated the potential of 2- and 4-hydroxylated estrogens to affect pituitary cell function. Hsueh *et al.* (1979) reported that 2-OH-E$_1$ stimulates basal LH release from dispersed rat pituitary cells. More recently, Franks *et al.* (1982a), using a similar cell culture system, demonstrated facilitatory effects of 2-OH-E$_2$ and 4-OH-E$_2$ on both basal and LHRH-induced LH release.

In addition to their acute "activational" effects on gonadotrophic release, CEs have also been shown to produce lasting developmental effects on the differentiation of the mechanisms controlling gonadotrophin secretion when administered during early postnatal life. It is now well established that estrogens play a major role in sexual differentiation of the rat brain (Naftolin *et al.*, 1975a; MacLusky and Naftolin, 1981). Thus, treatment of neonatal female rats with estrogen results in defeminization of the mechanisms regulating gonadotrophin release, resulting in anovulatory sterility in adulthood. Parvizi and Naftolin (1977) found that neonatal injections of 2-OH-$E_2$, but not 2-OH-$E_1$, were capable of eliciting a similar developmental effect. These observations were subsequently confirmed and extended by Mac-Lusky *et al.* (1983) who compared the potencies of $E_2$, 4-OH-$E_2$, and 2-OH-$E_2$ with respect to induction of anovulatory sterility. 2-OH-$E_2$ was far less potent with respect to this end point than $E_2$ itself. In contrast, 4-OH-$E_2$ was found to be at least as potent as $E_2$: as little as 100 ng/day of 4-OH-$E_2$ over the first 5 days of postnatal life was sufficient to produce anovulatory sterility in all of the animals to which it was administered.

## 2. Prolactin

Monophenolic estrogens stimulate the synthesis and release of prolactin from the pituitary gland (Franks, 1980). Pharmacologic CE administration has also been shown to influence circulating prolactin levels, but as with gonadotrophin release, controversy exists over the nature and the extent of the prolactin responses to CE treatment.

In immature male rats, Barbieri *et al.* (1980) reported that 2-OH-$E_1$ and 2-OH-$E_2$ both induced a transient fall in circulating prolactin levels. Other workers have, in general, observed rather mixed effects of CEs in this species. In adult male rats, 2-OH-$E_2$ and 4-OH-$E_2$ have both been reported to increase prolactin release (Franks and Naftolin, 1980). Similarly, in prepubertal females, Rodriguez-Sierra and Blake (1982b) found that 2-OH-$E_2$ injections resulted within 48 hours in a marked prolactin surge. The same authors reinvestigated the effects of 2-OH-$E_1$ on prolactin release in immature male rats and were unable to confirm the inhibitory effects seen by Barbieri *et al.* (1980) (see discussion of this problem in Section III,B). However, in cycling adult female rats, Katayama and Fishman (1982) found that appropriately timed injections of 2-OH-$E_1$ could completely block the normal periovulatory prolactin surge. Very recently, the effects of long-term, high-dose (100 μg/d) 2-OH-$E_1$ and 2-OH-$E_2$ treatments on normal rats and rats with estrogen-induced prolactinomas were investigated by Lamberts *et al.* (1982). Both catechol estrogens inhibited prolactinoma growth, although less efficiently than $E_2$ or $E_3$. In contrast, in nontumor-bearing rats 2-OH-$E_2$ exerted effects that were dependent on the estrogen status of the animal. In male rats, 2-OH-$E_2$ stimulated prolactin synthesis and release; while in females, it had no effect by itself and completely blocked the effects of simultaneously administered $E_2$.

In man, the available data present a similarly confused picture. In estrogen-primed hypogonadal women, Adashi *et al.* (1981) reported that 2-OH-E$_2$ induced a rise in circulating prolactin concentrations. In both normal-cycling (Fishman and Tulchinsky, 1980) and estrogen-primed hypogonadal (Schinfeld *et al.*, 1980a) women, 2-OH-E$_1$ was found to have the opposite effect of decreasing prolactin release. In contrast to these observations, Merriam and his collaborators were unable to detect any significant effect of 2-OH-E$_1$ infusions in either normal men (Merriam *et al.*, 1981) or normal cycling women (Merriam *et al.*, 1982). Similarly, in a group of hyperprolactinemic women, Franks *et al.* (1982b) were unable to detect any reduction in circulating prolactin levels after infusions of 2-OH-E$_1$.

The reasons for the disparities between these reports cannot be determined at the present time. As with CE effects on gonadotrophin secretion, in some cases impurities in the steroids used may have contributed to the results. A confounding factor in all of the above-mentioned studies is the inherent variability of circulating prolactin concentrations. It is quite possible that small, transient effects of steroid administration could be completely submerged by normal changes in prolactin levels. As Merriam has pointed out (Merriam *et al.*, 1982), considerable care is necessary in the construction of experiments designed to test for CE effects on prolactin release, so as to avoid mistaking circadian or stress-induced changes in prolactin concentrations as responses to CE treatment.

### 3. Reproductive Behavior

Estrogens, such as E$_1$ and E$_2$, potentiate the expression of reproductive behaviors in female rodents (Beyer *et al.*, 1971). Several reports have appeared showing that CEs exert similar effects. Luttge and Jasper (1977) tested the effects of 2-OH-E$_2$ on lordotic behavior in ovariectomized rats. Subcutaneous injections or preoptic area implants of this steroid failed to induce a significant increase in lordosis. However, a response was observed when the subcutaneous injections and preoptic area implants were given together. The weak effects of systemic 2-OH-E$_2$ administration on female sexual behavior were confirmed, in rats and guinea pigs, by Marrone *et al.* (1977). The 4-hydroxyestrogens, in contrast, appear to be powerful estrogen agonists with respect to female sex behavior. Thus, Naish and Ball (1981), using various routes of steroid administration (subcutaneous injection, subcutaneous infusion, and intravenous injection), found that the ability of 4-OH-E$_2$ to induce lordosis in ovariectomized female rats was similar to that of E$_2$ itself. Jellinck *et al.* (1981) found that an approximately 10-fold higher dose of 4-OH-E$_2$ than E$_2$ was required to obtain the same behavioral response.

## C. Effects of Catechol Estrogens on Lipid Metabolism

There are a number of intriguing reports indicating that CEs influence lipid metabolism. Cantrall *et al.* (1964) and Gordon *et al.* (1964) found that the 2-methoxy and 2-hydroxymetabolites of $E_1$, $E_2$, and $E_3$ all were capable of reducing serum cholesterol in rats. Subsequently, Patt *et al.* (1971) reported that 2-hydroxyestrogens also decrease circulating levels of free fatty acids and increase phosphatide concentrations. Ackerman *et al.* (1981) have investigated the effects of CEs on lipolysis in the rat epididymal fat pad under *in vitro* conditions. While CEs or methoxyestrogens did not affect lipolysis by themselves, $2\text{-OH-}E_1$ and $2\text{-OH-}E_2$ both potentiated the lipolysis induced by epinephrine, possibly by competitively inhibiting COMT methylation of the catecholamine.

## D. Contragestational Effects

The studies of Wotiz *et al.* (1978) revealed a significant effect of intra-uterine implantation of Silastic capsules containing $2\text{-OH-}E_1$ on the fertilized ovum in rabbits. More recently, in a study published in abstract form, Rajan *et al.* (1982) reported that $2\text{-MeO-}E_2$ and $4\text{-MeO-}E_2$ both decreased the number of viable fetuses when given to pregnant rats on day 7 of gestation. In contrast, $E_2$ and $4\text{-OH-}E_2$ under the same conditions produced only a modest contragestational effect. These observations suggest that CEs, and particularly the methoxyestrogens, may have a contragestational effect that is not directly related to their estrogenic potencies.

## E. Circulatory Effects of Catechol Estrogens

As might be expected from their ability to interfere with catecholamine metabolism, CEs have been shown to exert significant effects on blood pressure and the regulation of local blood flow. The effects of $2\text{-OH-}E_2$ on peripheral blood pressure in the cocaine-treated pithed rat was examined by Ball *et al.* (1972). In the presence of $2\text{-OH-}E_2$, the pressor effects of norepinephrine were significantly enhanced. Using electromagnetic flow probes, Rosenfeld and Jackson (1982) explored the effects of $E_1$, $E_2$, $2\text{-OH-}E_1$, and $2\text{-OH-}E_2$ on uterine blood flow in ovariectomized ewes. All of the estrogens tested elicited a vasodilator response, their rank order of potency being $E_2 > E_1 > 2\text{-OH-}E_2 > 2\text{-OH-}E_1$. When the 2-hydroxyestrogens were given in combination with $E_2$, a sustained partial inhibition of the vasodilation response to $E_2$ was observed, once again illustrating the potential for 2-

hydroxyestrogens to exhibit estrogen antagonist activities in some experimental situations.

## IV. MECHANISM OF ACTION OF THE CATECHOL ESTROGENS

The biochemical properties of the CEs are unique amongst steroidal estrogens in that they combine the ability to interact with estrogen receptors with the potential to directly influence catecholamine systems. These properties suggest that for any response to CEs, it is necessary to consider several different possible modes of action.

The binding affinities of CEs for estrogen receptors have been studied by a number of authors, in several estrogen target tissues. Overall, the results obtained in different laboratories are in excellent agreement. The first evidence for binding of CEs to estrogen receptors was obtained by Davies *et al.* (1975), who found that 2-OH-$E_1$ and 2-OH-$E_2$ were capable of displacing [$^3$H]$E_2$ from binding sites in soluble cytoplasmic fractions from the pituitary and anterior hypothalamus of the rat. Extensive studies of the competition between CEs and rat uterine cytoplasmic estrogen receptors were reported by Martucci and Fishman (1977, 1979; see Table III). Their results demonstrate that the effects of different A-ring substituents on receptor binding are dependent on both the nature and the position of the substituent. Thus, 2-

TABLE III
RELATIVE BINDING AFFINITIES (RBAs) FOR
BINDING OF ESTRADIOL METABOLITES TO RAT
UTERINE CYTOSOL ESTROGEN RECEPTOR[a]

| Compound | RBA |
|---|---|
| Estradiol-17β | 100 |
| 4-Hydroxyestradiol | 45 |
| 2-Hydroxyestradiol | 24 |
| Estrone | 11 |
| 4-Hydroxyestrone | 11 |
| 2-Hydroxyestrone | 1.9 |
| Estriol | 10 |
| 4-Methoxyestradiol | 1.3 |
| 4-Hydroxyestradiol-3-methyl ether | 0.6 |
| 2-Methoxyestradiol | 0.05 |
| 2-Methoxyestrone | 0.01 |

[a]Reprinted with permission from Martucci and Fishman (1977, 1979). © 1977, 1979 by the Endocrine Society, the Williams and Wilkins Company, agent.

hydroxylation reduces receptor affinity to a greater extent than 4-hydroxylation. Monomethylation of 4-OH-$E_2$ reduces its relative binding affinity by approximately 40-fold, while 2-methylation of 2-OH-$E_2$ or 2-OH-$E_1$ essentially abolishes binding to the estrogen receptor. This is of considerable physiologic importance, since methylation represents the predominant route of further CE metabolism.

There do not appear to be any major differences between the binding affinities of CEs for estrogen receptors from different estrogen target organs. Merriam *et al.* (1980b,c) compared the apparent equilibrium dissociation constants for binding of a number of CEs for cytoplasmic estrogen receptors from rat uterus, pituitary, and brain. No significant intertissue differences were observed. Qualitatively similar results were obtained by Kirchhoff *et al.* (1981) for rat pituitary and hypothalamic cytosol receptor, using a different receptor assay methodology. In the rat liver, Dickson and co-workers (1980) found that at a 50-fold molar excess, the 2- and 4-hydroxylated derivatives of $E_1$, $E_2$, and 17α-ethinyl estradiol were all capable of inhibiting the binding of [3H]$E_2$ to ammonium sulfate purified cytoplasmic receptor sites. In cytosols from rat dimethyl benzanthracene-induced mammary tumors, Abul-Hajj (1980) obtained estimates of RBA for 2-OH-$E_1$ and 2-OH-$E_2$ very close to those reported by Martucci and Fishman (1976) for rat uterine cytoplasmic receptors.

To our knowledge, there has only been one report of CE binding to estrogen receptors in nonrodent tissues. In pituitary cytosols from ovariectomized ewes, Clarke and Findlay (1981) obtained estimates of RBA for binding of $E_2$, 4-OH-$E_2$, 4-OH-$E_1$, and 2-OH-$E_2$ of 100, 30, 20, and 5%, respectively.

The catechol portion of the CE molecule also confers on these steroids the ability to directly influence several different aspects of catecholamine function. As we have already indicated, CEs are excellent competitive inhibitors of COMT (Breuer *et al.*, 1968; Ball *et al.*, 1972b). In addition, studies by Lloyd and Weisz (1978) and Foreman and Porter (1980) have shown that 2-OH-$E_1$ and 2-OH-$E_2$ are both capable of inhibiting the activity of tyrosine hydroxylase, the rate-limiting enzyme in the biosynthesis of catecholamines. The mechanism of this inhibition probably involves competition between the CEs and the enzyme's pterin cofactor (see Fig. 4).

Several authors have raised the possibility that CEs may interact with catecholamine receptors. From a purely theoretical standpoint, there are good reasons to suspect that such interactions might take place. Crystallographic studies (Duax *et al.*, 1982) have suggested that the molecular structural attributes of 2-OH-$E_2$ may facilitate binding to the dopamine receptor. Consistent with this hypothesis, Schaeffer and Hsueh (1979) found that 2-OH-$E_2$ was capable of inhibiting binding of the dopamine antagonist

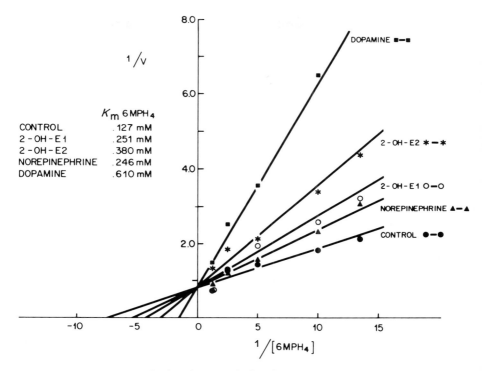

FIG. 4. Lineweaver–Burk plot of tyrosine hydroxylase activity in hypothalamic extracts in the presence of 50 μM dopamine, L-norepinephrine, 2-hydroxyestradiol (2-OH-E$_2$) or 2-hydroxyestrone (2-OH-E$_1$). The reaction mixtures contained 100 μM tyrosine, 10 mM ascorbic acid, and 50–800 μM 6MPH$_4$. Incubations were for 30 minutes at 37°C. Reaction velocity is expressed as nanomoles of tyrosine oxidized × hr$^{-1}$ × mg$^{-1}$ protein. Each symbol represents a mean of triplicate measurements. [From Foreman and Porter (1980).]

spiperone to putative dopamine receptors on rat pituitary cell membranes. Shortly afterward, Schaeffer *et al.* (1980) identified a high-affinity ($K_d$ 0.6 nM) binding site for [$^3$H]2-OH-E$_2$ in pituitary membranes. Binding of [$^3$H]2-OH-E$_2$ to this site was inhibited by unlabeled dopamine and spiperone. More recently, Paden *et al.* (1982) studied the effects of a number of estrogens (including 2-OH-E$_1$ and 2-OH-E$_2$) on the binding of several different specific neurotransmitter-receptor ligands to rat brain and pituitary membrane-binding sites. Both of the 2-hydroxyestrogens tested were found to interact with striatal as well as pituitary dopamine receptor sites (see Fig. 5). The inhibitory potencies of the two CEs with respect to [$^3$H]spiperone binding to these receptor sites were somewhat less than those reported by Schaeffer and Hsueh (1979), whereas Schaeffer and Hsueh reported a $K_i$ for

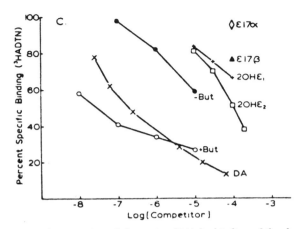

Fig. 5. Competition by steroids and dopamine (DA) for binding of the dopamine receptor "tag" [³H]ADTN. Results are expressed as percentage specific binding of 2.5 nM [³H]ADTN versus the log of the concentration of unlabeled competitors. Data are averages of three to five separate experiments. Abbreviations: +But, *d*-butaclamol; −But, I-Butaclamol. [From Paden *et al.* (1982).]

2-OH-E$_2$ and pituitary membranes of $8 \times 10^{-4}$ M. Interestingly, Paden *et al.* (1982) also found that 2-OH-E$_2$, but not 2-OH-E$_1$, was capable of inhibiting [³H]WB4101 binding to $\alpha_1$-adrenergic receptors with an inhibitory potency similar to that of noradrenaline itself. This inhibition was stereospecific and apparently dependent on the presence of a 17β-hydroxyl. Thus, 17β-E$_2$ but not 17α-E$_2$ was also capable of inhibiting WB4101 binding.

Yet another potential site of interaction between CEs and neurotransmitter systems was identified in a recent study by Caffrey (1982). *In vitro* enkephalin metabolism by rat brain homogenates was found to be inhibited to a greater extent by 2-hydroxyestrogens (2-OH-E$_1$ and 2-OH-E$_2$) than by catecholamines.

With the range of possible modes of interaction between CEs and estrogen target cells in the brain, determining the mechanism(s) by which CEs induce behavioral or neuroendocrine responses is not at all easy. In the case of the monophenolic estrogens, studies using estrogen-receptor antagonists and inhibitors of protein synthesis in general support the hypothesis that the central effects of these steroids involve at least an important contribution from estrogen-receptor mediated events (McEwen, 1981; Pfaff and McEwen, 1983; see section on Kinetics of Catechol Estrogen for further discussion). However, it remains uncertain whether the actions of CEs are mediated primarily through estrogen receptors or whether they also involve other "catechol-dependent" mechanisms.

A valuable experimental approach to this question was suggested by Merriam (Merriam *et al.*, 1980c), who noted that changing the stereochemistry of the 17-hydroxyl group in 2- and 4-OH-$E_2$ to the α-configuration results in a marked reduction in estrogen-receptor affinity, without significantly affecting the ability of the compounds to interact with COMT. Subsequent studies (Hersey *et al.*, 1982b; Pfeiffer *et al.*, 1982) have shown that 17α-$E_2$ is at least as good a substrate for CE biosynthesis as $E_2$-17β and is as potent as its 17-isomer with respect to inhibition of tyrosine hydroxylase activity. These results suggest that comparisons of the biologic potencies of 17α- and 17β-monophenolic estrogens and CEs may provide an indication of the relative importance of receptor and catechol-mediated cellular responses. This approach was used by Emons *et al.* (1981a) who compared the abilities of 4-OH-$E_2$ 17α and 4-OH-$E_2$ 17β to induce LH release in ovariectomized adult rats. Only the 17β isomer induced an LH surge, suggesting that with respect to this end point the actions of 4-OH-$E_2$ are more dependent on estrogen receptor-binding affinity than on the presence of a catechol structure. This conclusion must, however, be tempered with caution in view of the demonstration by Paden *et al.* (1982) that binding of estrogens to $α_1$-adrenergic receptors is *also* influenced by the stereochemistry of the 17-hydroxyl group. Thus, the failure of 17α CEs to elicity the same effects as their 17β isomers cannot be taken as definitive evidence that the estrogen receptor system is the most important factor in the response mechanism.

### Kinetics of Catechol Estrogen: Estrogen Receptor Interaction

An important factor in the mechanism of estrogen action is the stability of the estrogen–receptor complex. As the studies of Clark and his collaborators have shown, transient occupation of the estrogen receptor may not lead to a full estrogenic response. Many features of the response, in particular longer term effects, may only emerge if cell nuclear estrogen-receptor occupation is sustained for a period of at least several hours. Thus, estrogens such as $E_3$ that form rapidly-dissociating estrogen–receptor complexes are relatively weak estrogen agonists when given in the form of pulse injections because such injections produce only short-lived cell nuclear receptor occupation. In contrast, estrogens such as $E_2$ that dissociate from the receptor relatively slowly tend to induce much more powerful responses when administered in a similar fashion. Conversely, when $E_3$ and $E_2$ are injected simultaneously, the ability of the former to compete for estrogen receptor sites without eliciting a full response results in antagonism of the $E_2$ effects (Clark *et al.*, 1977; Bouton and Raynaud, 1979).

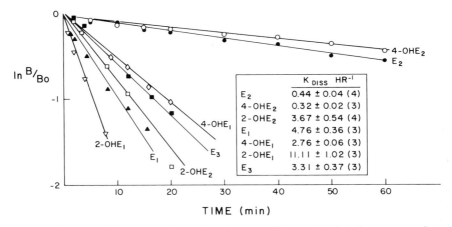

| | $K_{DISS}$ HR$^{-1}$ |
|---|---|
| $E_2$ | $0.44 \pm 0.04$ (4) |
| 4-OHE$_2$ | $0.32 \pm 0.02$ (3) |
| 2-OHE$_2$ | $3.67 \pm 0.54$ (4) |
| $E_1$ | $4.76 \pm 0.36$ (3) |
| 4-OHE$_1$ | $2.76 \pm 0.06$ (3) |
| 2-OHE$_1$ | $11.11 \pm 1.02$ (3) |
| $E_3$ | $3.31 \pm 0.37$ (3) |

FIG. 6. Kinetics of dissociation of complexes between different $^3$H-labeled estrogens and rat uterine cytoplasmic receptors. The $^3$H-labeled estrogens were either purchased from New England Nuclear or prepared by Fremy's salt oxidation (Gelbke *et al.*, 1973b) of the corresponding [6,7-$^3$H]monophenolic estrogen and purified by HPLC (Aten *et al.*, 1982). Cytosols prepared from uteri of rats ovariectomized 5–7 days previously were equilibrated with labeled estrogen (5 n*M*) overnight at 4°C, then raised to 25°C. At $t = 0$ a 1000-fold molar excess of the corresponding unlabeled estrogen was added. At various times thereafter receptor-bound radioactivity in samples of each incubate was determined by Sephadex LH-20 gel filtration (Ginsburg *et al.*, 1974). Results are expressed in terms of the log of the percentage of bound radioactivity remaining at each time point, to facilitate comparison between the different estrogens. (*Inset Table*) Apparent first-order dissociation-rate constants calculated by linear regression analysis of dissociation-rate plots like those presented in the figure. Results represent the means ($\pm$SEM) of data from the number of experiments given in parenthesis. Statistical analysis: $E_2$ vs. 2-OH-$E_2$; $E_1$ vs. 2-OH-$E_1$; $p < 0.01$ and $E_2$ vs. 4-OH-$E_2$; $E_1$ vs. 4-OH-$E_1$; $p < 0.05$ (Duncan's multiple range test).

Recent studies in our laboratory (Barnea *et al.*, 1983b) have demonstrated that similar factors may also contribute to the actions of 2- and 4-hydroxylated estrogens. As indicated previously, the 2-hydroxyestrogens are in general much weaker estrogen agonists than their 4-hydroxyisomers. These potency differences cannot be explained entirely on the basis of receptor affinity or metabolic clearance rate. Although the 4-hydroxyestrogens do have low MCRs and lower equilibrium dissociation constants for binding cytosol estrogen receptors than their 2-hydroxy counterparts, these differences are relatively slight (see Tables I and III). However, there are large differences between 2- and 4-hydroxyestrogens with respect to the rates of dissociation of their estrogen–receptor complexes. This is illustrated by Fig. 6, which depicts the *in vitro* dissociation of a number of monophenolic and catechol estrogens from rat uterine cytoplasmic estrogen receptors at 25°C. With both $E_1$ and $E_2$, 2-hydroxylation results in a marked increase in the rate of dissociation of the steroid from the receptor. This increase is roughly proportional to the change in equilibrium dissociation constant produced by 2-hydroxylation (Table III). In contrast, substitution of a 4-hydroxy results in a decrease in receptor dissociation rate; thus, 4-OH-E$_1$ and 4-OH-E$_2$ both dissociate at slightly but significantly slower rates than their parent compounds (Fig. 6).

These results suggest that the difference in estrogen-agonist activity between the 2- and 4-hydroxyestrogens is at least partly a function of the steroids' receptor-binding properties. The 2-hydroxyestrogens resemble E$_3$ in that they are capable of binding to the receptors but do not induce a sustained cell nuclear receptor occupation and therefore exert partial-agonist–partial-antagonist effects. The 4-hydroxyestrogens, however, form stable, long-lived receptor complexes and therefore induce full estrogenic responses (Naftolin and MacLusky, 1983).

Studies of the patterns of cell nuclear estrogen receptor occupation in the rat uterus after CE administration have provided evidence consistent with this hypothesis. Martucci and Fishman (1979) and Abul-Hajj (1980) have shown that cytosol estrogen receptor depletion and cell nuclear translocation are of shorter duration after 2-OH-E$_2$ than after E$_2$. We have confirmed these observations and in addition shown that 4-OH-E$_2$ induces a pattern of uterine cell nuclear estrogen-receptor translocation, which is indistinguishable from that of E$_2$ (Fig. 7).

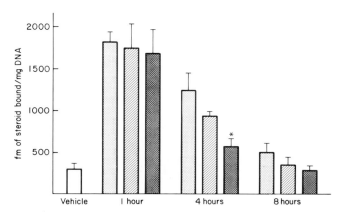

FIG. 7. Cell nuclear retention of E$_2$, 4-OH-E$_2$ and 2-OH-$_2$ receptor complexes in immature rat uteri. Twenty-five day-old rats were injected subcutaneously with subsaturating doses of unlabeled E$_2$ (10 μg/kg), 4-OH-E$_2$ (100 μg/kg) and 2-OH-E$_2$ (500 μg/kg). Nuclear estrogen receptors were extracted using 0.5 *M* KCl. The salt-extracted nuclear estrogen receptors were measured using the exchange assay described by Roy and McEwen (1977). Results are expressed as femtomoles per milligram DNA. The bars denote means (±SEM) of four observations. * Denotes significantly different from the results for E$_2$ at the same time point; $p < 0.05$, Duncan's multiple range test.

## V. CONCLUSIONS

### PHYSIOLOGIC ROLE OF CATECHOL ESTROGENS

Although it is clear that CEs are major estrogen metabolites, with varied and extensive biologic actions, their physiologic role remains something of an enigma. In the nonpregnant state, it is difficult to envisage them as circulating hormones, in view of their extremely rapid rates of metabolism and low concentrations in biologic fluids. Pharmacologic studies have shown that, in general, relatively large doses of CE must be administered in order to obtain a response. It seems inconceivable, given these findings, that the low endogenous concentrations of CEs in the bloodstream could exert important physiologic effects.

In addition to circulating CEs, however, there may also be effects mediated through locally formed 2- and 4-hydroxylated estrogens. This hypothesis is particularly attractive in the central nervous system (Naftolin *et al.*, 1975b) which not only synthesizes Es and CEs but also contains estrogen receptors as well as neurotransmitter systems with which the CEs could potentially interact. Studies in the rat liver have established that such local interactions may play a part in the actions of at least one synthetic estrogen, 17α-ethinyl estradiol ($EE_2$). Under both *in vitro* (Weinberger *et al.*, 1978; Dickson *et al.*, 1980) and *in vivo* (Aten *et al.*, 1982) conditions, $[^3H]EE_2$ is extensively converted to 2-hydroxylated metabolites. Some of the 2-OH-$EE_2$ produced in the liver cells binds to estrogen receptors and is translocated into the cell nucleus, raising the possibility that locally formed 2-hydroxyestrogens could play a significant part in the effect of $EE_2$ on liver function.

The role of local CE formation in the actions of the natural hormonal estrogens remains uncertain. A major problem that is still unclear is exactly how much CE is present in target tissues under physiologic circumstances. As indicated earlier, there is no consensus on this question in the literature, although radioimmunoassay measurements suggest that the free concentrations of 2-hydroxyestrogens are low (Fishman and Martucci, 1979). Recent studies in our laboratory on the metabolism of $[^3H]E_2$ in the rat also support the view that free CEs do not accumulate in estrogen target tissues. Using an HPLC procedure to separate the labile catechol metabolites and incorporating unlabeled authentic CE and methoxyestrogen standards to correct for any procedural losses, we have examined the retention of $[^3H]E_2$ and its metabolites in a number of tissues (hypothalamus, pituitary, liver, and uterus) from ovariectomized rats. In all cases, we have been unable to detect significant quantities of labeled CEs in the tissues. The majority of the nonconjugated radioactivity, in the bloodstream as well as in the tissues, represents $E_1$ and unchanged $E_2$ with somewhat lower concentrations of 2-MeO-$E_1$ (see Fig. 8).

The absence of measurable CE concentrations from estrogen target tissues does not, however, invalidate the hypothesis that local CE formation may be physiologically important. Even extremely small quantities of the steroids could have powerful effects if they were synthesized close to CE-sensitive cellular mechanisms. An analogous situation exists for local androgen-to-estrogen conversion in the central nervous system: even though the amounts

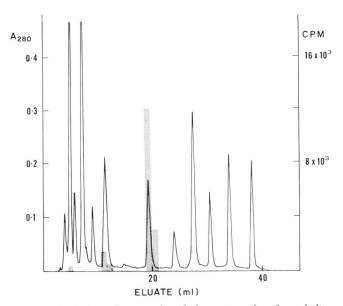

FIG. 8. Separation by high-performance liquid chromatography of metabolites retained in hypothalamic tissue of ovariectomized female rats 1 hour after the intravenous administration of 25 μg/kg [6,7-³H]estradiol. Radioactivity present in the tissue homogenate was extracted into toluene under the protection of ascorbic acid (Gelbke and Knuppen, 1972), partially purified by solvent partition and Sephadex LH-20 chromatography in methylene chloride methanol, 7:3, then separated by HPLC as described by Aten and co-workers (1982). Solid line; left vertical axis absorbance measured at 280 nM. The peaks represent unlabeled recovery estrogen standards, added immediately after homogenization to allow correction for procedural losses. From left to right these peaks correspond to the solvent front, 2-Me-$O_1$, 4-MeO-$E_1$, 2-MeO-$E_2$, 4-MeO-$E_2$, $E_1$, $E_2$, 4-OH-$E_1$, 2-OH-$E_1$, 4-OH-$E_2$, 2-OHE$_2$, and $E_3$. The recoveries of all 11 unlabeled estrogens, determined by integration of the A280 peak areas, exceeded 80% in this experiment. Histogram bars, right vertical axis (tritium counts per minute) recovered in 1-ml fractions of the eluate collected from the HPLC column. The only fractions found to contain significant amounts of radioactivity were those eluting coincident with authentic unlabeled estradiol-17β and with 2-MEO-$E_1$ and $E_1$.

of estrogen produced within the brain are minute, they have an enormous impact on both the adult and developing brain because the aromatase enzyme activity is closely associated with neural estrogen receptor systems (Naftolin *et al.*, 1975a; MacLusky and Naftolin, 1981; McEwen, 1981).

The notion that local CE formation may play a role in the mechanism of estrogen action is difficult to test experimentally. Unfortunately, there are as yet no specific inhibitors of 2- to 4-hydroxylase activity and thus it is not feasible to examine the effects or reproductive function of selectively blocking CE formation. Some insight into the importance of CE biosynthesis can, however, be obtained by examining the effects of structural modifications of the estrogen molecule. As indicated previously, altering the stereochemistry of the 17-hydroxyl to the $\alpha$-configuration results in a marked reduction in estrogen receptor-binding affinity. This modification does not, however, influence either the compound's ability to act as a substrate for A-ring hydroxylation or the interactions of the $17\alpha$-CE metabolites with COMT or tyrosine hydroxylase (Merriam *et al.*, 1980c; Hersey *et al.*, 1982b; Pfeiffer *et al.*, 1982b). Thus, $17\alpha$-$E_2$ provides a useful pharmacologic tool with which to explore the possible role of local CE formation with a reduced contribution from estrogen receptor-mediated responses. Conversely, structural modifications on the A or C rings of the estrogen molecule can lead to a marked reduction in CE biosynthesis without significant loss of estrogen receptor-binding affinity. For example, the potent synthetic estrogen, moxestrol ($11\beta$-methoxy, $17\alpha$-ethinyl estradiol) is a very poor substrate for 2-hydroxylation, presumably as a result of steric hindrance from the $11\beta$-methoxy group (Salmon *et al.*, 1979). Impairment of CE biosynthesis can also be achieved by substitution of a fluorine atom at C-2 or C-4, thereby effectively blocking further metabolism at these two positions (Pfeiffer *et al.*, 1982b).

Comparisons of the actions of $17\alpha$-$E_2$, $17\beta$-$E_2$, moxestrol, and 2- and 4-F-$E_2$ have been used by MacLusky and his collaborators to explore the role of local CE formation in the effects of circulating estrogens on gonadotrophin release and female sexual behavior in the rat (MacLusky *et al.*, 1982; Krey *et al.*, 1983). In these experiments, the steroids were infused over a period of 24 hours from Alzet osmotic pumps. The infusion rates for $E_2$, moxestrol, 2-F-$E_2$, and 4-F-$E_2$ were adjusted to give similar cell nuclear estrogen receptor concentrations in the brain and pituitary, thereby limiting the contribution to the results for these steroids from differences in receptor affinity. Estradiol-$17\alpha$ was infused at the same rate as its $17\beta$ isomer as well as at a 10-fold higher rate. Both of the $17\alpha$-$E_2$ infusion rates produced no response in the animals, in terms of either gonadotrophin release or sexual behavior. In contrast, all four of the other steroids tested exerted positive feedback effects on gonadotrophin release and facilitated feminine sex behavior despite their radically different abilities to act as substrates for 2- and 4-hydroxylation (MacLusky *et al.*, 1982; Krey *et al.*, 1983).

These observations suggest that, at least for ovariectomized rats, local CE formation is probably not an obligatory step in the mechanism of estrogen action on gonadotrophin release and sexual behavior. They do not, however, invalidate the concept that CEs might have a modulatory role, in conjunction with estrogen-receptor-mediated responses. It remains possible that CEs might have a specific role in the control of prolactin release. In addition, it would be wrong to extrapolate from the above-mentioned results to other physiologic states in which CE formation might play a considerably greater role.

One of the most interesting physiologic conditions from the point of new potential CE involvement is pregnancy. During the latter stages of pregnancy, circulating 2-hydroxyestrogen concentrations rise to far higher levels than in the nonpregnant condition. Conceivably, these high circulating CE concentrations could have a significant impact on the reproductive system and perhaps also on the circulatory system through alterations in the metabolism of catecholamines (Ball and Knuppen, 1980). At a local level, CE formation could play an important part in the physiology of the placenta. The placenta contains high levels of 2-hydroxylase (Milewich and Axelrod, 1971; Barnea and Naftolin, 1983) as well as high concentrations of COMT (Barnea *et al.*, 1983a). The role of these enzymes in normal placental function, however, remains uncertain, As mentioned earlier, circulating concentrations of 2-hydroxyestrogens increase dramatically during the latter part of pregnancy. Recent studies in our laboratory have shown that the levels of both 2-hydroxy and 2-methoxy estrogens in pregnancy fluids are very high at around the time of parturition. For example, at birth the concentrations of 2-$OHE_1$ in amniotic fluid and maternal serum are within the range of 100–300 pg/ml.; while 2-$MeOE_1$ concentrations can range as high as 2–3 ng/ml. (MacLusky, Barnea, and Naftolin, unpublished observations). These very high 2-substituted estrogen concentrations suggest that 2-hydroxyestrogen formation and metabolism might play an important role in normal placental physiology, as well as in pathophysiologic conditions of pregnancy in which placental function is impaired.

## ACKNOWLEDGMENTS

We are indebted to Marya Shanabrough and Christina Holdridge for technical assistance and to J. Fishman for providing us with copies of a manuscript prior to publication. Supported by Grant No. HD 13587 (F.N.) and postdoctoral fellowship No. HD 06324 (E.R.B.) from the

National Institute of Child Health and Human Development, National Institutes of Health, by Fogarty Senior International Fellowship No. TW00706 (F.N.), and by an Alfred P. Sloan Foundation fellowship (N.J.M.)

## REFERENCES

Abul-Hajj, T. J. (1980). *J. Steroid Biochem.* **13**, 83.
Acevedo, H. F., and Beering, S. C. (1965). *Steroids* **6**, 531.
Acevedo, H. F., and Goldzieher, J. W. (1965). *Biochem. Biophys. Acta.* **97**, 571.
Ackerman, G. E., MacDonald, P. C., Gudelsky, G., Mendelson, C. R., and Simpson, E. R. (1981). *Endocrinology (Baltimore)* **109**, 2084.
Adashi, E. Y., Fishman, J., and Yen, S. S. C. (1979). *Life Sciences* **25**, 2051.
Adlercreutz, H. and Luukainen, T. (1968). *In* "Gas Phase Chromatography of Steroids," (K. R. Eiknes and E. C. Horning, eds.), pp. 115–149. Springer-Verlag, Berlin and New York.
Adlercreutz, H., and Luukainen, T. (1970). *Ann. Clin. Res.* **2**, 365.
Adlercreutz, H., Ervast, H.-S., Tenhunen, A., and Tikkanen, M. J. (1973). *Acta Endocrinol. (Copenhagen)* **73**, 543.
Adlercreutz, H., Tikkanen, M. J., Wichmann, K., Svanborg, A., and Anberg, A. (1974). *J. Clin. Endocrinol. Metab.* **38**, 51.
Aten, R. F., Eisenfeld, A. J., MacLusky, N. J., and Hochberg, R. B. (1982). *J. Steroid Biochem.* **16**, 447.
Axelrod, J., and Tomchick, R. (1958). *J. Biol. Chem.* **233**, 702.
Ball, P. (1976). *Steroid Biochem.* **7**, 139.
Ball, P., and Knuppen, R. (1978). *J. Clin. Endocrinol. Metab.* **47**, 732.
Ball, P., and Knuppen, R. (1980). *Acta Endocrinol. (Copenhagen), Suppl 232* **93**, 1.
Ball, P., Knuppen, R., and Breuer, H. (1972a). *Eur. J. Biochem.* **26**, 560.
Ball, P., Knuppen, R., Haupt, M., and Breuer, H. (1972b). *J. Clin. Endocr. Metab.* **34**, 736.
Ball, P., Gelbke, H. P., and Knuppen, R. (1975). *J. Clin. Endocrinol. Metab.* **40**, 406.
Ball, P., Knuppen, R., Wennrich, W., and Breuer, H. (1972c). *Acta Endocrinol. Suppl.***159**, 85.
Ball, P., Stubenrauch, G., and Knuppen, R. (1977). *J. Steroid Biochem.* **8**, 989.
Ball, P., Emons, G., Haupt, O., and Knuppen, R. (1978a). *Steroids* **31**, 249.
Ball, P., Haupt, M., and Knuppen, R. (1978b). *Acta Endocrinol. (Copenhagen)* **87**, 1.
Ball, P., Reu. G., Schwab, J., and Knuppen, R. (1979). *Steroids* **33**, 563.
Ball, P., Emons, G., Klingebiel, T., Gruhn, K.-M., and Knuppen, R. (1981). *Endocrinology* **109**, 1037.
Barbieri, R. L., Canick, J. A., and Ryan, K. J. (1978). *Biochem. Pharmacol.* **29**, 83.
Barbieri, R. L., Todd, R., Morishita, H., Ryan, K. J., and Fishman, J. (1980). *Fertil. Steril.* **34**, 391.
Bardin, C. W., and Catterall, J. F. (1981). *Science* **211**, 1285.
Barnea, E. R., and Naftolin, F. (1983). *Proc. 65th Annu. Meet. Endocrine Soc.*, San Antonio, Texas.
Barnea, E. R., MacLusky, N. J., and Naftolin, F. (1983a). *Proc. Soc. Gynecol. Invest.* Washington, D.C., Abstract No. 349.
Barnea, E. R., MacLusky, N. J. and Naftolin, F. (1983b). *Steroids*, in press.
Bates, G. W., Edman, C. D., Porter, J. C., and MacDonald, P. C. (1977). *J. Clin. Endocrinol. Metab.* **45**, 1120.
Beyer, C., Morali, G., and Vargas, R. (1971). *Horm. Behav.* **2**, 273.

Bolt, H. M., Kappus, H. (1974). *J. Steroid Biochem.* **5**, 179.

Bouton, M. M., and Raynaud, J.-P. (1979). *Endocrinology (Baltimore)* **105**, 509.

Breuer, H., Lubrich, W., and Knuppen, R. (1968). *Hoppe-Seyler's Z. Physiol. Chem.* **349**, 3.

Caffrey, J. L. (1982). *Proc. 64th Annu. Meet. Endocrine Soc.*, San Francisco, California, Abstract No. 596.

Cantrall, E. W., Conrow, R. B., and Bernstein, S. (1964). *J. Am. Chem. Soc.* **86**, 2943.

Cecchini, D., Chattoraj, S. C., Farous, A. S., Nowroozi, K., and Edelin, K. (1980). *Proc. 62nd Annu. Meet. Endocrine Soc.*, Washimgton, D.C. Abstract No. 722.

Chattoraj, S. C., Fanous, A. S., Cecchini, D., Lowe, E. W. (1978). *Steroids* **31**, 375.

Clark, J. H., Paszko, Z., and Peck, E. J. (1977). *Endocrinology (Baltimore)* **100**, 91.

Clarke, I. J., and Findlay, J. K. (1981). *J. Endocr.* **85**, 503.

Cohen, S. L., Ho, P., Suzuki, Y., and Alspector, F. E. (1978). *Steroids* **32**, 279.

Conney, A. H. (1967). *Pharmacol. Rev.* **19**, 317.

Coombs, M. M. (1960). *Nature (London)* **188**, 317.

Crowley, L. G., Demetriou, J. A., Kotin, P., Dovovan, A. J., and Kushinsky, S. (1965). *Cancer Res.* **25**, 371.

Davies, I. J., Naftolin, F., Ryan, K. J., Fishman, J., and Siu, J. (1975). *Endocrinology (Baltimore)* **97**, 554.

Dickson, R. B., Aten, R. F., and Eisenfeld, A. J. (1980). *Mol. Pharmacol.* **18**, 215.

Duax, W. L., Griffin, J. F., Swenson, D. C., and Weisz, J. (1982). *Proc. 64th Annu. Meet. Endocrine Soc.*, San Francisco, California, Abstract No. 632.

Dunn, J. F., Merriam, G. R., Eil, G., Kono, S., Loriaux, D. L., and Nisula, B. C. (1981). *J. Clin. Endocrinol. Metab.* **51**, 404.

Emons, G., Knuppen, R., and Ball, P. (1981a). *Endocrinology (Baltimore)* **109**, 1799.

Emons, G., Schwarzlose, C., and Ball, P. (1981b). *Proc. 63rd Annu. Meet. Endocrine Soc.*, Cincinnati, Ohio, Abstract No. 363.

Engel, L. L., Baggett, B., and Carter, P. (1957). *Endocrinology (Baltimore)* **61**, 113.

Femino, A. M., Longcope, C., Patrick, J. E., and Williams, K. I. H. (1974). *Steroids* **24**, 849.

Fishman, J. (1963). *J. Clin. Endocrinol. Metab.* **23**, 207.

Fishman, J. and Dixon, D. (1967). *Biochemistry* **6**, 1683.

Fishman, J., and Norton, B. (1975). *Endocrinology (Baltimore)* **96**, 1054.

Fishman, J., and Hellman, L. (1976). *J. Clin. Endocrinol. Metab.* **42**, 365.

Fishman, J., and Martucci, C. (1979). *J. Clin. Endocrinol. Metab.* **49**, 940.

Fishman, J., and Martucci, C. (1980). *J. Clin. Endocrinol. Metab.* **51**, 611.

Fishman, J., and Tulchinsky, D. (1980). *Science* **210**, 73.

Fishman, J., and Norton B. (1983). *J. Steroid Biochem.* in press.

Fishman, J., Cox, R. J., and Gallagher, T. F. (1960). *Arch. Biochem. Biophys.* **90**, 318.

Fishman, J., Hellman, L., Zumoff, B., and Cassouto, J. (1966). *Biochemistry* **5**, 1789.

Fishman, J., Goldberg, S., Rosenfeld, R. S., Zumoff, B., Hellman, L., and Gallagher, T. F. (1969). *J. Clin. Endocrinol. Metab.* **29**, 41.

Fishman, J., Guzik, H., and Hellman, L. (1970). *Biochemistry* **9**, 1593.

Fishman, J., Boyar, R. M. and Hellman, L. (1975). *J. Clin. Endocrinol. Metab.* **41**, 989.

Fishman, J., Naftolin, F., Davies, I. J., Ryan, K. J., and Petro, Z. (1976). *J. Clin. Endocrinol. Metab.* **42**, 177.

Fishman, J., Norton, B. J., and Krey, L. C. (1980a). *Biochem. Biophys. Res. Commun.* **93**, 471.

Fishman, J., Norton, B. J., and Hahn, E. F. (1980b). *Proc. Natl. Acad. Sci. U.S.A.* **77**, 120.

Foreman, M. M., and Porter, J. C. (1980). *J. Neurochem.* **34**, 1175.

Frandsen, V. A. (1959). *Acta Endocrinol.* **32**, 603.

Franks, S. (1980). *In* "Endocrinology of Human Infertility: New Aspects," (P. G. Crosignani and B. L. Rubin, eds.), p. 27. Academic Press, New York.

Franks, S. and Naftolin, F. (1980). *Proc. 60th Annu. Meet. Endocrine Soc.*, Washington, D. C., abstract.
Franks, S., Ball, P., Naftolin, F., and Ruf, K. (1980). *J. Endocrinol.* **86**, 263.
Franks, S., MacLusky, N. J., Naish, S. J., and Naftolin, F. (1981). *J. Endocrinol.* **89**, 289.
Franks, S., MacLusky, N. J., and Naftolin, F. (1982a). *J. Endocrinol.*, **94**, 91.
Franks ,S., Lightman, S. L., MacLusky, N. J., Naftolin, F., Lynch, S. S., Butt, W. R., and Jacobs, H. S. (1982b). *Clin. Endocrinol.*, in press.
Gelbke, H. P., and Knuppen, R. (1972). *J. Chromatogr.* **71**, 465.
Gelbke, H. P., and Knuppen, R. (1973). *Acta Endocrinol. Suppl.* **173**, 110.
Gelbke, H. P., Haupt, O., and Knuppen, R. (1973b). *Steroids* **21**, 205.
Gelbke, H. P., Bottger, M., and Knuppen, R. (1975). *J. Clin. Endocrinol. Metab.* **41**, 744
Gethmann, U., and Knuppen, R. (1976). *Hoppe-Seyler's Z. Physiol. Chem.* **357**, 1011.
Ginsburg, M., Greenstein, B. D., MacLusky, N. J., Morris, I. D., Thomas, P. J. (1974). *Steroids* **23**, 773.
Gold, A. M., and Schwenk, E. (1958). *J. Am. Chem. Soc.* **80**, 5683.
Gordon, S., Cantrall, E. W., Cekleniak, W. P., Albers, H. J., Maurer, S., Stolar, S. M., and Bernstein, S. (1964). *Steroids* **4**, 267.
Gorski, J., and Gannon, F. (1977). *Ann. Rev. Physiol.* **38**, 425.
Gugler, R., Knuppen, R., and Breuer, H. (1970). *Biochem. Biophys. Acta.* **220**, 10.
Gurpide, E. (1978). *Pediatrics* **62**, 1114.
Hecker, E., and Walk, E. (1960). *Chem. Ber.* **93**, 2928.
Hecker, E., and Marks, F. (1965). *Biochem. Z.* **343**, 211.
Hellman, L., Zumoff, B., Fishman, J., and Gallagher, T. F. (1970). *J. Clin. Endocrinol. Metab.* **30**, 161.
Hellman, L., Zumoff, B., Fishman, J., and Gallagher, T. F. (1971). *J. Clin. Endocrinol. Metab.* **33**, 138.
Hersey, R. M., Gunsalus, P., Lloyd, T., and Weisz, J. (1981a). *Endocrinology (Baltimore)* **109**, 1902.
Hersey, R. M., Williams, K. I. H., and Weisz, J. (1981b). *Endocrinology (Baltimore)* **109**, 1912.
Hershey, R. M., Weisz, J. and Katzenellenbogen, B. S. (1982a). *Endocrinology (Baltimore)* **111**, 896.
Hershey, R. M., Lloyd, T., MacLusky, N. J., and Weiss, J. (1982b). *Endocrinology (Baltimore)* **111**, 1734.
Hobkirk, R., and Nilsen, M. (1963). *J. Clin Endocr. Metab.* **23**, 274.
Hoffman, A. R., Paul, S. M., and Axelrod, J. (1979a). *Biochem. Pharmacol.* **29**, 83.
Hoffman, A. R., Paul, S. M., and Axelrod, J. (1979b). *Cancer Res.* **39**, 4584.
Hoppen, H. O., Sickmann, L., and Breuer, H. (1974). *Hoppe-Seyler's Z. Physiol. Chem.* **355**, 1305.
Hsueh, A. J. W., Erickson, G. F., and Yen, S. S. C. (1979). *Endocrinology (Baltimore)* **104**, 806.
Jellinck, P. H. (1980). *Steroids*, 35, 579.
Jellinck, P. H., and Perry, G. (1967). *Biochim. Biophis Acta* **137**, 367.
Jellinck, P. H., and Elce, J. S. (1969). *Steroids* **13**, 711.
Jellinck, P. H., and Brown, B. J. (1971). *Steroids* **17**, 133.
Jellinck, P. H., and Newcombe, A. M. (1980). *J. Steroid Biochem.* **13**, 681.
Jellinck, P. H., Krey, L., Davis, P. G., Kamel, F., Luine, V., Parsons, B. P., Roy, E. J., and McEwen, B. S. (1981). *Endocrinology (Baltimore)* **108**, 1848.
Jensen, E. V., and DeSombre, E. R. (1973). *Science* **182**, 126.
Kanojia, R. M. (1977). *Steroids* **30**, 343

Kappus, H., Bolt, H. M., and Remmer, H. (1973). *Steroids* **22**, 203.
Katayama, S., and Fishman, J. (1982). *Endocrinology (Baltimore)* **110**, 1448.
Keith, W. B. (1977). *Assoc. Southeast. Biol. Bull.* **24**, 62.
Kelly, R. W., and Abel, M. H. (1980). *Prostaglandins* **20**, 613.
Kelly, R. W., and Abel, M. H. (1981). *J. Steroid Biochem.* **14**, 787.
Kirchhoff, J., Hornung, E., Ghraf, R., Ball, P., and Knuppen, R. (1981). *J. Neurochem.* **37**, 1540.
Knuppen, R., Lubrich, W., Haupt, O., Ammerlhahn, U., and Breuer, H. (1969). *Hoppe-Seyler's Z. Physiol. Chem.* **350**, 1067.
Knuppen, R., Haupt, O., and Breuer, H. (1970). *Biochem J.* **118**, 9.
Knuppen, R., Breuer, H., and Pangels, G. (1961). *Hoppe-Seyler's Z. Physiol. Chem.* **324**, 108.
Kono, K. S., Brandon, D., and Lipsett, M. B. (1981). *Proc. 63rd Annu. Meet. Endocrine Soc.*, Cincinnati, Ohio, Abstract No. 759.
Kono, S., Brandon, D., Merriam, G. R., Merriam, G. R., Loriaux, D. L., and Lipsett, M. G. (1980). *Steroids* **36**, 463.
Kono, S., Brandon, D. D., Merriam, G. R., Loriaux, D. L., and Lipsett, M. B. (1981). *Endocrinology (Baltimore)* **108**, 40.
Krachy, S., and Gallagher, T. F. (1957). *J. Biol. Chem.* **229**, 519.
Kreek, M. J., Lahita, R., Schaefer, R. A., Anderson, K. and Bradlow, H. L. (1982). *Proc. 64th Annu. Meet. Endocrine Soc.*, San Francisco, California Abstract No. 287.
Krey, L. C., MacLusky, N. J., Merriam, G., Naftolin, F., Parsons, B., and Pfeifer, D. (1983). In "Proceedings of the Fogarty International Center Workshop on Catechol Estrogens" (G. R. Merriam and M. R. Lipsett, eds.). Raven, New York.
Kuss, E. (1967) *Hoppe-Seyler's Z. Physiol. Chem.* **348**, 1707.
Lamberts, S. W. J., Nagy, I., Uitterlinden, P., and MacLeod, R. M. (1982). *Endocrinology (Baltimore)* **110**, 1141.
Lloyd, T., and Weisz, J. (1978). *J. Biol. Chem.* **253**, 4841.
Loke, K. H., and Marrian, G. F. (1958). *Biochim. Biophys. Acta* **27**, 213.
Longcope, C., Femino, A., Flood, C., and Williams, K. I. H. (1982). *J. Clin. Endocrinol. Metab.* **54**, 374.
Loudon, J. D., and Scott, J. A. (1953). *J. Chem. Soc.*, p. 265.
Luttge, W. G., and Jasper, T. W. (1977). *Life Sci.* **20**, 419.
McEwen, B. S. (1981). *Science* **211**, 1303.
MacLusky, N. J. and Naftolin, F. (1981). *Science* **211**, 1294.
MacLusky, N. J., Naftolin, F., Krey, L. C., and Franks, S. (1981). *J. Steroid Biochem.* **15**, 111.
MacLusky, N. J., Clark, C. R., Paden, C. M. and Naftolin, F. (1982b). *In* "Mechanisms of Steroid Action" (G. P. Lewis, ed.). Macmillan, New York.
MacLusky, N. J., Riskalla, M., Krey, L., Parvizi, N., and Naftolin, F. (1983). *Neuroendocrinology*, in press.
Marrone, B. L., Rodriguez-Sierra, J. F., and Feder, H. H. (1977). *Pharmacol. Biochem. Behav.* **7**, 13.
Martucci, C., and Fishman, J. (1976). *Steroids* **27**, 325.
Martucci, C., and Fishman, J. (1977). *Endocrinology (Baltimore)* **101**, 1709.
Martucci, C., and Fishman, J. (1979). *Endocrinology (Baltimore)* **105**, 1288.
Merriam, G. R., Naftolin, F., and Ryan, K. J. (1976). *In* "Hypothalamus and Endocrine Function" (F. Labrie, J. Meites, and G. Pelletier, eds.), p. 494. Plenum, New York.
Merriam, G. R., Brandon, D. D., Kono, S., Davis, S. E., Loriaux, D. L., and Lipsett, M. B. (1980a). *J. Clin. Endocrinol. Metab.* **51**, 1211.
Merriam, G. R., MacLusky, N. J., Johnson, L. S., and Naftolin, F. (1980b). *Steroids* **36**, 13.

Merriam, G. R., MacLusky, N. J., Picard, M. K., and Naftolin, F. (1980c). *Steroids* **31,** 1.

Merriam, G. R., Kono, S., Keiser, H. R., Loriaux, D. L., and Lipsett, M. B. (1981d). *J. Clin. Endocrinol. Metab.* **53,** 784.

Merriam, G. R., Kono, S., Loriaux, D. L., and Lipsett, M. B. (1982). *J. Clin. Endocrinol. Metab.* **54,** 753.

Milewich, L., and Axelrod, L. R. (1971). *Endocrinology (Baltimore)* **88,** 589.

Morishita, H., Adachi, H., Naftolin, F., Ryan, K. J., and Fishman, J. (1976). *Acta Obstet. Gynaecol. Jpn. (Engl. Ed.)* **23,** 325.

Mueller, G. C. (1955). *Nature (London)* **176,** 127.

Naftolin, F., and MacLusky, N. J. (1983). *In* "Prolactin and Prolactinomas," (G. Tolin, C. Stefanis, T. Mountopalakis, and F. Labrie, eds.), pp. 305–310. Raven, New York.

Naftolin, F., Morishita, H., Davies, I. J., Todd, R., Ryan, K. J., and Fishman, F. (1975a). *Biochem. Biophys. Res. Commun.* **64,** 905.

Naftolin, F., Ryan, K. J., Davies, I. J., Reddy, V. V., Flores, F., Petro, Z., Kuhn, M., White, R. J., Takaoka, Y., and Wolin, L. (1975b). *Recent Prog. in Horm. Res.* **31,** 295.

Naish, S. J., and Ball, P. (1981). *Neuroendocrinology* **33,** 225.

Neiderl, J. B., and Vogel, H. J. (1949). *J. Am. Chem. Soc.* **71,** 2566.

Paden, C. M., McEwen, B. S., Fishman, J., Snyder, L., and DeGroff, V. (1982). *J. Neurochem.* **39,** 512.

Parvizi, N., and Naftolin, F. (1977). *Psychoneuroendocrinology* **2,** 409.

Patt, V., Mollering, M., and Breuer, H. (1971). *Arzneim Forsch.* **21,** 308.

Paul, S. M., Axelrod, J., and Diliberto, E. J. (1977). *Endocrinology (Baltimore)* **101,** 1604.

Paul, S. M., and Axelrod, J. (1977). *Science* **167,** 657.

Pfaff, D. W., and McEwen, B. S. (1983). *Science* **219,** 808.

Pfeiffer, D. G., MacLusky, N. J., Emons, G., Ball, P., and Merriam, G. R. (1982a). *Int. Congr. Horm. Ster. VI.* Jerusalem.

Pfeiffer, D. G., Barnea, E. R., MacLusky, N. J., Krey, L. C., Loriaux, D. L., and Merriam, G. R. (1982b). *Proc. 11th Annu. Meet. Soc. Neurosci.*, Minneapolis, Minnesota, Abstract No. 18.7.

Rajan, R., Kaufman, S., and Reddy, V. V. R. (1982). *Proc. Soc. Gynecol. Invest.*, Dallas, Texas, Abstract No. 39.

Rao, P. N., and Axelrod, L. R. (1960). *Tetrahedron* **10,** 144.

Rodriguez-Sierra, J. F., and Blake, C. A. (1980). *Life Sci.* **26,** 743.

Rodriguez-Sierra, J. F., and Blake, C. A. (1982a). *Endocrinology (Baltimore)* **110,** 318.

Rodriguez-Sierra, J. F., and Blake, C. A. (1982b). *Endocrinology (Baltimore)* **110,** 325.

Rosenfeld, C. R., and Jackson, G. M. (1982). *Endocrinology (Baltimore)* **110,** 1333.

Roy, E. J. and McEwen, B. S. (1977). *Steroids* **30,** 657.

Salmon, J., Coussediere, D., Cousty, C., Delaroff, V., and Raynaud, J.-P. (1979). *Steroids* **34,** 381.

Schaeffer, J. M., and Hsueh, A. J. W. (1979). *J. Biol. Chem.* **254,** 5606.

Schaeffer, J. M., Stevens, S. R., and Smith, R. G. (1980). *Proc. 62nd Annu. Meet. Endocrine Soc.*, Washington, D.C., Abstract No. 317.

Scheike, O., Svenstrup, B., and Frandsen, V. A. (1973). *Steroid Biochem.* **4,** 489.

Schinfeld, J. S., Tulchinsky, D., Schiff, I., and Fishman, J. (1980a). *J. Clin. Endocrinol. Metab.* **50,** 408.

Smith, S. W., and Axelrod, L. R. (1969). *J. Clin. Endocrinol. Metab.* **29,** 85.

Stubenrauch, G., and Knuppen, R. (1976). *Steroids,* **28,** 733.

Tagatz, G. E., Gurpide, E. I. (1973). *In* "Handbook of Physiology, Section 7: Endocrinology" Vol. II. (R. O. Greep and E. B. Astwood, eds.), pp. 603–613. Williams & Wilkins, Baltimore, Maryland.

Tapper, C. M., Naftolin, F. and Brown-Grant, K. (1972). *J. Endocrinol.* **53,** 47.

Tsibris, J. C. M. (1979). *Ann. Clin. Lab. Sci.* **9,** 236.

Tsibris, J. C. M., Shees, E. E., and Spellacy, W. N. (1982). *Proc. Soc. Gynecol. Invest.*, Dallas, Texas, Abstract No. 278.

Weinberger, M. J., Aten, R. F., and Eisenfeld, A. J. (1978). *Biochem. Pharmacol.* **27,** 2469.

Westerfield, W. W. (1940). *Biochem. J.* **34,** 51.

Williams, M. C., and Goldheizer, J. W. (1979). *Chromatogr. Sci.* **12,** 395.

Williams, J. G., Longcope, E., and Williams, K. J. H. (1974). *Steroids* **24,** 8.

Wotiz, H. H., and Chatoraj, S. C. (1964). *Anal. Chem.* **36,** 1466.

Wotiz, H. H., Chatoraj, S. C., Kudisch, M., and Mueller, R. E. (1978). *Cancer Res.* **38,** 4012.

Yoshizawa, I., Tamura, M., and Kimura, M. (1972). *Chem. Pharmacol. Bull. (Tokyo)* **20,** 1842.

Yoshizawa, I., and Fishman, J. (1971). *J. Clin. Endocrinol. Metabol.* **32,** 3.

Yoshizawa, I., and Fishman, J. (1970). *J. Clin. Endocrinol. Metab.* **31,** 324.

Zumoff, B., Fishman, J., Cassouto, J., Hellman, L., and Gallagher, T. F. (1966). *J. Clin. Endocrinol. Metab.* **26,** 960.

Zumoff, B., Fishman, J., Gallagher, T. F., and Hellman, L. (1968). *J. Clin. Invest.* **47,** 20.

Zumoff, B., Fishman, J., Levin, J., Gallagher, T. F., and Hellman, L. (1970). *J. Clin. Endocrinol. Metab.* **30,** 598.

# CHAPTER 11

# Peroxidase: A Marker for Estrogen Expression

*Eugene R. DeSombre*

Ben May Laboratory for Cancer Research
The University of Chicago
Chicago, Illinois

## I. INTRODUCTION

Research over the last 25 years has led to major advances in our understanding of how hormones effect their biologic responses. Long before there was any appreciation of the details of the interaction of estrogenic hormones with their target tissues, the potent action of these steroids could be readily

BIOCHEMICAL ACTIONS OF HORMONES, VOL. XI

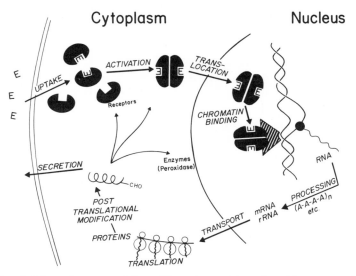

Fɪɢ. 1. Schematic representation of the estrogen interaction with a target cell.

appreciated by the dramatic uterine growth seen on administration of estrogen to an immature or ovariectomized rodent. This provided a sensitive
biological endpoint, which was essential for studies designed to establish the
mechanism of estrogen action. It is now clear, as indicated in Fig. 1, that
estrogen interacts with its target cell in a sequential pathway dependent on
the presence, or unique concentration, of the specific estrogen-receptor
proteins in the cytoplasm of the estrogen target cell. The association of
estrogen with the cytoplasmic-receptor protein leads to an activation of the
receptor complex, giving a receptor form that shows enhanced uptake by
nuclei and increased affinity for chromatin and DNA. While there is some
evidence, mainly from studies of glucocorticoid receptors, that the differences between the activated and the native state of the steroid–receptor
complex may relate to the state of phosphorylation of the receptor protein,
studies on the activation of the estrogen receptor suggest that a dimerization
of subunits may be involved, as shown in Fig. 1 (Little *et al.*, 1975; Notides
*et al.*, 1975). Even when the nature of the significant change in the receptor
complex, effected by the activation process, is understood, it will be necessary to elucidate how this change can give rise to the hormonal responses,
such as the increase in expression of specific proteins and, in the case of
estrogens, tissue growth as well. To be able to investigate the molecular
details of the tissue responses, it is important to have convenient, readily
measurable biologic endpoints for the hormones. While uterine growth is a
dramatic consequence of estrogen action, it represents the culmination of a

cascade of molecular events in which a late blockage could complicate the interpretation of the results of a productive receptor interaction at the chromatin level. Furthermore, it is unlikely that the uterine growth response can be easily reproduced *in vitro*, as indicated by the long controversy over whether estrogen really stimulates "growth" of the MCF-7 cell, the estrogen-receptor-containing, human breast cancer cell line. There has been an attraction to study hormone action in cell lines, uncomplicated by the uncertainties of metabolism and nutrition concomitant with studies in the whole animal. However, in addition to a concern that regulation in the transformed cells, which can be studied in continuous culture, may have certain anomalies, one would like to study an endpoint that can be applied to subsequent studies of both normal and neoplastic tissues in the whole animal.

Quite a few proteins whose concentration increases after estrogen administration *in vivo* have been identified. Probably best known is the protein referred to as IP, or induced protein, first reported by Notides and Gorski (1966) and studied by the laboratories of Gorski, Katzenellenbogen, Kaye, Lindner, and others (see Beato, 1980, for a comprehensive review of this work). While IP, recently identified as an isoenzyme of creatine kinase (Reiss and Kaye, 1981), is synthesized early after estrogen treatment, it has a relatively high rate of constitutive synthesis in the uterus and the extent of the hormonal stimulation is only severalfold, not optimal characteristics for a marker to be used for studying the hormonal control of gene expression in the uterus. The progesterone receptor content of the uterus is increased by estrogen *in vivo* (Leavitt and Blaha, 1972; Rao *et al.*, 1973; Milgrom *et al.*, 1973), and progesterone receptor is clearly important to the hormonal regulation of various normal and neoplastic target tissues (McGuire *et al.*, 1977). Like estrogen receptor, progesterone receptor is present in target tissues in extremely minute concentrations, somewhat limiting its usefulness as a gene marker until appropriate, sensitive probes are available, probably through gene cloning. Hence, there is some attraction in studying a marker, like an enzyme, which is present in high concentration in the estrogen-stimulated state but is absent in the atrophic condition. While a number of enzymes involved in carbohydrate metabolism have been found to increase in concentration in the uterus after estrogen treatment (Baquer and McClean, 1972), many show only severalfold increases after estrogen. The rate of *de novo* synthesis of uterine glucose-6-phosphate dehydrogenase has been shown to increase some 12- to 18-fold after estrogen administration to the rat (Smith and Barker, 1974), and, despite its expression in the unstimulated uterus, it has been a useful marker of estrogen action.

Because of the very dramatic increases in the uterine level of the enzyme peroxidase (donor:hydrogen peroxide oxidoreductase, EC 1.11.1.7) reported in the literature and, equally important, the low or undetectable amounts of the enzyme in the unstimulated animal, it seemed to be an excellent candidate for a marker of estrogen action in the uterus. This chapter will present the studies of the hormonal regulation of this marker enzyme in the uterus and other tissues carried out in our laboratory as well as reports of work performed in other laboratories. As will become evident, the initial hopes to be able to use this marker for detailed study of the hormonal regulation of gene expression in the uterus have not yet come to fruition due to the complication arising from both exogenous and endogenous sources of the enzyme in the uterus. Nonetheless, it will be seen that peroxidase can provide a useful tool to document important endocrine changes that influence the uterus, although a combination of biochemical and histochemical methods must be employed for a full appreciation of the modulation of this enzyme.

## II. THE ATROPHIC UTERUS

### A. HORMONE REGULATION

#### 1. Estrogen

The first report of increases in the uterine content of peroxidase in the rat following estrogen administration came in 1955 (Lucas *et al.*, 1955). Although what would now be considered hyperphysiologic doses of DES and estradiol were used (50–500 μg), very dramatic increases in the uterine concentration of peroxidase, up to several hundredfold, were reported to occur between 24 and 96 hours after administration of estrogen to ovariectomized female rats. This report was followed (Martin *et al.*, 1958) by a comparison of the uterine peroxidase activity with various, previously reported, peroxidases in which similarity to lactoperoxidase was noted. In 1965, Klebanoff reported that uterine peroxidase activity was absent in the immature animal but could be extracted with 1.2 *M* NaCl from uteri of estrogen-treated rats. Figure 2 shows that the magnitude of the response in uterine peroxidase after administering a physiologic dose of 1 μg of estradiol to the immature female rat is also substantial. As indicated by Klebanoff, little or no peroxidase is seen in the untreated uterus. One can first detect increases in biochemically assayed peroxidase activity at 4–8 hours after estradiol treatment. The maximum activity appears at 20–24 hours following a single injection of the hormone and is followed by a decline in activity thereafter. When assayed histochemically in tissue sections, peroxidase is first seen at about 12 hours, even after the very large dose of 200 μg of

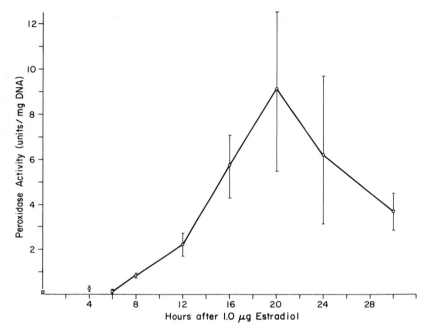

F<small>IG</small>. 2. Time course for estrogen induction of rat uterine peroxidase. Twenty-one-day-old female rats were given 1.0 μg estradiol and, at the times indicated, groups of five animals were sacrificed for assay of peroxidase in 0.5 *M* calcium chloride extracts of individual uteri. [Results, representing mean values ± SD, taken from DeSombre and Lyttle (1980b).]

estradiol (Brokelman and Fawcett, 1969), and it appears to increase thereafter. Even on continued daily treatment with estrogen, not all of the endometrial epithelial cells appear to contain the enzyme (Anderson *et al.*, 1975a). The peroxidase reaction product in the epithelium was found in the endoplasmic reticulum and nuclear envelope (Brokelman and Fawcett, 1969) and, especially in the glandular epithelium, also within the Golgi cisternae, in Golgi-derived condensing vacuoles, and secretory granules (Churg and Anderson, 1974).

When the subcellular localization of estrogen-induced, rat uterine peroxidase was examined by sucrose density gradient centrifugation, the activity was localized in a region of reticular membrane-bound vesicles that were distinct from peroxisomes, mitochondria, and lysosomes (Lyttle and Jellinck, 1976). Subsequent treatment of the vesicles with detergent solubilized the enzyme. Hosoya and Saito (1981) also observed only minor (<5%) peroxidase activity in the soluble fraction after homogenization of rat uteri in buffered 0.25 *M* sucrose. The largest amount of peroxidase activity was reported by these workers to be in the microsomal fraction, although activity appeared in mitochondrial and lysosomal fractions. However, enzyme markers showed the various fractions were not pure.

Even though the response to the administration of a single dose of estradiol is very dramatic, continued daily treatment with estrogen causes continued increases in the uterine content of peroxidase, in parallel to the increases in uterine weight (Fig. 3). By 5–7 days of treatment with 1 μg of estradiol, the uterus, which has now nearly reached the size and peroxidase content of the uterus of the mature animal, no longer showed significant increases in weight or peroxidase. Similar dramatic increases in peroxidase in the rat uterus following up to 6 days of treatment with estradiol or the nonsteroidal estrogen, DES, were observed using histochemical techniques (Anderson *et al.*, 1975a).

The estrogen-induced increase in uterine peroxidase occurs in a number of laboratory animals (Table I). The rodent seems to be most sensitive, showing the most substantial increases in this marker after administration of estradiol. Interestingly, when equivalent body weight doses of estradiol were administered to the species shown in Table I, there was a parallel between the relative uterine weight gain and the relative increase in uterine

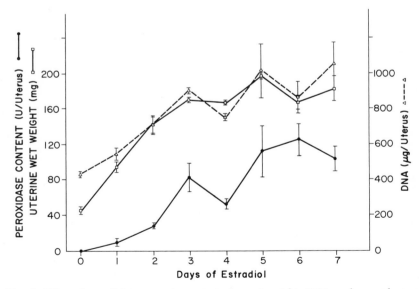

FIG. 3. Effect of estradiol treatment on rat uterine wet weight, DNA, and peroxidase content. Ovariectomized rats were given 1 μg of estradiol per day and groups of five animals were sacrificed 20 hours after the last dose of estrogen. [From DeSombre and Lyttle (1979).]

TABLE I

ESTRADIOL STIMULATION OF THE UTERUS OF VARIOUS SPECIES

| Animal (age/wt) | Group[a] | Uterine wt (mg) | Units (per g ± SEM) | mUnits per uterus |
|---|---|---|---|---|
| | | | Uterine peroxidase activity | |
| Hamster | C | 45.8 | 0.064 ± 0.018 | 2.9 |
| (25 days/46 g) | E | 62.4 | 0.132 ± 0.016 | 8.2 |
| | (E/C) | (1.36) | (2.06) | (2.9) |
| Guinea pig | C | 232 | 0.18 ± 0.04 | 42 |
| (23 days/210 g) | E | 534 | 0.83 ± 0.17 | 443 |
| | (E/C) | (2.30) | (4.61) | (10.5) |
| Rat | C | 25.2 | 0.27 ± 0.09 | 6.8 |
| (30 days/54 g) | E | 84.3 | 24.6 ± 7.3 | 2074 |
| | (E/C) | (3.35) | (91.1) | (305) |
| Mouse | C | 7.8 | 0.1 ± 0.04 | 0.78 |
| (28 days/19 g) | E | 35.0 | 29.3 ± 10 | 1026 |
| | (E/C) | (4.49) | (293) | (1315) |

[a]Animals (4–10 per group) received subcutaneous injections of vehicle (C) or estradiol (E) 40 µg kg$^{-1}$ body weight, 44 and 20 hours before killing. E/C is ratio of weight or peroxidase of estrogen treated to control uteri. [Reprinted by permission from Lyttle and DeSombre (1977b), *Nature (London)* **268**, 337. Copyright © 1977 Macmillan Journals Ltd.]

peroxidase. Nonetheless, while the estrogen-induced increase in uterine weight ranged from 1.3- to 4.5-fold, the peroxidase increases ranged from 3- to 1300-fold with only 2 days of treatment. While a significant part of the impressive magnitude of the peroxidase increase in the rodent uterus is derived from the low baseline concentration in the immature animal, this marker probably shows one of the largest increases seen on estrogen treatment. A recent report, however, suggests that the pig uterus contains low concentrations of peroxidase. This organ may also be less sensitive to estrogen-dependent increases of peroxidase than is the rat uterus (Hosoya and Saito, 1981).

The response in uterine peroxidase to estradiol is clearly dose dependent, as indicated in Fig. 4. The dose response was unlike other commonly studied uterine responses, such as IP or glycolytic enzymes, since the response continued beyond the dose levels usually considered physiologic. As can be seen in Fig. 4, there was clearly a significant increase in uterine peroxidase comparing a 10-µg and 100-µg dose of estradiol. Nonetheless, the differences in biologic potency for various estrogens seemed to be similar for the peroxidase response and other biologic endpoints. For example, as shown in Fig. 5 when single doses of estrone, estradiol, and estriol were compared, estradiol was clearly seen to be the most potent. It would appear

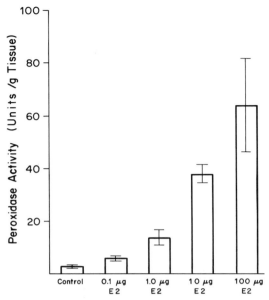

FIG. 4. Dose dependence of estradiol stimulation of peroxidase activity in immature rat uteri. Animals injected subcutaneously with the indicated amount of estradiol ($E_2$) in saline or vehicle alone were sacrificed at 20 hours and the uteri assayed for peroxidase activity. [From Lyttle and DeSombre (1977a).]

to require at least 10 times more estrone or estriol to elicit the same response. These results were confirmed by Hosoya and Saito (1981) after studying 3-day treatment protocols. Furthermore, a relationship between the quantity of nuclear–receptor complex and the amount of peroxidase induced in the immature rat uterus has been noted (McNabb and Jellinck, 1976).

A good correlation between the uterotrophic activity and the ability to increase uterine peroxidase in the immature rat uterus has been reported for a series of hexestrol analogs (Jellinck and Newcombe, 1980a). However, these investigators also found that the catechol estrogen 2-hydroxy estradiol, which did not reduce the uterine weight response to estradiol administration, did cause a significant decrease in the peroxidase activity of the uteri of estradiol-treated animals. On the other hand, 2-hydroxyestrone, used in 50-fold excess, was not found to inhibit the uterine response to estradiol (Jellinck and Newcombe, 1980b). This latter report also confirmed our earlier observation that estriol was required in higher doses than estradiol in order to give comparable increases in uterine peroxidase activity.

Brokelman and Fawcett (1969) were unable to demonstrate histo-

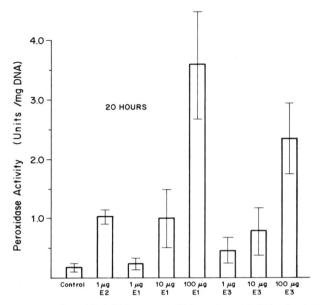

FIG. 5. Comparison of estradiol ($E_2$), estrone ($E_1$), and estriol ($E_3$) stimulation of uterine peroxidase activity in the immature rat, 20 hours after administration of the steroids. [From Lyttle and DeSombre (1977a).]

chemically identifiable peroxidase in the untreated castrate animal but did see activity in uteri of estrogen-treated castrate adult rats. Both our laboratory (DeSombre and Lyttle, 1980c) and that of Jellinck (Jellinck and Lyttle, 1972; Jellinck and Newcombe, 1977) have found similar sensitivities to estrogen-induced increases in peroxidase in uteri of immature and castrate rats. These reports also indicate a consensus that the uterus of the hypophysectomized rat is initially less sensitive to estrogen stimulation of peroxidase content, as well as weight gain, than is the uterus of the ovariectomized rat. However, on multiple-day estradiol treatment protocols, the uterus of the hypophysectomized rat does show a more substantial increase in weight and peroxidase content. It is probable that more time is needed for preparing the necessary biochemical capacity (i.e., polysomes) to respond fully to estrogen because of the more complete hormone deprivation in the hypophysectomized animal. It is also possible, as has been suggested by Sonnenschein and Soto (1977), that the pituitary is directly responsible for part of the initial response to estrogen.

As indicated earlier, Klebanoff (1965) had studied the estrogen-inactivating function of uterine peroxidase. Brokelman (1969) suggested that by mediating the binding of estrogens to protein, peroxidase could function as an initial step in a mechanism to eliminate excess amounts of estrogen in the uterus. Jellinck *et al.* (1979) discussed the possibility that uterine peroxidase could metabolize estradiol exiting the nucleus, thus preventing the recycling of hormone back to the cytosol. However, despite evidence that uterine peroxidase *in vitro* can convert estradiol to water-soluble and protein-bound products (Lyttle and Jellinck, 1972), it was concluded that such a role does not appear to occur *in vivo* with physiologic concentrations of estradiol (Jellinck *et al.*, 1979). Other roles for this enzyme have been proposed, such as bactericidal (Klebanoff, 1967) or spermicidal (Smith and Klebanoff, 1970) action or the cross-linking of tyrosyl residues of uterine proteins (Jellinck *et al.*, 1979). However, as indicated by the aminotriazole inhibition of uterine peroxidase activity but not uterine growth (cf. Section II,B), the role of peroxidase would not appear to be obligatory for estrogen-induced uterine growth.

## 2. Antiestrogens

In the 24 years since the first report of the activity of a nonsteroidal antiestrogen (Lerner *et al.*, 1958), numerous triphenylethylene derivatives, with a range of antiestrogenic activities, have been studied (for a recent review see Sutherland and Jordan, 1981). In general, antiestrogens are found to act as weak to moderately strong estrogens (agonists) when administered by themselves but effectively block expression of the full potency of estrogens when given concomitantly (antagonists). In general, this combination of agonist/antagonist behavior of antiestrogens is also found when uterine peroxidase is used as the marker of estrogenic activity. Using electron microscopy to detect the diamino-benzidine reaction product of endogenous rat uterine peroxidase, Churg and Anderson (1974) found clear evidence for substantial endometrial epithelial peroxidase expression after treatment with one of the more effective antiestrogens, Parke Davis CI628. Our studies of the activity of CI628 using biochemical assay of peroxidase, extracted from whole rat uterine homogenates by 0.5 $M$ calcium chloride, indicated a measurable agonist activity but a more dramatic antagonism of the estradiol-induced increase in uterine peroxidase (Fig. 6). While concomitant treatment with CI628 and estradiol reduced the biochemically assayed peroxidase activity to about one-half of that found after a dose of estradiol alone, the same amount of CI628 given 24 hours prior to treatment with estradiol entirely prevented the estrogen-dependent increase in uterine peroxidase 20 hours after estrogen. However, McNabb and Jellinck (1976) reported the pretreatment with the antiestrogen nafoxidine was less effective than coadministration with estrogen for preventing the estrogen-dependent increase in uterine peroxidase. Further study of the time dependence of the antagonist activity of CI628 (Fig. 7)

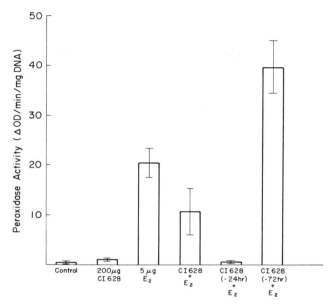

Fig. 6. CI628 modulation of the estrogen-dependent stimulation of uterine peroxidase activity. Groups of five ovariectomized female rats were treated as indicated and uteri removed in each case 20 hours after estradiol treatment. [From DeSombre and Lyttle (1978a), *in* "Hormones, Receptors and Breast Cancer" (W. L. McGuire, ed.), Raven Press, New York.]

showed complete inhibition of estrogen-dependent increases in peroxidase for the first 12 hours followed by a gradual release from this CI628-dependent inhibition, such that by about 48 hours after CI628 treatment the uterus was again competent to respond to estrogen with increased peroxidase activity. Interestingly, as seen in both Figs. 6 and 7, there appears to be an increased sensitivity for estrogen-dependent increases in uterine peroxidase at later times such that if estradiol is administered 72 hours after CI628 there is a significantly greater level of uterine peroxidase 20 hours later than if no antiestrogen were given. The results shown in Figs. 6 and 7 are consistent with effects of CI628 on the uterine concentration of estrogen receptor (DeSombre and Lyttle, 1978a) since up to at least 12 hours after CI628 there is a complete depletion of cytosol estrogen-receptor content, and the receptor content is gradually recovered by 24–48 hours. Interestingly, there is often an overshoot in cytosol estrogen-receptor recovery that could explain the enhanced sensitivity to estrogen at later times. It is also possible that an increased synthetic capability of the antiestrogen-treated uterus, due to the agonist activity of CI628, allows more effective responses when receptors are

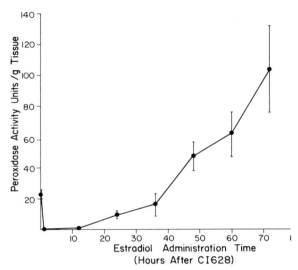

Fig. 7. Time independence of CI628 inhibition of estradiol-dependent uterine peroxidase activity. At various times after administration of 200 μg of CI628, groups of five ovariectomized female rats were given 5 μg of estradiol and 20 hours later the uteri were assayed for peroxidase activity. [From DeSombre and Lyttle (1978a), *in* "Hormones, Receptors and Breast Cancer" (W. L. McGuire, ed.), Raven Press, New York.]

available. Indeed, dramatic hypertrophy of endometrial epithelial cells is found after treatment with antiestrogens (Churg and Anderson, 1974; Kang *et al.*, 1975).

Studying the activity of the antiestrogen tamoxifen, Keeping and Lyttle (1981) reported that a single dose of 100 μg of tamoxifen administered to the immature rat led to a delayed peak of uterine peroxidase activity, found at 36 hours rather than around 20 hours, which is seen after estradiol, and this activity remained high for the 72-hour period studied. In contrast, the Lilly antiestrogen LY 117018, at the same dose, did not give an increase in either uterine weight or peroxidase activity. Levy *et al.* (1980) also found a significant increase in uterine peroxidase activity on administering 40 μg of Tamoxifen but, probably due to the large ratio of estrogen to antiestrogen, did not see Tamoxifen antagonism of either estrogen-dependent uterine weight gain or uterine peroxidase when the two were given together. Studies in the Katzenellenbogens' laboratories of the agonist-antagonist activities of the separate *cis*- and *trans*-tamoxifens showed parallel effects of these isomers on inhibition of uterine growth and peroxidase activities (Robertson *et al.*, 1982). The cis isomer showed full estrogenic growth potency by itself and did not inhibit the estrogenic stimulation of uterine growth. *cis*-Tamoxifen showed no antiestrogenic activity with regard to estrogen-induced peroxidase activity when given along with estradiol and only at the highest dose caused a significant increase in peroxidase by itself. On the other hand, the *trans*-tamoxifen, which showed partial agonist activity for both uterine weight gain and peroxidase, caused a dose-dependent inhibition of the estrogenic effect on both of these parameters when given concurrently with estrogen for 3 days.

Because of the increased affinity of the hydroxy metabolites of the antiestrogens for the estrogen receptor, there is a growing consensus that the hydroxy metabolites of antiestrogens may be the biologically active compounds. Recently Vass and Green (1982) compared the activities of hydroxytamoxifen and tamoxifen and reported that in a short-term protocol (18 hours), hydroxytamoxifen showed more potency in stimulating increases in uterine peroxidase than did tamoxifen itself; when both tamoxifen and its hydroxy metabolite were administered, the uterine peroxidase concentration corresponded to the lower level elicited by tamoxifen alone.

Studying the biologic potencies of hydroxy (i.e., demethylated) derivatives of CI628 and the Upjohn triphenylethylene antiestrogen, U23469, Rorke and Katzenellenbogen (1981) found that both the parent methoxy and the derivative hydroxy antiestrogens reduced the uterine peroxidase activities of tumor-bearing rats treated for 25–30 days at either 25 or 100 μg/day. On such chronic treatment, the hydroxy antiestrogens were not superior to the parent. However, further studies with these antiestrogens (Hayes *et al.*, 1981) showed that while 3-day *in vivo* dose studies showed similar potencies of the methoxy and hydroxy forms, *in vitro* studies of IP response indicated the expected greater potency of the hydroxy metabolites. Obviously, the actions of antiestrogens are complicated by the varying agonist/antagonist ratios as well as the *in vivo* pharmacodynamics of their metabolism and clearance. To understand how antiestrogens act and to make maximum use of their potential in treating endocrine disorders and neoplasia will require careful study *in vivo* and *in vitro*, using a variety of biologic endpoints. As described above, the marker peroxidase appears to be a useful parameter to help clarify the action of antiestrogens.

## 3. Other Hormones

In general, nonestrogenic hormones do not themselves effect an increase in the uterine content of peroxidase. The only exception to this is pregnant mare serum gonadotrophin (PMSG) (Lyttle and Jellinck, 1972), which, as a gonadotrophin, stimulates the ovary to increase the endogenous levels of estrogen. As would be expected, the response to PMSG is considerably prolonged (up to 9 days), compared to the response to a single dose of estrogen. Even rather large quantities of progestins, androgens, glucocorticoids, or thyroid hormones do not cause significant increases in uterine peroxidase (Anderson *et al.*, 1975a; DeSombre and Lyttle, 1979; Hosoya and Saito, 1981; Keeping *et al.*, 1982). However, a number of these hormones have been found to have dramatic affects on the estrogen stimulation of uterine peroxidase activity.

Even with the massive 1-mg dose of estradiol, used in the early study by Klebanoff (1965), 2 mg of progesterone decreased the "estradiol inactivating" activity of uterine extracts, activity found to be associated with peroxidase. Our results show a clear dose dependence for the progesterone-dependent inhibition of estrogen-stimulated increases in uterine peroxidase activity (Fig. 8). In view of the known effect of progestins to increase the level of the uterine enzyme 17β-hydroxysteroid dehydrogenase (Tseng and Gurpide, 1974) and the previously indicated diminished activity of estrone relative to estradiol regarding peroxidase stimulation, it was of interest to see if progesterone would be able to inhibit the peroxidase increase effected by estrone. If the activity of progesterone were mediated by its ability to cause increases in uterine 17β-hydroxysteroid dehydrogenase, one would not expect to see progesterone inhibition of the increase in uterine peroxidase following treatment with estrone. As seen in Fig. 9, progesterone is a potent inhibitor of the peroxidase increase due to estrone and DES, as well as estradiol. Thus, it would seem that progesterone action on peroxidase is not

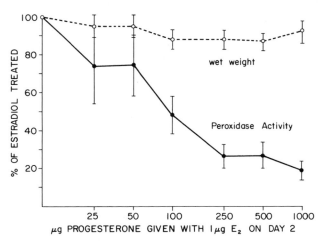

FIG. 8. Dose dependence of progesterone inhibition of estrogen-stimulated uterine peroxidase. Groups of five immature female rats were treated with 1 μg estradiol alone on day 1 and the indicated doses of progesterone along with 1 μg of estradiol on day 2. Uteri were removed 20 hours later and assayed for wet weight and peroxidase activity. Results presented as percent of the mean value found for uteri of rats which only received estradiol on both days.

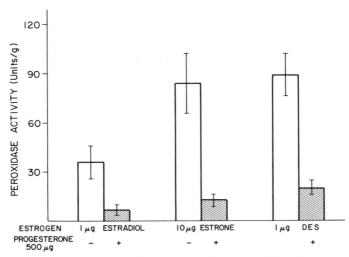

FIG. 9. Progesterone antagonism of uterine peroxidase activity effected by various estrogens. Groups of five immature rats were treated with one of the three estrogens alone or with 500 µg of progesterone. Twenty hours later uteri were assayed for peroxidase activity. [From De-Sombre and Lyttle (1979).]

mediated by its effect on the dehydrogenase enzyme. In addition, as recently reported by Keeping and Lyttle (1981), progesterone inhibits the tamoxifen-induced increase in uterine peroxidase as well. The inhibitory activity is not limited to progesterone, as a number of progestins show such activity (Table II). The highly active progestins, R5020 and norethindrone, not only showed greater activity at an equivalent dose than did progesterone, but they also seemed to be able to effect a more complete inhibition of estrogen-induced peroxidase increases. The progestin clogestone, 3β,17α-diacetoxy-6-chloropregna-4,6-diene-20-one, which has been reported to be an effective progestin in the rabbit but practically inactive in the rat (Revesz *et al.*, 1967), showed little inhibitory activity with regard to estrogen-dependent increases in rat uterine peroxidase. Hence, there seemed to be a fair correlation of the structure–activity relationship of various progestins in standard assays and their effects on uterine peroxidase stimulation by estrogens. Furthermore, as shown in Fig. 10, similar effects on estrogen-dependent increases in uterine weight and uterine peroxidase were found. The progestin-induced changes in uterine peroxidase can be seen to be of the same direction, but of much greater magnitude, than the changes in uterine weight. It can be seen in Fig. 10 that giving progesterone along with estradiol on the second day of the protocol reduced the uterine weight gain somewhat but dramatically inhibited the peroxidase activity of

TABLE II
INHIBITION OF ESTROGEN-INDUCED UTERINE PEROXIDASE BY VARIOUS PROGESTINS[a]

| | Peroxidase activity (% of $E_2$ alone) | | |
|---|---|---|---|
| | 100 μg[b] | 500 μg[b] | 1000 μg[b] |
| Progesterone | 48.4 | 26.7 | 19.0 |
| R5020 | 31.9 | 9.4 | 9.6 |
| Norethindrone | 31.7 | 4.2 | 3.7 |
| Medrogestone | 72.8 | 36.1 | 40.1 |
| Clogestone | 72.2 | 73.0 | 71.1 |

[a]Immature rats received 1 μg estradiol ($E_2$) on day 1 and either 1 μg estradiol alone or 1 μg estradiol simultaneous with progestin 24 hours later. Twenty hours after the second injection, the animals were sacrificed and uteri assayed for peroxidase. (From DeSombre and Lyttle, 1979.)

[b]Dose of progestin given along with the estradiol on day 2.

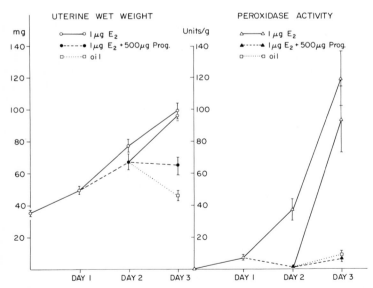

FIG. 10. Progesterone modulation of estrogen-dependent changes in uterine wet weight and peroxidase activity. Groups of five immature female rats were treated with 1 μg of estradiol alone or with 500 μg of progesterone in oil or vehicle alone. Each day, 20 hours after the last injection, groups of rats were sacrificed for assay of uterine wet weight (after expressing luminal fluid) and uterine peroxidase activity.

the estradiol-treated animals. If such animals were treated with both estradiol and progesterone on the next day, the uterine weight stayed about the same and the peroxidase activity did not rise dramatically. However, if on the third day the animals were treated with estradiol alone, both the uterine weight and the uterine peroxidase increased dramatically, indicative of the release from the apparent progestin block. This type of release was also reported by Anderson *et al.* (1977) to occur on treatment of progesterone-primed mature animals with estrogen alone.

Further study of the nature of the progestin inhibition has shown a rather unexpected time course for the inhibition (Table III). It can be seen that the maximum activity of progesterone is found when it is given 2–4 hours after estrogen. While it is conceivable that the progestin could act after the estrogen receptor has gone to the nucleus, for example by reducing the nuclear content or residence time of estrogen receptor, the RNA and protein-synthesis inhibitor studies (cf. Section II,B) indicated that emetine and actinomycin D were most effective at blocking estrogen-dependent increases in peroxidase when given at the same time as estrogen or shortly thereafter. While the explanation of the nature of this delayed action of progestin is not certain, more recent studies in our laboratory have led us to believe that the time dependence of the progestin effect may relate in part to its activity as a weak glucocorticoid.

When we began comparing the effects of glucocorticoids and progestins on

TABLE III

Time Course of Progesterone-Dependent Inhibition of Estrogen Induction of Uterine Peroxidase[a]

| Treatment time[b] (hours after E2) | Peroxidase activity[d] | |
|---|---|---|
| | Units/g | % of E2 alone |
| Control[c] | 11.95 ± 4.8 | 100.0 |
| 0 | 4.14 ± 1.6 | 34.6 |
| 1 | 2.02 ± 1.9 | 16.9 |
| 2 | 0.70 ± 0.4 | 5.9 |
| 4 | 1.03 ± 0.5 | 8.6 |
| 6 | 4.62 ± 2.3 | 38.7 |
| 11 | 11.57 ± 3.6 | 96.0 |

[a]Reprinted by permission from Table 4, page 261, in *The Endometrium* by Frances A. Kimball (ed.). Copyright 1980, Spectrum Publications, Inc., Jamaica, New York.

[b]Treatment time is the time, in hours, after administration of 1 μg estradiol (E2) that 500 μg progesterone was administered. In each case, all animals were sacrificed 20 hours after E2 for assay of uterine peroxidase.

[c]Control animals received no progesterone.

[d]Peroxidase activities given as mean values of five uteri per group ± SEM.

TABLE IV

EFFECT OF DEXAMETHASONE ON ESTRADIOL-STIMULATED UTERINE PEROXIDASE

| Treatment[a] | Uterine wet weight (mg) | Uterine peroxidase (units/g) |
|---|---|---|
| Saline | $27.2 \pm 2.0$ | $1.2 \pm 0.36$ |
| 5 μg $E_2$ | $44.8 \pm 3.1$ | $11.2 \pm 2.3$ |
| 5 μg $E_2$ + 2.5 μg dex | $47.0 \pm 1.8$ | $8.1 \pm 3.1$ |
| 5 μg $E_2$ + 10 μg dex | $43.2 \pm 3.2$ | $1.36 \pm 0.6$ |
| 5 μg $E_2$ + 30 μg dex | $39.0 \pm 2.2$ | $0.17 \pm 0.07$ |
| 5 μg $E_2$ + 100 μg dex | $46.2 \pm 2.6$ | 0 |

[a] Estradiol ($E_2$) alone or along with dexamethasone was injected subcutaneously at time 0 and animals were sacrificed at 20 hours for determination of uterine wet weight and calcium chloride extractable uterine peroxidase by published methods (Lyttle and DeSombre, 1977a).

the estrogen-dependent increases in uterine peroxidase, it became apparent, as seen in Table IV, that the glucocorticoid dexamethasone was a more effective inhibitor at any of the doses compared (see also Fig. 8). While it was difficult to administer any dose of progestins that completely inhibited the estrogen-induced increases in uterine peroxidase, even quite small doses of glucocorticoids completely abolished the estrogen stimulation. Although dexamethasone was most active, triamcinolone acetonide was also a more effective inhibitor than progesterone. This relationship could be understood by the knowledge that progestins, while often active as glucocorticoids, seldom display the complete activity of the latter. As will be seen later, it is probable that at least part of this activity of glucocorticoids relates to the eosinophil peroxidase component of uterine peroxidase.

Recently, Keeping and Jellinck (1980) reported that when iodide was administered in the drinking water for some days, the level of estrogen-induced rat uterine peroxidase was increased. The effect was specific for iodide since neither chloride, bromide, thiocyanide, or perchlorate were active. Further studies (Keeping et al., 1982) showed that iodide caused the effect in both normal and thyroidectomized rats. In addition, administration of T3 or T4 produced a large decrease in the estradiol-induced level of uterine peroxidase. The actual basis of these iodide and thyroid hormone-related effects is not clear, and the results seem paradoxical to the usual permissive action of the thyroid hormones in a variety of other responses. It may be necessary to clarify the effects of these substances on the sequestration of eosinophils, the exogenous source of uterine peroxidase, as well as on the endogenous enzyme in order to understand the nature of this regulation of uterine peroxidase activity. It has recently been reported, for example, that both T3 and T4 decrease the number of eosinophils in the blood and the uterine eosinophilia induced by estrogen (Steinsapir *et al.*, 1982).

## B. Effects of Inhibitors of Macromolecular Synthesis

In the original study of histochemically detected, estrogen-induced rat endometrial peroxidase, Brokelman and Fawcett (1969) found that administration of the protein-synthesis inhibitor acetoxycycloheximide completely prevented the appearance of the endogenous, epithelial uterine peroxidase. From studies of the time dependence of the cycloheximide suppression of estrogen-induced uterine peroxidase, McNabb and Jellinck (1975) concluded that the half life of the sodium-chloride extracted, biochemically assayed enzyme was about 4 hours. We reported the essentially complete suppression of the estrogen-dependent increase in uterine peroxidase by administration of the protein-synthesis inhibitors cycloheximide and emetine, as well as the RNA-synthesis inhibitor, actinomycin D (Lyttle and De-Sombre, 1977a; DeSombre and Lyttle, 1980a,b). When we studied the time dependence of the effects of emetine and actinomycin D (DeSombre and Lyttle, 1980b), we found that, as expected for a genomic response, the time for the required RNA synthesis preceded that for protein synthesis (Fig. 11). With regard to the estrogen-induced increase in uterine peroxidase measured biochemically at the 20-hour time point, the data shown in Fig. 11 indicate that 50% of the required RNA synthesis has occurred by about 8 hours while 50% of the required protein synthesis has taken place by 10–12 hours. While the difference in the time for required RNA and protein synthesis may be larger than expected, the rather large standard errors usually found when studying a time course of peroxidase increase (see Fig. 2) suggests that there is a significant uncertainty in the exact timing. It should be noted that the large animal-to-animal variations in uterine peroxidase have been characteristics of the variability of the response and not indicative of assay reproducibility. It would appear that there is significant variability of response among cells in the same uterus (Brokelman and Fawcett, 1969; Anderson *et al.*, 1977) as well as among animals. Interestingly, in a recent study (King *et al.*, 1981) we found that very large animal-to-animal variation was found with regard to estrogen-induced uterine eosinophilia as well. In this study we also found that a dose of actinomycin D, which inhibited more than 95% of the incorporation of radioactive uridine into RNA, completely inhibited the uterine eosinophilia and the biochemically assayed uterine peroxidase 20 hours after 5 μg of estradiol. Therefore, it would appear that macromolecular synthesis may be required for both the expression of endog-

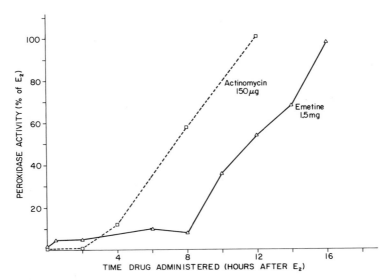

FIG. 11. Time-dependent inhibition of estrogen-dependent uterine peroxidase by emetine and actinomycin D. One μg of estradiol was administered subcutaneously to immature female rats at time zero, and at various times thereafter 1.5 mg emetine or 150 μg actinomycin D was administered to groups of the estrogen-treated rats. All animals were sacrificed 20 hours after estradiol administration and uteri assayed for peroxidase activity, which is expressed as a percent of the activity from animals which received only estradiol. [Data from DeSombre and Lyttle (1980b).]

enous uterine peroxidase and the uterine eosinophilia effected by estrogen. However, it must be kept in mind that the toxicity-induced stress often associated with agents like actinomycin D could be responsible for the inhibition. Such stress would be expected to increase the circulating levels of glucocorticoids which, as shown above, are potent inhibitors of estrogen-dependent increases in peroxidase and probably cause the sequestration of eosinophils into peripheral lymph nodes (Porter, 1954; Tchernitchin, 1979).

Finally, as shown in Fig. 12, aminotriazole, an inhibitor of heme biosynthesis, also can prevent the estrogen-induced increase in the heme-containing peroxidase enzyme activity in the uterus (C. R. Lyttle and E. R. DeSombre, unpublished observations). Although aminotriazole also is a direct inhibitor of peroxidase activity, such direct inhibition does not appear to be the basis of the inhibition shown in Fig. 12, since addition of uterine extracts of aminotriazole-treated animals did not reduce the assayed peroxidase activity of the uteri of estrogen-treated animals. A more likely basis is a block of the biosynthesis of the heme-containing active center of the en-

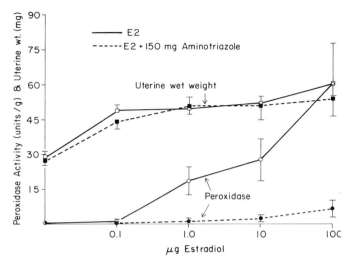

FIG. 12. Effect of aminotriazole on uterine responses to estradiol. Immature female rats were treated with one of the indicated doses of estradiol alone or along with 150 mg of aminotriazole. Uteri were removed at 20 hours for assay of wet weight and peroxidase activity. [From C. R. Lyttle and E. R. DeSombre (unpublished observations).]

zyme. Interestingly, this inhibition represents one of the few conditions in which estrogen-induced rat uterine growth occurs without a major increase in peroxidase. While it is possible that there is an increase in protein corresponding to an inactive peroxidase, lacking its necessary heme, specific antibodies to rat uterine peroxidase, which would allow testing such a possibility, are not available at present.

## C. Ontogeny during Development

There has been considerable interest in the ontogeny of the hormone responsiveness of the uterus of the developing rat since such information could help one understand differences between hormone-responsive and hormone-insensitive tissues, as well as providing a basis for understanding important developmental processes. It was therefore of interest to us to study the ontogeny of the estrogen-dependent stimulation of rat uterine peroxidase content during development. As shown in Fig. 13, up to 11 days of age the rat uterus does not show a significant response to administered estrogen. The hormone does not stimulate a significant increase in uterine weight and no peroxidase activity can be found. In this experiment, treat-

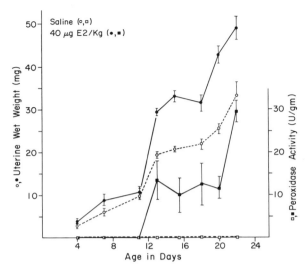

FIG. 13. Effect of estradiol on uterine wet weight and uterine peroxidase concentration in the postnatal female rat. Estradiol (closed symbols) or saline vehicle (open symbols) was administered subcutaneously to five pups each of the same age from the same foster-mother-fed litter and the pups were sacrificed 20 hours later for assay of uterine wet weight (circles) and uterine peroxidase (squares). Values given as means ± S.E.M. [Reprinted with permission from Lyttle *et al.* (1979a), *J. Steroid Biochem.* **10**, 359. Copyright 1979, Pergamon Press, Ltd.]

ment of 13-day-old rats with the same body-weight dose of estradiol elicited significant increases in both uterine weight and peroxidase, as did similar treatment of rats between 13 and 22 days of age. Since Raynaud (1973) had reported that the substantial amounts of a circulating, estradiol-binding serum protein, probably α-fetoprotein, altered the availability of free estradiol to the uterus of young, postnatal rats, it was important to study estrogens that had only low affinity for α-fetoprotein. As shown in Fig. 14, a similar experiment with R2858, the 11-methoxy derivative of ethinylestradiol and a very potent estrogen, showed essentially the same pattern of postnatal development of estrogen sensitivity. Again, the parallel between estrogen-induced increases in uterine peroxidase activity and uterine weight was striking. A similar response pattern was also found with DES, another potent estrogen with low affinity for α-fetoprotein (Lyttle *et al.*, 1979a). It appears, therefore, that around 13 days of age the Sprague–Dawley rat develops the ability to respond to estrogen and this change does not simply result from the greater availability of the hormone due to the decreasing circulating quantities of α-fetoprotein. Furthermore, this change does not simply relate to the synthesis of estrogen receptor since the 1-day-old rat uterus contains estrogen receptor (Clark and Gorski, 1970), and by 9 or 10 days of age the receptor content (DeSombre and Lyttle, 1980c) and receptor characteristics (Clark and Gorski, 1970; Kaye, 1978) are indistinguishable from those of the fully responsive, 21-day-old animal.

It would appear that the developmental changes that are manifested by about 13 days of age do not only involve estrogen responsiveness but sensitivity to other hormones as well. As shown in Fig. 15, at the same time the uterus is responsive to estradiol it is also sensitive to the progesterone inhibition of the response to estrogen. In this experiment, the estrogen response was not very dramatic at 12 days, but a distinct inhibition of uterine weight and peroxidase increases due to estrogen were seen when progesterone was also given. By 14 days of age, striking inhibition of estrogen-dependent increases in weight and peroxidase were evident (Fig. 15). While it is not yet clear what the nature of the developmental changes are that correspond to the acquisition of hormone sensitivity, it would appear that in a period of only several days the uterus changes from an organ that is totally insensitive to hormones to one that responds in the same way as that of the 21-day-old animal.

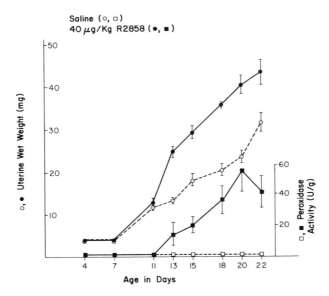

FIG. 14. Effect of the synthetic estrogen, R2858, on uterine wet weight and uterine peroxidase concentration in the postnatal female rat. Protocol, symbols, and procedures as described in Fig. 13 except that R2858 rather than estradiol was used. [Reprinted by permission from Figure 9, page 263, in *The Endometrium* by Frances A. Kimball (ed.). Copyright 1980, Spectrum Publications, Inc., Jamaica, New York.]

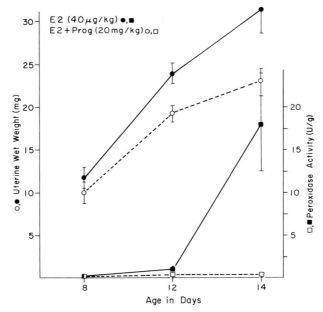

Fɪɢ. 15. Progesterone antagonism of estradiol action in the postnatal rat uterus. Estradiol (E₂) alone, solid lines, or combined with progesterone (Prog), dashed lines, was administered according to the experimental protocol described for Fig. 13. [Reprinted with permission from Lyttle *et al.* (1979a), *J. Steroid Biochem.* **10**, 359. Copyright 1979, Pergamon Press, Ltd.]

## III. THE MATURE UTERUS

Our studies on the variation of rat uterine peroxidase content with the stage of the estrous cycle are shown in Fig. 16. Consistent with the estrogen stimulation discussed earlier, higher levels of peroxidase are found in proestrus and estrus than in metestrus and diestrus. These results in the rat were recently confirmed by Hosoya and Saito (1981). However, these investigators were unable to find a cycle-dependent variation of peroxidase in the pig, where the peroxidase levels were generally very low. As also shown in Fig. 16, estrogen administration to metestrous or diestrous rats increased the uterine peroxidase content but the already higher levels in estrus and proestrus do not seem to be further increased by estrogen treatment. Rorke and Katzenellenbogen (1980) found no further stimulation of uterine peroxidase activity in the uteri of cycling, tumor-bearing rats given estrogen. A recent study (Myatt *et al.*, 1980) reported that placement of an intrauterine device (IUD) into one horn of the rat uterus for 18 days resulted in higher average peroxidase content in the IUD-containing horn than in the contralateral control horn, although both horns demonstrated the previously referred to cyclic variation of peroxidase.

Study of the postpartum rat uterus (Woessner and Ryan, 1980) showed that there was a substantial concentration of peroxidase in the uterus at day 0 postpartum and that with the subsequent decrease in uterine weight, the total peroxidase content decreased but its uterine concentration increased by day 2 or 4 postpartum. Administration of a large dose of estrogen at days 1 or 3 postpartum significantly increased the peroxidase concentration but, if administered along with cortisol, the estrogen-induced increase was prevented. Histochemical studies (Brokelman and Fawcett, 1969) had not been able to demonstrate endogenous uterine peroxidase in the early pregnant or lactating rat uterus. Our studies with lactating rats also indicated a suppression of biochemically assayable uterine peroxidase.

Lucas *et al.* (1964) assayed the peroxidase content of human endometrial brushings from 150 women and found a cyclic variation which, unlike the variation in the rat, reached a peak during the progesterone-dominant period. Using a method that effected a physical separation of excised human endometrium into stromal and glandular elements, Gurpide's laboratory (Holinka and Gurpide, 1980) found the peroxidase activity limited to the glandular tissue and confirmed the maximum peroxidase content during the secretory stage of the menstrual cycle. Our initial studies detected biochemically assayable, salt-extractable peroxidase activity throughout the

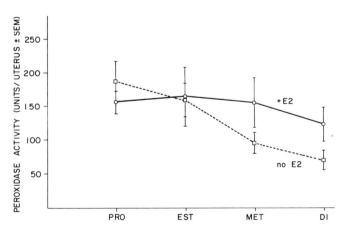

FIG. 16. Variation of rat uterine peroxidase content during the estrous cycle and after estradiol treatment. Groups of 5 to 10 female rats for each stage of the estrous cycle were assayed for uterine peroxidase activity directly (dashed line) or given an injection of 5 μg estradiol and their uterine peroxidase activity assayed 20 hours later (solid line). [From DeSombre and Lyttle (1979).]

menstrual cycle, with generally higher content evident in secretory endo-
metria. Our recent results (Press *et al.*, 1983a), combining biochemical and
morphological assays for peroxidase, indicate that there is a major exogenous
source of enzyme, the biochemical quantity of which is directly proportional
to the number of granulocytes in the endometrial sample; there is also a
second endogenous source evident essentially only in secretory-stage samples, which is found in the endometrial epithelial cells. Tsibris *et al.* (1982)
recently reported results of a study to determine the peroxidase activity in
human uteri as a function of location from the oviductal end to the endocervix. These workers, using only biochemical assay of salt-extractable activity,
found the highest activity in the sections closest to the endocervix. A recent
study in our laboratory (Press *et al.*, 1983b) confirms these results by biochemical assay and suggests that such a distribution, in fact, correlates well
with the distribution of peroxidase associated with granulocytes present in
the uterus. When the peroxidase activity was studied in sections along the
mature rat uterus (Affleck *et al.*, 1981), the highest activity was also found
near the cervical end of the uterus, consistent with our observations (King *et
al.*, 1981) that there tended to be more eosinophils in this region of the rat
uterus as well. Despite the complications due to granulocytic peroxidase in
the uterus, we have found endogenous peroxidase in endometrial hyper-
plasia and carcinoma (Press *et al.*, 1983b).

Several studies have attempted to measure the peroxidase concentration
of human cervical mucus as a putative, readily assayed marker of ovulation.
It would appear that while there are dramatic variations in the peroxidase
concentration in cervical mucus, it does not appear to be a reliable marker of
ovulation (Shindler *et al.*, 1977) nor does it show a consistent variation with
the stage of the menstrual cycle (Blain *et al.*, 1975). Despite the difficulty in
obtaining large quantities of peroxidase from this source, Shindler *et al.*
(1977) carried out a characterization of the enzyme from cervical mucus and
found its properties to be similar to a classical hemoprotein, peroxidase. A
preliminary report based on data from 14 menstrual cycles of 6 women
suggested that the concentration of salivary peroxidase may rise at about the
time of ovulation (Cockle and Harkness, 1978).

## IV. OTHER TISSUES AND TUMORS

### A. MAMMARY GLAND

While it is obvious that other tissues, like the spleen and thyroid, contain
substantial concentrations of peroxidase, their content is generally independent of estrogen modulation (Lyttle and DeSombre, 1977b). Likewise, nei-

ther the pituitary (Anderson *et al.*, 1975a; Lyttle and DeSombre, 1977b) nor the hypothalamus (Anderson *et al.*, 1975a) showed peroxidase activity, leading to the suggestion that peroxidase may be a marker for tissues showing growth dependence on estrogen (Anderson *et al.*, 1975a).

Peroxidase activity associated with bovine milk and mammary gland has been known for some time, and the purification of the enzyme from milk was reported in 1963 (Morrison and Hultquist). More recently, by using antibodies to purified bovine peroxidase and immunofluorescence, it was shown that there was an antigenic relationship of the peroxidases of the bovine mammary gland, sublingual gland, and lacrimal gland as well as peripheral leukocytes (Harada *et al.*, 1973). The peroxidase was found in the ductal epithelia of these glands. Using ultrastructural methods with the diaminobenzidine reaction product, Anderson *et al.* (1975b) demonstrated that the subcellular localization of peroxidase in the rat mammary gland is similar to that found in the uterus. These workers found peroxidase staining in the mammary glands of prelactating and lactating rats and reported that the staining was diminished or absent in mammary glands of hypophysectomized or ovariectomized rats as well as during early pregnancy and in nonpregnant rats. These results were confirmed by Strum (1978b), who tried to elicit increased peroxidase activity in mammary glands by administration of hormones. Although she observed some peroxidase activity in mammary glands of a few rats injected with estrogen, mouse mammary glands in organ culture appeared to respond to combinations of dexamethasone and insulin alone or with prolactin. Chan and Shyamala (1981), who studied the regulation of mouse mammary gland peroxidase by biochemical assay of salt extracts, found an entirely different pattern of incidence of peroxidase since they reported activity in mammary glands of intact virgin mice. This activity was reduced by ovariectomy and elevated greater than threefold by administration of estradiol. In fact, these workers found little or no activity in mammary glands of lactating mice and no change when such animals were ovariectomized or estrogen treated. Obviously, further studies, preferably using both biochemical and morphological techniques, will be needed to clarify this conflict. Strum (1978a) also reported iodination occurring in late pregnant and lactating mammary glands of rats to which radiolabeled iodide had been administered, activity that correlated with cytochemical evidence for peroxidase in the glands.

## B. MAMMARY TUMORS

There has been considerable interest as to whether peroxidase might provide a useful marker for hormone dependence in breast cancer. Our original studies of the DMBA-induced rat mammary cancer suggested that, with histochemical techniques, the hormone-dependent tumors in intact and estrogen-treated rats showed peroxidase localization similar to what had been seen in the rodent uterus (Anderson *et al.*, 1975a; DeSombre *et al.*, 1975). Although the concentration of peroxidase extractable from such tumors varied widely, it provided a good source of the enzyme for purification (DeSombre and Lyttle, 1978b). Strum and Becci (1979) found that only some of the apparently hormone-dependent, DMBA-induced rat mammary tumors they studied contained histochemically detectable peroxidase, and they reported that all of the NMU-induced rat mammary tumors were peroxidase negative. Penney *et al.* (1980) found a higher peroxidase activity, as well as higher estrogen and progestin receptor concentrations, in the ovary-dependent, DMBA-induced rat mammary tumors than in several ovary-independent transplantable rat mammary tumor cell lines. Several authors, studying the effects of various antiestrogens on DMBA-induced mammary tumors, reported opposite effects of the antiestrogens on tumor growth and biochemically assayed tumor peroxidase activity. Rorke and Katzenellenbogen (1981) found that both the antiestrogens, CI628 and U23469, and their demethylated metabolites administered to DMBA-induced, tumor-bearing rats for 25–30 days were able to cause tumor regression and, on average, appeared to cause increased peroxidase activity in the tumors that showed very large individual variations in peroxidase concentration. Studying the effect of tamoxifen in the same tumor system, Levy *et al.* (1981b) reported that tumor peroxidase content increased substantially, while the tumors regressed and the tumor estrogen- and progestin-receptor concentrations decreased. In fact, these workers (Levy *et al.*, 1981a) indicate that in DMBA-induced tumors there is an inverse relationship between tumor peroxidase, on the one hand, and tumor growth, estrogen, and progestin receptors on the other.

A recent study compared the biochemical and histochemical assays of density-banded cells from DMBA-induced rat mammary tumors as well as from normal and lactating rat mammary glands (Brightwell and Tseng, 1982). These investigators found that with increasing cell density there was a greater percentage of histochemically peroxidase-positive cells, an increased biochemically assayable peroxidase activity, and an increased proportion of granulocytes. These results suggest that some of the divergent results reported for peroxidase activity in the mammary tumors and mammary glands may relate to the presence or amounts of granulocytic peroxidase.

In the transplantable R3230AC rat mammary tumors, Rorke and Katzenellenbogen (1980) found that both estrogen and antiestrogen, U11100A, separately administered stimulated tumor peroxidase activity. With concomitant estrogen and U11100A treatment, the somewhat lower tumor-peroxidase content effected by the antiestrogen alone was found.

Although the total peroxidase activity found in the hormone-responsive GR mouse tumor by biochemical assay was significantly lower than the activity found in the DMBA-induced rat tumors, we found that both the peroxidase activity and the iodide uptake of the hormone-independent counterpart was significantly lower yet (Lyttle *et al.*, 1979b). However, using a cytochemical method, Strum and Becci (1979) were unable to demonstrate endogenous peroxidase in any of the mouse mammary tumors they examined, including the GR mouse tumors. It is not clear at present whether the differences between the biochemical and cytochemical studies of peroxidase relate to different sensitivities, different sources of enzyme (i.e., exogenous versus endogenous), or to destruction of enzyme during fixation. The latter suggestion was made by Anderson *et al.* (1975b) from their study of the cytochemical localization of peroxidase in the rat mammary gland, where they indicated that the formaldehyde–glutaraldehyde fixation may not allow optimal visualization of endogenous peroxidase.

Human breast cancers also have biochemically detectable peroxidase activity (Lyttle and DeSombre, 1977b). Although initial studies (Duffy and Duffy, 1977) correlating the presence of estrogen receptor and peroxidase activity in breast cancer looked promising, more recent results indicate that biochemically assayed peroxidase activity does not correlate with estrogen or progestin receptor content (Collins and Savage, 1979; Keenan *et al.*, 1979a,b). In fact, our more recent studies indicate that in the human breast cancer samples, biochemical assay of salt-extractable peroxidase seemed to correlate better with tumors lacking both estrogen and progestin receptor (E. R. DeSombre, J. Leinen, and C. R. Lyttle, unpublished observations). This would be consistent with exogenous enzyme predominating, since there is some evidence that leukocyte infiltration may occur more frequently in receptor-negative breast cancers.

## C. OVARY

Peroxidase has been identified in the rat ovary by both biochemical and histochemical methods. Agrawal and Laloraya (1977) reported an inverse relationship between ascorbate depletion and peroxidase in a time-course study of LH treatment. Since ascorbate is an inhibitor of peroxidase activity, modulation of ascorbate could give the appearance of peroxidase activity changes. However, using a histochemical procedure, these same investigators (Agrawal and Laloraya, 1978) found peroxidase activity in the corpus luteum but not in the growing follicles of immature or mature rats.

### D. HAMSTER KIDNEY

The hamster kidney has been known for some time to be susceptible to induction of hormone-responsive tumors on chronic treatment, especially of male animals, with high doses of DES (Kirkman, 1959). An hypothesis was proposed that the organospecific activity of DES in the kidney may relate to the bioactivation of DES by the enzyme peroxidase (Metzler and McLachlan, 1978b). In this regard it has been reported that the kidney of the hamster, in contrast to that of the rat or mouse, does possess peroxidase activity (McLachlan *et al.*, 1978). Moreover, hamster kidney peroxidase levels were higher in the male, the susceptible animals, than in females. In the female hamster the renal peroxidase activity was lower in the late pregnant hamster than in the nonpregnant; this is at least consistent with the progesterone suppression of peroxidase expression seen in the rat. Combined with the evidence that rodent uterine, as well as horseradish, peroxidase oxidizes DES to β-dienestrol, a major, reactive *in vivo* metabolite of DES, the proposed role of peroxidase in the mediation of DES-induced hamster renal carcinoma seems tenable (Metzler and McLachlan, 1978a).

## V. UTERINE EOSINOPHILIA

Uterine eosinophilia is a well-documented phenomenon (Bjersing and Borglin, 1964; Brokelman and Fawcett, 1969; Tchernitchin *et al.*, 1976), and the estradiol inactivating capability of extracts containing uterine peroxidase was also reproduced by extracts of eosinophils (Klebanoff, 1965). Despite the early recognition of the presence of eosinophils in the uterus and despite the recognition of the dramatic increase in eosinophils in the rat uterus after estrogen administration (Tchernitchin *et al.*, 1974), there was little quantitative data on the proportion of the total uterine peroxidase that comes from eosinophils and that resulting from the estrogen-dependent increase in the endogenous enzyme of the uterine epithelium. We studied this problem recently (King *et al.*, 1981) and concluded that by far the greater part of the total, biochemically assayed rat uterine peroxidase activity can be ascribed to the exogenous enzyme brought to the uterus by eosinophils. Experiments were carried out with rats treated under a variety of conditions which modulate biochemically assayable peroxidase activity, comparing the biochemically assayable peroxidase of one uterine horn with the number of eosinophils found in the contralateral horn (Fig. 17). Despite the widely differing total peroxidase activities found under the variety of conditions tested, there was very good agreement between these parameters. After determining the average peroxidase activity per rat eosinophil by assay of

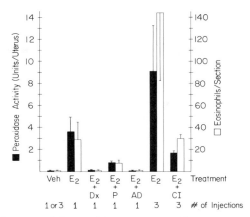

FIG. 17. Effect of various inhibitors of the uterine peroxidase response to estradiol on uterine eosinophilia. Immature female rats were treated with 5 μg estradiol ($E_2$) alone or in combination with 100 μg progesterone (P), 100 μg dexamethasone (Dx), 150 μg actinomycin D (AD), or 200 μg CI628 (CI). Twenty hours after the last injections, the animals were sacrificed and the uterus from each animal separated into the two individual horns, one of which was assayed histologically for eosinophil content (open bars) and the other assayed biochemically for peroxidase (solid bars). [From King *et al.* (1981).]

the peroxidase activity of a preparation of eosinophils purified from peritoneal lavage, the calculated peroxidase due to eosinophils, obtained from eosinophil counts in one uterine horn, was compared with the quantity of biochemically assayable peroxidase in the other horn in animals treated with estrogen alone or with estrogen and the antiestrogen CI628. The results showed a good quantitative relationship between the two peroxidase amounts (King *et al.*, 1981). Furthermore, when several methods were used to separate rat uterine epithelium from the stroma and the myometrium, we found the major amounts of peroxidase were associated with the stroma–myometrium fraction, where the infiltrating eosinophils are found, and less than 5% of the total peroxidase activity remained with purified epithelium under conditions where >95% of the peroxidase activity of the intact uterus could be accounted for. These data, especially when considered with previously mentioned phenomena such as the substantial effects of corticoids on the inhibition of uterine eosinophilia (Tchernitchin *et al.*, 1975; see Section II,A,3), lead us to conclude that the major part of the biochemically assayable uterine peroxidase is due to hormone-regulated changes in the uterine content of eosinophils. It is still necessary to elucidate the nature of this hormone modulation of uterine eosinophilia. It is entirely possible that under estrogen control the uterus may synthesize a chemotactic agent that is directly responsible for the attraction of eosinophils to the uterus. The results, described earlier, indicating the emetine and actinomycin D inhibition of estrogen-dependent increases in uterine peroxidase, would be consistent with such a mechanism.

## VI. PEROXIDASE PURIFICATION

Several laboratories have purified peroxidases extracted from rat uterus or mammary tumors. Jellinck's laboratory purified the portion of uterine peroxidase extractable with 1.2 $M$ NaCl, reporting a molecular weight of about 40,000 and an approximate 40-fold increase in specific activity after salt precipitation and gel filtration (McNabb and Jellinck, 1975; Jellinck *et al.*, 1976). After finding that uterine peroxidase activity could be more completely solubilized with 0.5 $M$ calcium chloride (Lyttle and DeSombre, 1977a), we were able to achieve about a 6000-fold purification of rat uterine peroxidase by a combination of Con A–Sepharose affinity chromatography, hydrophobic interaction chromatography on phenyl Sepharose, and gel filtration on G200 (DeSombre and Lyttle, 1980c). Due to an approximately fourfold increase in the total assayable uterine peroxidase on calcium chloride extraction, we were able to obtain a greater than 50% recovery of the apparent initial activity in the uterine homogenate. Despite the high degree of purification and the largely single band of protein-stained product on SDS electrophoresis under denaturing conditions, the enzyme still aggregated when exposed to low salt under nondenaturing conditions. In the presence of calcium chloride, the molecular weight by gel filtration appeared to be around 50,000 (Lyttle and DeSombre, 1977a). Like Jellinck *et al.* (1976), who found that CETAB could replace salt with the NaCl-extracted rat uterine enzyme, Hosoya and Saito (1981) purified both the rat uterine enzyme and a NaCl-extracted peroxidase from rat eosinophils by CM-cellulose chromatography in the presence of CETAB. They found similar elution characteristics and molecular weights (about 40,000) for the extracted uterine and eosinophil enzymes, consistent with observations described in the previous section. Interestingly, these workers found that the CM-cellulose elution pattern of the peroxidase found in uterine luminal fluid was different than the salt-extracted uterine or eosinophil enzymes. The cyanide difference spectra found for these three sources of enzyme were found to be similar, although the molecular weight of the uterine fluid peroxidase (90,000) was larger and the enzyme was less resistant to excess peroxide than that of the salt-extracted enzymes (Hosoya and Saito, 1981). Further study of the purified uterine fluid enzyme (Hosoya *et al.*, 1981) indicated that while the spectral properties were similar to those of lactoperoxidase, the uterine enzyme had distinctly .different substrate specificity, pH optima, and isoelectric point. When the uterine fluid enzyme was studied by microelectrophoresis (Burnett *et al.*, 1978), up to about 10 peaks in the pH range 4.5–5.9 were found. These workers also reported that the native enzyme, of molecular weight around 100,000, could be separated into two subunits of about 70,000 and less than 20,000. Like the extracted enzyme, the uterine fluid enzyme was found to bind to Con A–Sepharose (Burnett *et al.*, 1978).

Olsen and Little (1979), using calcium chloride extraction of uteri of estradiol-treated mature Wistar rats, found two molecular-weight forms (92,000 and 40,000) of uterine peroxidase in the presence of CETAB. Despite the different molecular weights, the two enzymes showed similar properties. Subsequently, these investigators purified the smaller of these two uterine enzymes some 300-fold (Olsen and Little, 1981). They report that the final product, purified by methods identical to those we reported (DeSombre and Lyttle, 1980c), was >95% homogenous, had a molecular weight of about 48,000, and had an absorption maximum and specific activity similar to other hemoprotein peroxidases. Using similar methods, we had earlier obtained a 600-fold purification of the calcium chloride extracted enzyme from DMBA-induced rat mammary cancers (DeSombre and Lyttle, 1978b). This enzyme also had an apparent molecular weight of about 50,000.

In view of the earlier discussion of the probably significant contributions of eosinophil peroxidase to both rat uterine and tumor peroxidase extracted with salt and assayed biochemically, it is apparent that the above purifications must have contained both endogenous uterine epithelial enzyme and exogenous eosinophilic enzyme. The data available (Hosoya and Saito, 1981) suggest that the enzyme extracted from rat uteri and eosinophils are very similar. Recent data (Keeping and Lyttle, 1982) indicated that monoclonal antibody prepared against purified calcium chloride extracted rat uterine peroxidase reacted with peroxidase extracted from rat spleen. This result would imply that either the enzyme purified from the uterus was an eosinophilic peroxidase or at least it showed antigenic similarity to the enzyme from the spleen.


## VII. SUMMARY

Estrogens effect dose-dependent increases in the peroxidase activity in the uterus and certain other tissues of experimental animals. There appears to be a good correlation between the uterotrophic activity of various estrogens and the extent of the increases in uterine peroxidase. Antiestrogens show some agonist activity but in general are potent inhibitors of the estrogen-dependent increases in uterine peroxidase. Both progestins and glucocorticoids are effective inhibitors of estrogen-dependent increases in uterine peroxidase, and the dose dependence suggests that the less-effective progestins may be acting as weak glucocorticoids. During early postnatal development, the rat shows its first response to estrogen with increases in both uterine weight and peroxidase at exactly the same time (12–13 days). In the mature animal, cyclic changes in uterine peroxidase occur during the estrous cycle, with the highest content present during proestrus and estrus. Similar concentrations of uterine peroxidase to those of the mature rat can be elicited in the castrate rat by daily administration of estradiol for 5–7 days.

Hormone-regulated peroxidase activity is also found in the normal and the neoplastic rodent mammary gland, in rat ovary, and in the hamster kidney. Biochemically assayable peroxidase, also found in human breast cancer, does not appear to be a reliable marker for hormone responsiveness in rodent or human mammary cancer, however. The often-elevated peroxidase content of receptor-negative cancers may relate to granulocyte infiltration, thus complicating simple interpretation of extractable peroxidase activity.

Although it has been recognized for some time that estrogens effect substantial eosinophilia in the rodent uterus, recent studies suggest that uterine eosinophils constitute the major source of biochemically detected uterine peroxidase. Morphologic studies, which can clearly identify the endogenous epithelial enzyme, have confirmed an estrogen-dependent stimulation of endogenous uterine enzyme in the rodent but suggest a progestin dependence in the human. While peroxidase activity has been found in human cervical mucus, it does not appear to be a usable indicator of ovulation.

Rat uterine peroxidases have been purified by several investigators. While several forms have been isolated from extracts of uterine tissue and somewhat different forms identified in uterine fluids, all appear to share general characteristics of hemoprotein peroxidases. While the role of the enzyme in hormone-responsive tissues is unknown at the present time, the clear hormonal modulation of both endogenous and exogenous forms of uterine peroxidase make it a marker enzyme of interest.

## ACKNOWLEDGMENTS

The investigations in our laboratory were supported by grants from the American Cancer Society (RD84 and BC279), the National Cancer Institute (CA09183, CA21525, and CA27476), and the National Institute of Child Health and Human Development (HD15513).

## REFERENCES

Affleck, A., Keeping, H. S., Newcombe, A. M., and Jellinck, P. H. (1981). *Acta Endocrinol. (Copenhagen)* **98**, 609.
Agrawal, P., and Laloraya, M. M. (1977). *Biochem. J.* **166**, 205.

Agrawal, P., and Laloraya, M. M. (1978). *Acta Anat.* **102,** 94.
Anderson, W. A., Kang, Y., and DeSombre, E. R. (1975a). *J. Cell Biol.* **64,** 668.
Anderson, W. A., Trantalis, J. and Kang, Y. (1975b). *J. Histochem. Cytochem.* **23,** 295.
Anderson, W. A., DeSombre, E. R., and Kang, Y. (1977). *Biol. Reprod.* **16,** 409.
Baquer, N. Z., and McClean, P. (1972). *Biochem. Biophys. Res. Commun.* **48,** 729.
Beato, M. (ed.) (1980). *In* "Steroid Induced Uterine Proteins." Elsevier, New York.
Bjersing, L., and Borglin, N. E. (1964). *Acta Pathol. Microbiol. Scand.* **60,** 27.
Blain, J. A., Heald, P. J., Mack, A. E., and Shaw, C. E. (1975). *Contraception* **11,** 677.
Brightwell, J., and Tseng, M. T. (1982). *Cancer Res.* **42,** 4562.
Brokelman, J. (1969). *J. Histochem. Cytochem.* **17,** 394.
Brokelman, J. and Fawcett, D. W. (1969). *Biol. Reprod.* **1,** 59.
Burnett, C. C. P., Anderson, W. A., and Ruchel, R. (1978). *J. Histochem. Cytochem.* **26,** 382.
Chan, J. K., and Shyamala, G. (1981). *Proc. 72nd Annu. Meet. Am. Assoc. Cancer Res.,*
    Washington, D.C., p. 12 (Abstract).
Churg, A., and Anderson, W. A. (1974). *J. Cell Biol.* **62,** 449.
Clark, J. H., and Gorski, J. (1970). *Science* **169,** 76.
Cockle, S. M., and Harkness, R. A. (1978). *Br. J. Obstet. Gynecol.* **85,** 776.
Collins, J. R., and Savage, N. (1979). *Br. J. Cancer* **40,** 500.
DeSombre, E. R., and Lyttle, C. R. (1978a). *In* "Hormones, Receptors and Breast Cancer" (W.
    L. McGuire, ed.), p. 181. Raven, New York.
DeSombre, E. R., and Lyttle, C. R. (1978b). *Cancer Res.* **38,** 4086.
DeSombre, E. R., and Lyttle, C. R. (1979). *In* "Steroid Hormone Receptor Systems" (W. W.
    Leavitt and J. H. Clark, eds.), p. 157. Plenum, New York.
DeSombre, E. R., and Lyttle, C. R. (1980a). *In* "Perspectives in Steroid Receptor Research"
    (F. Bresciani, ed.), p. 167. Raven, New York.
DeSombre, E. R., and Lyttle, C. R. (1980b). *In* "Steroid Induced Uterine Proteins" (M. Beato,
    ed.), p. 283. Elsevier, New York.
DeSombre, E. R., and Lyttle, C. R. (1980c). *In* "The Endometrium" (F. A. Kimball, ed.), p.
    247. Spectrum, New York.
DeSombre, E. R., Anderson, W. A., and Kang, Y. (1975). *Cancer Res.* **35,** 173.
Duffy, M. J., and Duffy, G. (1977). *Biochem. Soc. Trans.* **5,** 1738.
Harada, T., Baba, M., and Morikawa, S. (1973). *J. Histochem. Cytochem.* **21,** 804.
Hayes, J. R., Rorke, E. A., Robertson, D. W., Katzenellenbogen, B. S., and Katzenellen-
    bogen, J. A. (1981). *Endocrinology (Baltimore)* **108,** 164.
Holinka, C. F., and Gurpide, E. (1980). *Am. J. Obstet. Gynecol.* **138,** 599.
Hosoya, T., and Saito, T. (1981). *J. Biochem. (Tokyo)* **89,** 203.
Hosoya, T., Sasaki, K., and Wagai, N. (1981). *J. Biochem. (Tokyo)* **89,** 1453.
Jellinck, P. H., and Lyttle, C. R. (1972). *In* "Advances in Enzyme Regulation" (G. Weber, ed.),
    Vol. 11, p. 17. Pergamon, New York.
Jellinck, P. H., and Newcombe, A. (1977). *J. Endocrinol.* **74,** 147.
Jellinck, P. H., and Newcombe, A. M. (1980a). *Biochem. Pharmacol.* **29,** 3031.
Jellinck, P. H., and Newcombe, A. M. (1980b). *J. Steroid Biochem.* **13,** 681.
Jellinck, P. H., McNabb, T., Cleveland, S., and Lyttle, C. R. (1976). *In* "Advances in Enzyme
    Regulation" (G. Weber, ed.), Vol. 14, p. 447. Pergamon, New York.
Jellinck, P. H., Newcombe, A., and Keeping, H. S. (1979). *In* "Advances in Enzyme Regula-
    tion" (G. Weber, ed.), Vol. 17, p. 325. Pergamon, New York.
Kang, Y., Anderson, W. A., and DeSombre, E. R. (1975). *J. Cell Biol.* **64,** 682.
Kaye, A. M. (1978). *In* "Biochemical Action of the Hormones" (G. Litwack, ed.), Vol. V, p. 149.
    Academic Press, New York.
Keenan, E. J., Bacon, D. R., and Garrison, L. B. (1979a). *Pro. West. Pharmacol. Soc.* **22,** 277.

Keenan, E. J., Garrison, L. B., Kemp, E. D., Porter, J. M., Moseley, H. S., and Fletcher, W. S. (1979b). *Surg. Forum* **30**, 547.

Keeping, H. S., and Jellinck, P. H. (1980). *Biochim. Biophys. Acta* **632**, 150.

Keeping, H. S., and Lyttle, C. R. (1981). *Proc. 63rd Annu. Meet. Endocrine Soc.*, Cincinnati, Ohio, p. 158 (Abstract).

Keeping, H. S., and Lyttle, C. R. (1982). *Proc. 64th Annu. Meet. Endocrine Soc.*, San Francisco, California, p. 303 (Abstract).

Keeping, H. S., Newcombe, A., and Jellinck, P. H. (1982). *J. Steroid Biochem.* **16**, 45.

King, W. J., Allen, T. C., and DeSombre, E. R. (1981). *Biol. Reprod.* **25**, 859.

Kirkman, H. (1959). *Natl. Cancer Inst. Monogr.* **1**, 59.

Klebanoff, S. J. (1965). *Endocrinology (Baltimore)* **76**, 301.

Klebanoff, S. J. (1967). *J. Exp. Med.* **126**, 1063.

Leavitt, W. W., and Blaha, G. C. (1972). *Steroids* **19**, 263.

Lerner, L. J., Hothaus, F. J., Jr., and Thompson, C. R. (1958). *Endocrinology (Baltimore)* **63**, 295.

Levy, J., Burshell, A., Marbach, M., Afllalo, L., and Glick, S. M. (1980). *J. Endocrinol.* **84**, 371.

Levy, J., Liel, Y., and Glick, S. M. (1981a). *Isr. J. Med. Sci.* **17**, 970.

Levy, J., Liel, Y., Feldman, B., Afllallo, L., and Glick, S. (1981b). *Eur. J. Cancer Clin. Oncol.* **17**, 1023.

Little, M., Szendro, P., Teran, C., Hughes, A., and Jungblut, P. W. (1975). *J. Steroid Biochem.* **6**, 493.

Lucas, F. V., Neufeld, H. A., Utterback, J. G., Martin, A. P., and Stotz, E. (1955). *J. Biol. Chem.* **214**, 775.

Lucas, F. V., Carnes, V. M., Schmidt, H. J., Sipes, D. R., and Hall, D. G. (1964). *Am. J. Obstet. Gynecol.* **88**, 965.

Lyttle, C. R., and Jellinck, P. H. (1972). *Biochem. J.* **127**, 481.

Lyttle, C. R., and Jellinck, P. H. (1976). *Biochem. J.* **160**, 237.

Lyttle, C. R., and DeSombre, E. R. (1977a). *Proc. Natl. Acad. Sci. U.S.A.* **74**, 3162.

Lyttle, C. R., and DeSombre, E. R. (1977b). *Nature (London)* **268**, 337.

Lyttle, C. R., Garay, R. V., and DeSombre, E. R. (1979a). *J. Steroid Biochem.* **10**, 359.

Lyttle, C. R., Thorpe, S. M., DeSombre, E. R., and Daehnfeldt, J. L. (1979b). *J. Natl. Cancer Inst.* **62**, 1031.

McGuire, W. L., Raynaud, J. P., and Baulieu, E. E. (eds.) (1977). *In* "Progesterone Receptors in Normal and Neoplastic Tissues." Raven, New York.

McLachlan, J. A., Metzler, M., and Lamb, J. C. (1978). *Life Sci.* **23**, 2521.

McNabb, T., and Jellinck, P. H. (1975). *Biochem. J.* **151**, 275.

McNabb, T., and Jellinck, P. H. (1976). *Steroids* **27**, 681.

Martin, A. P., Neufeld, H. A., Lucas, F. V., and Stotz, E. (1958). *J. Biol. Chem.* **233**, 206.

Metzler, M., and McLachlan, J. A. (1978a). *Biochem. Biophys. Res. Commun.* **85**, 874.

Metzler, M., and McLachlan, J. A. (1978b). *J. Environ. Pathol. Toxicol.* **1**, 531.

Milgrom, E., Thi, L., Atger, M., and Baulieu, E. E. (1973). *J. Biol. Chem.* **248**, 6366.

Morrison, M., and Hultquist, D. E. (1963). *J. Biol. Chem.* **238**, 2847.

Myatt, L., Chaudhuri, G., Elder, M. G., and Lim, L. (1980). *J. Endocrinol.* **87**, 357.

Notides, A., and Gorski, J. (1966). *Proc. Natl. Acad. Sci. U.S.A.* **56**, 230.

Notides, A., Hamilton, D. E., and Auer, H. E. (1975). *J. Biol. Chem.* **250**, 3945.

Olsen, R. L., and Little, C. (1979). *Eur. J. Biochem.* **101**, 333.

Olsen, R. L., and Little, C. (1981). *Acta Chem. Scand. B* **35**, 1.

Penney, G. C., Scott, K. M., and Hawkins, R. A. (1980). *Br. J. Cancer* **41**, 648.

Porter, R. W. (1954). *Recent Prog. Horm. Res.* **10**, 1.

Press, M., Talerman, A., and DeSombre, E. R. (1983a), *J. Clin. Endocrinol. Metab.* **56**, 254.
Press, M., King. W., and DeSombre, E. R. (1983b), in preparation.
Rao, B. R., Wiest, W. G., and Allen, W. M. (1973). *Endocrinology (Baltimore)* **92**, 1229.
Raynaud, J. (1973). *Steroids* **21**, 249.
Reiss, N. A., and Kaye, A. M. (1981). *J. Biol. Chem.* **256**, 5741.
Revesz, C., Banik, U. K., and Herr, F. (1967). *Steroids* **10**, 291.
Robertson, D. W., Katzenellenbogen, J. A., Long, D. J., Rorke, E. A., and Katzenellenbogen, B. S. (1982). *J. Steroid Biochem.* **16**, 1.
Rorke, E. A., and Katzenellenbogen, B. S. (1980). *Cancer Res.* **40**, 3158.
Rorke, E. A., and Katzenellenbogen, B. S. (1981). *Cancer Res.* **41**, 1257.
Shindler, J. S., Haworth, K., Axon, A., Bardsley, W. G., Tindall, V. R., and Laing, I. (1977). *J. Reprod. Fertil.* **51**, 413.
Smith, E. R., and Barker, K. L. (1974). *J. Biol. Chem.* **249**, 6541.
Smith, D. C., and Klebanoff, S. J. (1970). *Biol. Reprod.* **3**, 229.
Sonnenschein, C., and Soto, A. M. (1977). *J. Steroid Biochem.* **9**, 533.
Steinsapir, J., Rojao, A. M., Mena, M., and Tchernitchin, A. N. (1982). *Endocrinology (Baltimore)* **110**, 1773.
Strum, J. M. (1978a). *Anat. Rec.* **192**, 235.
Strum, J. M. (1978b). *Tissue Cell* **10**, 505.
Strum, J. M., and Becci, P. J. (1979). *Virchows Arch. B.* **31**, 135.
Sutherland, R. L., and Jordan, V. C. (eds.) (1981). *In* "Non-Steroidal Antiestrogens: Molecular Pharmacology and Antitumor Activity." Academic Press, New York.
Tchernitchin, A. (1979). *J. Steroid Biochem.* **11**, 417.
Tchernitchin, X., Tchernitchin, A., and Galand, P. (1976). *Differentiation* **5**, 151.
Tchernitchin, A., Roorijck, J., Tchernitchin, X., Vandenhende, J., and Galand, P. (1974). *Nature (London)* **248**, 142.
Tchernitchin, A., Roorijck, J., Tchernitchin, X., Vandenhende, J., and Galand, P. (1975). *Mol. Cell. Endocrinol.* **2**, 331.
Tseng, L., and Gurpide, E. (1974). *Endocrinology (Baltimore)* **94**, 419.
Tsibris, J. C. M., Trujillo, Y. P., Fernandez, B. B., Bardawil, W. A., Kunigk, A., and Spellacy, W. N. (1982). *J. Clin. Endocrinol. Metab.* **54**, 991.
Vass, M. A., and Green, B. (1982). *J. Steroid Biochem.* **16**, 125.
Woessner, J. F., and Ryan, J. N. (1980). *J. Endocrinol.* **85**, 387.

# CHAPTER 12

# Inactivation, Activation, and Stabilization of Glucocorticoid Receptors

*Paul R. Housley, Joseph F. Grippo, Mary K. Dahmer, and William B. Pratt*

Department of Pharmacology
The University of Michigan School of Medicine
Ann Arbor, Michigan

BIOCHEMICAL ACTIONS OF HORMONES, VOL. XI
Copyright © 1984 by Academic Press, Inc.
ISBN 0-12-452811-2

There is now considerable evidence that unoccupied glucocorticoid receptors exist in at least two forms, an active steroid-binding form and an inactive nonbinding form. Unoccupied receptors can be inactivated and reactivated in both intact cells and cytosol preparations, and the active binding state of the receptor in cytosol is affected by Group VIA transition metal oxides, like molybdate and vanadate, and by two endogenous heat-stable activities. It is our purpose in this chapter to briefly review the role of phosphorylation and sulfur reduction in maintaining the steroid-binding state of the receptor and to summarize our studies on molybdate and the endogenous heat-stable factors.

It is important to note at the outset that we will use the term "activation" throughout this chapter to describe the process whereby the receptor is converted from a nonbinding form to a form that binds steroids. This is different from the use of the term "activation" to describe the process whereby the steroid-bound receptor is converted to a form that binds to nuclei, DNA cellulose, etc. We use the term "transformation" to describe this latter process.

## I. ALTERATION OF SPECIFIC BINDING CAPACITY IN INTACT CELLS

### A. ENERGY DEPENDENCE OF GLUCOCORTICOID-BINDING CAPACITY

In the first report demonstrating the existence of glucocorticoid receptors, Munck and Brinck-Johnsen (1968) showed that specific glucocorticoid binding in intact rat thymic lymphocytes is reduced by deprivation of oxygen and glucose and returns to normal when aerobic conditions are restored. The alterations in binding are accompanied by a similar loss and reappearance of cellular ATP. Thymocytes regain specific binding even in the presence of cycloheximide (Bell and Munck, 1973), suggesting that new protein synthesis is not required for receptor reactivation. On the basis of these obser-

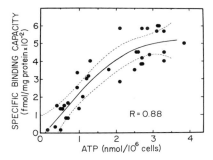

FIG. 1. Relationship between specific glucocorticoid-binding capacity and the amount of ATP in IM-9 human lymphocytes. The specific glucocorticoid-binding capacity assayed in low speed (27,000 g) supernatants prepared from cells incubated with or without glucose and oxygen has been plotted against the ATP content assayed in the same cell suspensions. The solid line represents a least-squares regression of the data and the dashed lines represent the 95% confidence limits for the regression. [From Wheeler *et al.* (1981).]

vations, Munck *et al.* (1972) proposed that the glucocorticoid receptor in thymocytes exists in two states and that energy (ATP) is required to convert the nonbinding form to the steroid-binding form.

This proposal is supported by other observations made in intact cells. When mouse fibroblasts (Ishii *et al.*, 1972), rat thymocytes (Rees and Bell, 1975), or chick embryo retina cells (Chader, 1973) are exposed to 2,4-dinitrophenol, glucocorticoid binding is lost. When the inhibitor is removed, steroid binding is restored, even if protein synthesis is inhibited (Ishii *et al.*, 1972; Chader, 1973; Sloman and Bell, 1976). It is clear from a recent study of glucocorticoid binding in IM-9 human lymphoblasts that the unoccupied receptor is readily inactivated and reactivated (Wheeler *et al.*, 1981). The striking correlation between glucocorticoid-binding capacity and ATP concentration in IM-9 cells is shown in Fig. 1. The fact that binding capacity can be altered raises the possibility that glucocorticoid receptors may be switched on and off in a rapid, reversible manner; and it is possible that a cell's capacity to respond to glucocorticoid could be modulated by altering the fraction of active receptors.

## B. THE MODEL OF THE RECEPTOR CYCLE

As the glucocorticoid receptor can be inactivated and activated in the absence of steroid and as steroid is required for association of the receptor with the nucleus, it is reasonable to infer that both inactivation and activation can take place in the cytoplasm of intact cells. When steroid is present,

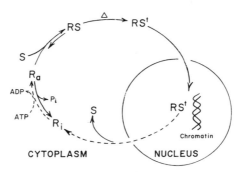

FIG. 2. Hypothetical cycle of events controlling the binding state and cellular location of the glucocorticoid receptor proposed by Munck *et al.* (1972) and Ishii *et al.* (1972). $R_i$, dephosphorylated form of the receptor that is inactive and cannot bind steroid; $R_a$, phosphorylated form of the receptor that binds steroids in the cytoplasm of the cell; RS, steroid–receptor complex; $RS^t$, transformed form of the steroid–receptor complex that can bind to nuclear components; S, steroid.

the bound glucocorticoid–receptor complex is transformed and translocated to the nucleus. The receptor can subsequently recycle back into the cytoplasm, but the rate at which binding capacity appears in the cytoplasmic fraction lags behind the rate at which specific binding is lost from the nucleus (Ishii *et al.*, 1972; Munck and Foley, 1976). This suggests that the receptor may exit from the nucleus in a form that does not bind steroid and be subsequently recycled into a steroid-binding form. Reappearance of binding capacity in the cytoplasm occurs even if protein synthesis is blocked, supporting the notion that the reappearance of glucocorticoid-binding capacity in the cytoplasm reflects receptor recycling and not new receptor synthesis.

These observations and the observation that glucocorticoid binding in intact cells is dependent on energy have led to the model of the receptor cycle presented in Fig. 2 (Munck *et al.*, 1972; Ishii *et al.*, 1972). In the model it is suggested that a receptor may participate in more than one cycle of gene activation. The model has been derived from studies in glucocorticoid-responsive systems and only a few studies with other steroids address the predictions of the model. Many investigators have felt that estrogen receptors, for example, are not recycled to the cytoplasm and that reappearance of cytoplasmic binding necessarily represents new receptor synthesis (Jungblut *et al.*, 1976; Horwitz and McGuire, 1978). It has recently been shown, however, that estrogen-receptor recycling can occur in intact uterine cells (Kassis and Gorski, 1981).

As Munck and Leung (1977) have noted, if the binding capacity in the cell is regenerated cyclically with an input of energy, that energy must be released cyclically through an irreversible step. Several years ago we suggested (Nielsen *et al.*, 1977a) that the energy-dependent step in the receptor cycle might represent phosphorylation of the inactive receptor to yield the active steroid-binding form. If this is the case, then receptor dephosphorylation must occur somewhere in the cycle. The site of receptor dephosphorylation has not been indicated in the model. We have proposed that the steroid–receptor complex may be dephosphorylated in the cytoplasm during temperature-mediated transformation (Sando *et al.*, 1979a), but it is also possible that dephosphorylation occurs in the nucleus and is related to release of the receptor from this compartment (Auricchio and Migliaccio, 1980). Glucocorticoid receptors must be reduced in order to bind steroids (Rees and Bell, 1975; Granberg and Ballard, 1977), and the sulfhydryl group requirement for binding is not indicated in the model of Fig. 2. As cellular metabolism is required to produce reducing equivalents, however, sulfur reduction is another potential energy-dependent process that is required for maintenance of the steroid-binding state in intact cells.

Before discussing our cell-free experiments on the roles of phosphorylation and sulfur reduction in determining binding capacity, we will review the evidence that steroid receptors are phosphorylated by intact cells. It is now clear that at least two steroid receptors are phosphoproteins.

## II. RECEPTOR PHOSPHORYLATION BY INTACT CELLS

### A. PHOSPHORYLATION OF THE GLUCOCORTICOID RECEPTOR

The glucocorticoid receptor from mouse L cells is a 92,000 dalton protein that can be readily identified by covalent labeling of the receptor site with [³H]dexamethasone 21-mesylate and separation of cytosol proteins on sodium dodecyl sulfate–polyacrylamide gel electrophoresis (SDS–PAGE). Dexamethasone 21-mesylate is a glucocorticoid derivative developed by Simons *et al.* (1980) that contains a reactive C-21 methanesulfonyl group. Dexamethasone mesylate has been demonstrated to be an affinity label for the glucocorticoid receptor of HTC cells (Simons and Thompson, 1981). In the experiment shown in Fig. 3, cytosol prepared from L929 mouse fibroblasts was incubated at 0° with radiolabeled dexamethasone 21-mesylate in the presence and absence of competing unlabeled dexamethasone and submitted to SDS–PAGE. The competing steroid completely prevents covalent labeling of the major receptor species migrating at $M_r$ 92,000.

In the experiment shown in Fig. 4, L cells in monolayer culture were grown in the presence of [³²P]orthophosphate for 18 hours prior to harvest. The glucocorticoid-binding proteins in cytosol were purified by affinity chro-

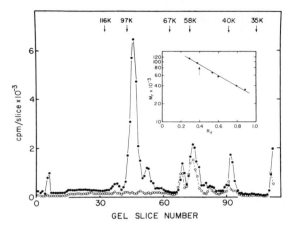

FIG. 3. SDS-polyacrylamide gel electrophoresis of [³H]dexamethasone mesylate labeled L cell cytosol. Cytosol was incubated at 0–4°C with 50 nM [³H]dexamethasone mesylate and either vehicle (●) or 50 μM unlabeled dexamethasone (○) and submitted to SDS gel electrophoresis. Sample lanes were cut into 1-mm slices, digested, and radioactivity was determined by liquid scintillation counting. The inset illustrates the standard curve used to obtain the $M_r$ of the covalently-labeled receptor using proteins of known $M_r$. [From Housley and Pratt (1983).]

matography on a column of deoxycorticosterone-agarose (G-K Biochemicals, Somerset, N.J.) and submitted to SDS–PAGE. In lane 1 the affinity column was eluted with 11α-cortisol, which has no glucocorticoid activity (Hackney *et al.*, 1970), and in lane 2 the active isomer 11β-cortisol was present. It is clear that the presence of the active glucocorticoid results in increased elution of the predominant phosphorylated band at $M_r \sim 92,000$. A small amount of a slightly larger phosphoprotein is also seen in lane 2 and this corresponds to the minor species of $M_r \sim 100,000$ that binds dexamethasone mesylate in a specific manner (Fig. 3). In addition to binding glucocorticoids in a stereospecific manner, these two phosphoproteins also bind them with high affinity. In lane 3, cytosol was incubated with 50 nM triamcinolone acetonide to occupy the binding sites prior to passage through the affinity column and elution with 11β-cortisol. This potent ligand in low concentration inhibits subsequent binding to the affinity column, and very little 92K phosphoprotein is obtained when the column is eluted with steroid-containing buffer. A cloned steroid-resistant L cell line that contains only 10% of the specific binding capacity of the parent strain was also incubated with [³²P]orthophosphate and the cytosol proteins were submitted to affinity chromatography. It is clear from lanes 4 and 5 that the resistant cells contain little of the 92K band and that none of the 100K species is detected with either isomer of cortisol.

Thus, L cells have been shown to produce a major phosphoprotein at 92K and a minor species at 100K. Both of these phosphoprotein species bind glucocorticoids in a high-affinity, stereospecific manner and both are

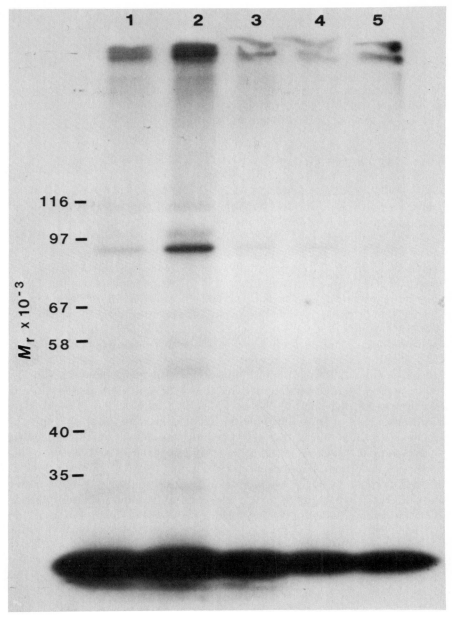

FIG. 4. Stereospecific elution of [32]P-labeled glucocorticoid receptor from deoxycorticosterone agarose. [32]P-labeled L cell cytosol was incubated with the affinity agarose to bind receptor and the column was eluted with the indicated isomer of cortisol. Following SDS-polyacrylamide gel electrophoresis, the [[32]P]phosphoproteins were visualized by autoradiography. Lane 1, elution with the physiologically inactive compound 11α-cortisol. Lane 2, elution with the active glucocorticoid 11β-cortisol. Lane 3, cytosol was preincubated with 50 n$M$ triamcinolone acetonide and then incubated with the affinity column and eluted with 11β-cortisol. Lane 4, 11α-cortisol elution of [32]P-labeled cytosol from glucocorticoid-resistant L cells. Lane 5, 11β-cortisol elution of [32]P-labeled cytosol from resistant L cells. [From Housley and Pratt (1983).]

markedly diminished in the glucocorticoid-resistant subline. As these proteins have the same $M_r$ and p$I$ as receptor identified by a site-specific affinity label, it is reasonable to conclude that the glucocorticoid receptor is a phosphoprotein. The receptor is phosphorylated on serine moieties, but it is not yet known how many phosphates there are per steroid-binding unit.

## B. PHOSPHORYLATION OF THE PROGESTERONE RECEPTOR

Weigel *et al.* (1981) first demonstrated that a steroid receptor could be phosphorylated by using the catalytic subunit of bovine cAMP-dependent protein kinase to phosphorylate purified hen progesterone receptor A and B subunits. Dougherty *et al.* (1982), however, have shown that the avian progesterone receptor is naturally phosphorylated. Progesterone receptor was purified by affinity chromatography, gel filtration, and DEAE–Sephadex chromatography from a tissue mince of hen oviduct incubated with [$^{32}$P]orthophosphate or from oviducts from chickens injected with [$^{32}$P]orthophosphate. Two progesterone-binding peaks are recovered from the DEAE column. The peak eluting at lower salt contains a major $^{32}$P-labeled protein of $M_r \sim$ 90–92K. The peak eluting at higher salt contains both the 90–92K phosphoprotein and a second species that migrates in SDS–PAGE at about 109K. The 90–92K phosphoprotein species that copurifies with the hen oviduct progesterone-binding activity is similar (and perhaps identical) in size to the 92K phosphoprotein that copurifies with the major glucocorticoid-binding activity of mouse fibroblasts. Like the glucocorticoid receptor, the progesterone receptor is phosphorylated on serine moieties. It is not known if the larger $M_r$ species in either system is a precursor of the 92K form or if it is the product of a different gene.

In the remainder of this chapter we will review studies in cell-free preparations that may contribute to an understanding of the role of phosphorylation and sulfur reduction in determining the steroid-binding state.

## III. RECEPTOR INACTIVATION IN CYTOSOL PREPARATIONS

### A. LABILITY OF GLUCOCORTICOID RECEPTORS

Unoccupied glucocorticoid receptors in cytosol preparations are extremely labile [e.g., rat liver (Koblinsky *et al.*, 1972), rabbit lung (Giannopoulos, 1976), rat thymocytes (Bell and Munck, 1973), mouse lymphosarcoma (Kirkpatrick *et al.*, 1972)]. The receptors are stabilized considerably when they are bound by glucocorticoids (Pratt and Ishii, 1972; Kirkpatrick *et al.*, 1972; Pratt *et al.*, 1975; Kaine *et al.*, 1975), and the degree of stabilization is roughly proportional to the binding affinity of the steroid (Nielsen *et al.*, 1977b). The rapid loss of binding activity in cytosol preparations prompted several early attempts at receptor stabilization. Because inactivation at higher temperatures is fast, all of the early studies were carried out at 0–4°C. At low temperature, the half-life of glucocorticoid-binding capacity in the very labile cytosol system prepared from rat thymocytes was increased somewhat by addition of EDTA (Bell and Munck, 1973) and high concentrations of glycerol (Schaumburg, 1972), and substantial stabilization was obtained with sulfhydryl protecting reagents (Rees and Bell, 1975). Some slowing of receptor inactivation in mouse fibroblast cytosol was obtained with phosphorylated sugars (Ishii and Aronow, 1973).

In papers published prior to 1975, it was suggested that glucocorticoid receptor inactivation reflected proteolysis, denaturation of the receptor protein (Ishii and Aronow, 1973; Schaumburg, 1972; Kirkpatrick *et al.*, 1972), or oxidation of one or more sulfhydryl groups required for binding (Rees and Bell, 1975). As will be described in subsequent sections of this chapter, oxidation of sulfhydryl moieties is an important component of temperature-mediated receptor inactivation. In some systems, like cytosol prepared from rat liver or mouse fibroblasts, however, the endogenous reducing activity is high, the rate of receptor inactivation is slower, and addition of sulfhydryl protecting reagents does not slow the rate further. As most of our work had been carried out with cytosols in which binding was not affected by addition of dithiothreitol (DTT), in our initial studies of binding lability we did not appreciate the role of sulfhydryl group oxidation in receptor inactivation. The first question we asked was whether the receptor was being inactivated enzymatically.

## B. Evidence for Phosphatase-Mediated Inactivation

### 1. Endogenous Receptor-Inactivating Enzyme Activity

As the activation energy for receptor inactivation is high for an enzymatic process (circa 20 kcal mol$^{-1}$; Schaumburg, 1972; Ishii and Aronow, 1973; Nielsen *et al.*, 1977b), investigators in this field had not looked for a receptor-inactivating enzyme. It had been known for some time that unoccupied glucocorticoid receptors in low-speed supernatants from broken cells were inactivated much more rapidly than receptors in high-speed supernatants (100,000 $g$ and greater). This suggested the existence of a membrane-associated receptor-inactivation process, and mixing experiments using membrane preparations as a source of inactivating activity and high-speed cytosol preparations as a source of receptor confirmed the existence of a membrane-bound glucocorticoid receptor-inactivating activity (Nielsen *et al.*, 1977b,c). The enzyme activity was partially purified from rat thymocyte membranes by lubrol solubilization followed by fractional polyethylene glycol precipitation and DEAE-cellulose chromatography. Neither the solubilized enzyme activity from thymocytes nor the membrane-associated activity from rat liver was affected by protease inhibitors, but their ability to inactivate the receptor was inhibited by a variety of phosphatase inhibitors, including fluoride, low-molecular-weight phosphorylated compounds, and molybdate (Nielsen *et al.*, 1977b,c; Sando *et al.*, 1979a).

Our crude membrane-containing fraction was prepared from rat thymocyte or liver cells, which had been ruptured by a method that also ruptures nuclei. We never determined whether the activity present in our crude microsomal preparation was possibly of nuclear origin. In this light, it is interesting to note that an estrogen receptor-inactivating enzyme activity has been identified in a crude nuclear pellet prepared from mouse and calf uteri (Auricchio and Migliaccio, 1980; Auricchio *et al.*, 1981c). The estrogen receptor-inactivating activity is not affected by protease inhibitors but is inhibited by a variety of inhibitors of phosphatase action. This enzyme activity has been reported to inactivate both unoccupied and estradiol-bound estrogen receptors but not receptors that are complexed with the nonsteroidal estrogen antagonists, nafoxidine and tamoxifen (Auricchio *et al.*, 1981a).

## 2. Inhibition of Inactivation by Phosphatase Inhibitors

Although the receptor-inactivating enzyme activity was first identified in a crude membrane fraction, it appears that similar or identical activity is also present in the soluble fraction of the cell. This is inferred from the observation that phosphatase inhibitors also stabilize the unbound receptor to endogenous inactivation in cytosol preparations. The relative effectiveness of several of these compounds in rat liver cytosol is illustrated in Fig. 5. Although molybdate is a phosphatase inhibitor, its ability to stabilize steroid receptors is due to a direct interaction with the receptor itself and its effects will be discussed in the next section. Fluoride produces significant stabilization of glucocorticoid-binding activity in cytosols prepared from a variety of sources, including rat liver (Nielsen *et al.*, 1977b,c), rat thymus (Sando *et al.* (1979a), mouse L cells (Nielsen *et al.*, 1977b), and human IM-9 lymphoblasts (Wheeler *et al.*, 1981). Fluoride also stabilizes the progesterone receptor in chick oviduct cytosol (Grody *et al.*, 1980) and prevents inactivation of the calf

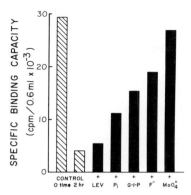

FIG. 5. Comparison of the effects of various inhibitors on the inactivation of the soluble glucocorticoid receptor of rat liver at 25°. Aliquots (0.45 ml) of rat liver cytosol were incubated for 2 hours at 25° with 1 m$M$ levamisole HCl (LEV), 10 m$M$ sodium phosphate ($P_1$), 10 m$M$ glucose-1-phosphate (G1P), 100 m$M$ sodium fluoride ($F^-$), 100 m$M$ sodium molybdate ($MoO_4^{2-}$), or vehicle (hatched bars). At zero time (control) and 2 hours (all conditions) specific binding capacity for triamcinolone acetonide was determined. [From Nielsen *et al.* (1977b).]

uterine estrogen receptor by the nuclear receptor-inactivating enzyme (Auricchio *et al.*, 1981a). We have presumed that fluoride stabilizes receptors via its ability to inhibit phosphatase activity, but this has not been proven and it is possible that fluoride interacts directly with the receptor itself (cf. Grody *et al.*, 1980).

When present at an optimal concentration of about 5 m$M$, several phosphorylated sugars and nucleotides inhibit glucocorticoid receptor inactivation in cytosol (Ishii and Aronow, 1973; Nielsen *et al.*, 1977b,c; Sando *et al.*, 1979a,b; Wheeler *et al.*, 1981). In general, we have not found these low $M_r$ phosphorylated compounds to be as effective at inhibition as 100 m$M$ sodium fluoride and the degree of inhibition varies somewhat according to the tissue or cell type that is used for preparing cytosol. ATP slows the rate of inactivation of glucocorticoid receptors better than the other nucleotides we have tested, and it has also been shown to inhibit progesterone receptor inactivation in chick oviduct cytosol (Toft and Nishigori, 1979). It is not clear why ATP is effective at stabilizing binding capacity over a significant length of time because it is being very rapidly hydrolyzed in both the glucocorticoid and progesterone receptor systems (Sando *et al.*, 1979b; Grody *et al.*, 1980). Inorganic phosphate produces some stabilization in rat liver cytosol, but it is not as effective as ATP, ADP, or AMP (Wheeler *et al.*, 1981). Both inorganic phosphate and pyrophosphate have been reported to prevent inactivation of the calf uterine estrogen receptor by the nuclear receptor-inactivating enzyme (Auricchio *et al.*, 1981a). Levamisole, an inhibitor of some alkaline phosphatases, does not affect glucocorticoid- or progesterone-receptor inactivation.

The low $M_r$ phosphorylated compounds may be acting as competitive inhibitors of a receptor-inactivating phosphatase, but that has not been proven. In the absence of confirmatory evidence using other approaches, the experiments with phosphatase inhibitors do not in themselves provide strong evidence that receptor inactivation in cytosol preparations is due largely, or in part, to phosphatase action. But when these experiments are considered together with confirmatory evidence based upon receptor inactivation by purified protein phosphatases and ATP-dependent reactivation of binding capacity in cytosol, a more convincing argument for a relationship between dephosphorylation and receptor inactivation emerges.

## 3. Inactivation by Purified Alkaline Phosphatase

It seems clear that the binding capacity of cytosols can be inactivated by phosphatase action. This was demonstrated by adding highly purified (but not homogeneous) alkaline phosphatase from calf intestine to L cell and rat liver cytosols and inactivating the glucocorticoid-binding capacity (Nielsen *et al.*, 1977a). Three observations suggested that the inactivation was due to phosphatase activity: (1) alkaline phosphatase activity (assayed with *p*-nitrophenyl phosphate as substrate) and receptor-inactivating activity coeluted on DEAE-cellulose purification of the enzyme; (2) calf intestinal alkaline phosphatase is a zinc-dependent enzyme and its ability to inactivate the receptor is entirely zinc dependent; and (3) the inactivation can be blocked by arsenate, a competitive inhibitor of this enzyme. Like the endogenous receptor-inactivating enzyme, the alkaline phosphatase preparation inactivated the unbound receptor but did not release steroid from the prebound glucocorticoid–receptor complex. Calf intestinal alkaline phosphatase also inactivates the estradiol-binding capacity of cytosol prepared from rabbit corpus luteum, rat uterus, or human breast tumor tissues (Yuh and Keyes, 1981; Abou-Issa *et al.*, 1982).

As the phosphatase has been added to cytosol and not to purified receptors, there is no direct evidence that the enzyme is inactivating the binding capacity by dephosphorylating the receptor protein itself. A variety of indirect mechanisms could be proposed. For example, the enzyme might be dephosphorylating NADPH, which could be required to donate reducing equivalents that are needed to maintain the receptor in the active steroid-binding state.

## 4. ATP-Dependent Reactivation of Receptors

As we had shown that the rate of receptor inactivation in L cell cytosol is inhibited by phosphatase inhibitors, we asked if receptors in this system could be reactivated by addition of ATP (Sando *et al.*, 1979b). At the time this work was carried out, we thought that molybdate was acting purely as a phosphatase inhibitor. The approach we took was to partially inactivate glucocorticoid-binding capacity by incubating L cell cytosol at 25°C and then add both molybdate, to prevent further inactivation by phosphatase, and ATP, to permit reactivation by a kinase. As shown in Fig. 6, L cell binding capacity is partially reactivated, and, at earlier times, it can be completely reactivated. The reactivation is temperature dependent and specific for ATP. Essentially the same protocol has been reported to reactivate estrogen-binding capacity after thermal inactivation of receptors in cytosol prepared from rat or mouse uterus (Abou-Issa *et al.*, 1982; Auricchio *et al.*, 1981b). In the latter case, a $Mg^{2+}$ ATP-dependent receptor-activating enzyme activity has been partially purified from cytosol.

These observations suggest that there is an ATP-dependent enzyme activity in cytosols that affects steroid binding capacity. The mechanism of ATP-dependent restoration of binding activity is not known. It has not been demonstrated that reactivation is due to phosphorylation of the receptor by a

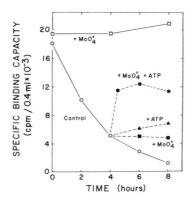

FIG. 6. Reactiviation of L cell glucocorticoid receptor with ATP and molybdate. L cell cytosol was incubated at 25°C with no addition (○) or with 10 m*M* molybdate (□), and aliquots were removed at the indicated times and assayed for glucocorticoid-binding capacity. After 4 hours of incubation of the control, 10 m*M* molybdate (■), 10 m*M* ATP (▲) or 10 m*M* molybdate plus 10 m*M* ATP (●) were added to portions of the supernatant. Again, aliquots were removed at the indicated times and assayed for glucocorticoid-binding capacity. [From Sando *et al.* (1979b).]

protein kinase. The conclusion that we draw from all of the information reviewed above is that the glucocorticoid-binding capacity of cytosol preparations is affected by a phosphorylation–dephosphorylation process. As the receptor is a phosphoprotein, it is possible that phosphorylation is required to maintain the active binding state.

## IV. RECEPTOR STABILIZATION BY MOLYBDATE

### A. INHIBITION OF STEROID RECEPTOR INACTIVATION AND TRANSFORMATION BY GROUP VIA TRANSITION METAL OXIDES

Molybdate, tungstate, and vanadate are group VIA transition metal oxyanions that inhibit a variety of phosphatases (Nordlie and Arion, 1964; VanEtten *et al.*, 1974; Paigen, 1958; Roberts and Brazer, 1976; Poietta and Sands, 1978; Lopez *et al.*, 1976) and some phosphohydrolases like. $Na^+, K^+$-AT-Pases (Cantley *et al.*, 1978; Simons, 1979; Karlish *et al.*, 1979). Because of its reported activity as a phosphatase inhibitor, we added molybdate to cytosols prepared from several tissues and cultured cells and found that it produced a profound inhibition of temperature-mediated inactivation of glucocorticoid receptors (Nielsen *et al.*, 1977b,c). Molybdate has subsequently been found to stabilize receptors for androgens (Noma *et al.*, 1980), estrogens (Anderson *et al.*, 1980), progestins (Toft and Nishigori, 1979), mineralocorticoids (Marver, 1980), and dihydroxycholecalciferol (Feldman *et al.*, 1979). At pH 7.35, sodium molybdate is maximally effective at a concentration of 10 m$M$. At concentrations less than 1 m$M$ vanadate is somewhat more potent than molybdate, but at higher concentrations we have found that its stabilizing effect on the glucocorticoid receptor actually decreases (Wheeler *et al.*, 1981). We had previously reported that tungstate was a very poor inhibitor of receptor inactivation (Leach *et al.*, 1979), but we have subsequently found that it is almost as potent as molybdate. Nishigori and Toft (1980) have shown that the effect of molybdate on progesterone receptor transformation is highly pH dependent (half-maximal inhibition is achieved with 1 m$M$ molybdate at pH 8.0 and 0.1 m$M$ at pH 7.0), and the weak stabilization of the glucocorticoid receptor that we originally observed with tungstate may reflect a problem with pH. Inhibition of receptor inactivation by Group VIA transition metal oxyanions is readily reversible (Leach *et al.*, 1979). In addition to inhibiting inactivation of steroid receptors, molybdate reversibly blocks transformation of the bound steroid–receptor complex to the DNA-binding state. Inhibition of transformation was first reported for the avian progesterone receptor by Toft and Nishigori (1979) and has been reported for glucocorticoid (Leach *et al.*, 1979), androgen (Noma *et al.*, 1980), and estrogen (Shyamala and Leonard, 1980) receptors.

### B. Evidence That Molybdate Stabilizes via a Direct Interaction with the Receptor

Although molybdate, vanadate, and tungstate inhibit a number of phosphatases, it is now clear that this action does not acccount for their ability to stabilize steroid receptors and to inhibit receptor transformation. Several observations support this proposal. Nishigori and Toft (1980), for example, examined the effect of a number of compounds on both progesterone receptor transformation and endogenous phosphatase activity (assayed with *p*-nitrophenyl phosphate as substrate) in chick oviduct cytosol and found that some compounds, like chromate and arsenate, inhibited phosphatase activity but not transformation. Although molybdate, vanadate, and tungstate inhibited both phosphatase activity and receptor transformation, the results obtained with other inhibitors suggested that these two activities might not be related. Leach *et al.* (1979) found that molybdate inhibited inactivation and transformation of glucocorticoid receptors caused by salt or ammonium sulfate precipitation at 0–4°C. As these are physical methods of receptor inactivation and transformation that are unlikely to involve phosphatase action, it seemed likely that molybdate was acting in a more direct way, possibly by interacting with the receptor itself.

Molybdate has a profound affect on the physical behavior of glucocorticoid and estrogen receptors submitted to ammonium sulfate precipitation. In the absence of molybdate, receptor is precipitated at 30% of ammonium sulfate saturation and is transformed, while in the presence of molybdate the receptor is precipitated at 40–55% ammonium sulfate saturation and is not transformed (Dahmer *et al.*, 1981; Mauck *et al.*, 1982). Grody *et al.* (1980) have shown that the ability of molybdate to stabilize the progesterone–receptor complex in cytosol to thermal inactivation is lost if the receptor is precipitated with ammonium sulfate prior to incubating it at 30°C. These data suggest that molybdate interacts directly with the receptor and possibly exclusively with the untransformed form.

Molybdate also prevents both transformation of glucocorticoid- or estrogen-bound receptors and the shift of these complexes to a less negatively charged state, which takes place during DEAE-cellulose chromatography (Dahmer *et al.*, 1981; Redeuilh *et al.*, 1981). As molybdate prevents the transformation of steroid receptors that occurs with many purification procedures, one of its most useful applications may be to permit purification of untransformed receptors so that the transformation process can be studied in greater detail. The use of both molybdate and the corticosterone affinity gel developed by Grandics *et al.* (1982) has recently permitted extensive purification of untransformed progesterone and glucocorticoid receptors (Puri *et al.*, 1982; Grandics and Litwack, 1982).

It is clear that in addition to stabilizing receptors and inhibiting their transformation, molybdate affects the size of the steroid-binding complex. In the presence of 10 m$M$ sodium molybdate, steroid receptors remain in a very large complex with a sedimentation value of 8–10 $s$. This stabilization of the apparent size of the binding complex has been demonstrated with glucocorticoid (McBlain *et al.*, 1981), estrogen (Sherman *et al.*, 1980; Miller *et al.*, 1981), and progesterone (Grody *et al.*, 1980; Puri *et al.*, 1982) receptors. These three effects of molybdate have been synthesized into a general model, suggesting that steroid receptors may normally be present as large units ($M_r$ circa 350,000, M. Sherman, personal communication) that bind steroid and that are subsequently dissociated during transformation to the DNA-binding state. Molybdate may prove to be a useful tool in probing several questions raised by the model. For example, is the large $M_r$ species composed of similar or dissimilar units? Why would a dissociation after steroid binding be highly temperature dependent? What triggers dissociation? Can both dissociation and transformation be reversed? Is dissociation both necessary and sufficient for transformation?

## C. The Molybdate Effect May Reflect a Weak Interaction with Functional Groups on the Receptor Protein

The observations made to date strongly suggest that molybdate interacts directly with the receptor or perhaps another component of a large $M_r$ receptor complex. This interaction must be a weak one, as a concentration of 0.5 to 1 m$M$ molybdate or 0.2 m$M$ vanadate is required to produce a half-maximal stabilization of receptors at pH 7.35 (Wheeler *et al.*, 1981). It is unlikely that the interaction between steroid receptors and group 6A transition metal oxyanions is the same as the interaction between vanadate and $Na^+, K^+$-ATPases, as these enzymes are inhibited at several orders of magnitude lower vanadate concentration (Cantley *et al.*, 1978; Wallick *et al.*, 1979). The transition metal oxyanions inhibit phosphatase enzymes by binding quite specifically at the phosphate-binding site on the enzyme (Van Etten *et al.*, 1974; Lopez *et al.*, 1976). In the case of acid phosphatases, there is evidence that molybdate complexes with a histidyl residue in the active site of the enzyme functioning as an analog of the transition state (Van Etten *et al.*, 1974). Again, the concentration of metal ion required for inhibition of these enzymes is in the order of $10^{-8}$ to $10^{-6}$ $M$, and this effect is probably quite different from the weak interaction occurring with steroid receptors.

It is interesting to note that molybdate is a reversible activator of adenylate cyclase in rat liver plasma membranes and the apparent $K_a$ for molybdate activation is 4.5 m$M$, with maximal activation being achieved at 50 m$M$ (Richards and Swislocki, 1979). The range of molybdate concentration required for the effect on the adenylate cyclase system is similar to that required for its effects on steroid receptors, and it is likely that these weak interactions will prove to be different from those occurring in the micromolar range and lower.

We do not know what type of functional groups are required for the proposed molybdate-receptor interaction. Molybdate, vanadate, and tungstate can form chelates with a variety of functional groups, including oxygen, nitrogen, and sulfur ligands (Van Etten *et al.*, 1974). We have previously proposed that phosphate and sulfur moieties on the receptor protein (or on some other component of a receptor complex) are two sites of interaction that should be considered for molybdate (Leach *et al.*, 1979). In the last section of this chapter we will discuss some observations that lead us to think that interactions with sulfur may be of particular importance for understanding molybdate effects on steroid receptors.

## D. Molybdate Stabilizes Receptors Even When Steroid-Binding Activity Is Not Present

When we studied the conditions that permit receptor activation in rat thymocyte cytosol, we began to appreciate the role of reduction in determining binding capacity. When thymocyte cytosol is incubated at 25°C, the unbound receptor is rapidly inactivated. Addition of molybdate provides no stabilization and dithiothreitol (DTT) stabilizes only slightly, but binding capacity is stabilized for many hours when both molybdate and DTT are present (Sando *et al.*, 1979a). To examine in further detail the interaction between DTT and molybdate in activation of thymocyte receptors at 25°C, the experiment illustrated in Fig. 7 was carried out. Control thymocyte cytosol was incubated at 25°C with no addition, with 2 m$M$ DTT, or with 10 m$M$ molybdate, and various additions were made after several times of receptor inactivation under the three control conditions. As shown in panel A, addition of molybdate during the receptor inactivation occurring in the presence of DTT results in stabilization of whatever binding capacity is present at the time of molybdate addition. The addition of more DTT with the molybdate does not give any more binding capacity than addition of only molybdate, showing that the receptor inactivation occurring in the presence

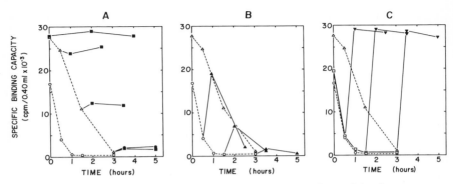

Fig. 7. Dithiothreitol reactivation of molybdate-stabilized and unstabilized receptors at 25°C. Thymocyte cytosol was divided into several portions and incubated at 25°C under the following conditions: A: ○- - -○, control incubation in buffer without additions; △- - -△, incubation in the presence of 2 mM dithiothreitol; ■, dithiothreitol-containing samples to which 10 mM molybdate was added at the indicated times; ●, samples to which both molybdate and additional dithiothreitol were added after they had been incubated in the presence of dithiothreitol for 3 hours. In B, the control and dithiothreitol curves are repeated, and ▲ shows the binding capacity in samples that were exposed to dithiothreitol after incubation for 0.5, 1.5, or 3 hours in the presence of buffer alone. In C, □ represents the binding capacity in samples containing 10 mM molybdate and ▼ represents molybdate-containing samples to which dithiothreitol was added at 0.5, 1.5, or 3 hours. All values represent the average of duplicate assays expressed as counts per minutes per 0.4 ml of incubation. [From Sando *et al.* (1979a).]

of DTT is not merely a function of loss of DTT from the system. Figure 7B shows that addition of DTT after varying times of the receptor inactivation occurring in the absence of DTT and molybdate results in activation of the binding capacity to the level that exists in samples to which DTT was added at time zero. This is the same effect observed by Rees and Bell (1975) and by Granberg and Ballard (1977) for addition of DTT at 0°C to partially inactivated glucocorticoid receptors in thymocyte and lung cytosols, respectively. Fig. 7C shows that if thymocyte glucocorticoid receptors were inactivated in the presence of molybdate, which, as shown, has no stabilizing effect by itself, addition of DTT results in total reactivation of the binding capacity to the maximum time zero value no matter how little active receptor remains at the time of addition.

At the time this experiment was carried out, we were making the assumption that molybdate was acting in this system as a phosphatase inhibitor. Fluoride, another well-known phosphatase inhibitor, also stabilizes the thymocyte receptor in the presence of DTT, and this led us to suggest that there were two processes responsible for thymocyte receptor inactivation, sulfhydryl group oxidation and receptor dephosphorylation. The fact that phosphatase inhibitors were ineffective in the absence of DTT indicated that the oxidation process is more rapid than the dephosphorylation and that both a reduced sulfhydryl moiety and a phosphorylated moiety are required for glucocorticoid-binding capacity. These two requirements were presented in the model illustrated in Eq. (1):

$$R \underset{R_{SH}}{\overset{{}^{P}R}{\diamondsuit}} {}^{P}R_{SH} + S \rightleftharpoons {}^{P}R_{SH}S \tag{1}$$

The active form of the receptor that binds steroid (S) is presented here as ${}^{P}R_{SH}$. Three possible inactive states of the receptor are presented: a dephosphorylated form ($R_{SH}$), an oxidized form (${}^{P}R$), and a form that is both dephosphorylated and oxidized (R).

As we thought that molybdate was acting by preventing a dephosphorylation, we interpreted the observations made in the experiment of Fig. 7 in the following way. When molybdate is present to prevent dephosphorylation and DTT is present to stabilize the appropriate sulfhydryl moieties, the binding capacity remains constant. Addition of DTT to receptor that had been inactivated in the absence of molybdate yields constantly decreasing amounts of reactivation because the receptor is being dephosphorylated and less ${}^{P}R$ is available to be converted to ${}^{P}R_{SH}$. We thought that if the phosphate had been stabilized by molybdate (as in Fig. 7C), however, the conversion of ${}^{P}R$ to R is prevented and complete reactivation can be achieved with the reducing agent alone. As we will describe in the last section of this chapter, binding capacity can be inactivated by dephosphorylation in the presence of molybdate and our interpretation of the molybdate effect has changed considerably. The observations and the model are important, however, for indicating the four potential forms of the receptor and for underlining the importance of understanding receptor reduction in order to understand steroid binding. In the next section we will review our knowledge of the endogenous factors that reduce and stabilize glucocorticoid receptors.

## V. ROLE OF ENDOGENOUS, HEAT-STABLE FACTORS IN RECEPTOR ACTIVATION AND STABILIZATION

### A. ACTIVATION OF GLUCOCORTICOID RECEPTORS WITH BOILED CYTOSOL

In 1977 we showed (Sando *et al.*, 1977) that glucocorticoid receptors in thymocyte cytosol could be slowly activated at 0°C by a heat-stable activity in mouse L cell cytosol that was eluted in the macromolecular peak on Sephadex G-25 chromatography. At the same time, Granberg and Ballard (1977) reported that boiled cytosol from rat liver activated glucocorticoid receptors in rat lung cytosol. The lung receptors could also be activated by DTT, and these investigators proposed that the activation was due to sulfhydryl reducing activity in the boiled liver extract. In a later study in which we examined the role of reducing agents, ATP, molybdate, and endogenous heat-stable factors on thymocyte receptor activation, we found (Sando *et al.*, 1979a) that boiled cytosol from rat liver or L cells had receptor-activating activity, whereas boiled cytosol prepared from rat thymocytes did not. All of the boiled cytosol preparations had the ability to stabilize receptors that had been activated by DTT. This observation suggested that there might be two endogenous heat-stable activities that affected glucocorticoid-binding capacity, one that activates and one that stabilizes.

## B. Identification of the Endogenous Glucocorticoid Receptor-Activating Factor

We have recently examined in some detail the ability of boiled rat liver cytosol to activate and stabilize unbound glucocorticoid receptors in rat thymocyte cytosol (Leach *et al.*, 1982b). Rat thymocyte cytosol has a comparatively low content of nonprotein sulfhydryl groups (Granberg and Ballard, 1977) and the ability of freshly prepared high-speed cytosol preparations to bind glucocorticoids can be approximately doubled by adding either DTT (2 to 10 m$M$) or an equal volume of a boiled rat liver cytosol preparation (Leach *et al.*, 1982b). It subsequently became clear that the receptor-activating activity in the boiled liver cytosol preparation is eliminated by charcoal extraction. This is in contrast to the stabilizing activity, which is not adsorbed to charcoal. As the receptor-activating activity could be adsorbed to charcoal, we were able to ask if the glucocorticoid-binding activity of rat liver cytosol is comparatively stable because it is in the continuous presence of the activating factor. It is clear that this is the case. If rat liver cytosol containing unoccupied glucocorticoid receptor is extracted for 30 minutes at 0° with 10% charcoal, all binding activity is eliminated and the binding capacity can be restored by adding DTT. We concluded from this observation that glucocorticoid receptors in a normally stable cytosol are rapidly inactivated, even at 0–4°C, when endogenous sulfhydryl reducing activity is eliminated.

The charcoal-extracted liver cytosol has provided us with an excellent system for assaying the endogenous heat-stable-activating activity (Grippo *et al.*, 1983). In this receptor-activating assay we have taken advantage of the fact that molybdate stabilizes the receptor to thermal inactivation even when steroid-binding activity is not present. If liver cytosol is first inactivated by extraction with 10% charcoal and then passed through Sephadex G-50 (in buffer containing 10 m$M$ molybdate) to eliminate endogenous NADPH, reduced glutathione, and thioredoxin, it can be reactivated in a tempera-

TABLE I

REQUIREMENT FOR NADPH AND THE HEAT-STABLE ACTIVITY IN SEPHADEX G-25
MACROMOLECULAR PEAK FOR RECEPTOR ACTIVATION BY REDUCTION[a]

| Additions to inactive receptor preparation | Specific-binding capacity (cpm/aliquot) |
|---|---|
| None | 580 |
| DTT | 24,800 |
| NADPH | 5,780 |
| EAF | 600 |
| Thioredoxin | 610 |
| EAF plus NADPH | 21,500 |
| Thioredoxin plus NADPH | 16,800 |

[a]Rat liver cytosol was extracted for 30 minutes at 0–4°C with 10% charcoal and chromatographed on a column of Sephadex G-50 in buffer containing 10 m$M$ sodium molybdate. The macromolecular peak was returned to original volume by Amicon filtration and used as the source of inactive receptor. The heat-stable-activating factor was prepared by boiling liver cytosol, passing the heat-stable components through a Sephadex G-25 column, and concentrating the fractions containing the macromolecular peak. This material is referred to as the endogenous-activating factor (EAF). After the indicated additions were made, mixtures were incubated for 2 hours at 20°C, and the specific binding capacity was assayed with [$^3$H]triamcinolone acetonide. The inactive-receptor preparation and the heat-stable-activating factor were present in a ratio of 3:2 (v:v). The concentration of NADPH is 100 μ$M$, and dithiothreitol (DTT) is present at 10 m$M$. The thioredoxin has been purified to homogeneity from *Escherichia coli* and is present at 45 μ$M$.

ture-dependent manner by a boiled liver cytosol preparation. We have taken this activating system apart and found that two components of boiled cytosol are required for receptor reactivation, NADPH and a heat-stable entity that elutes with the macromolecular material from Sephadex G-25. As shown in Table I, the heat-stable macromolecular factor is required for complete receptor activation, and it can be replaced with 45 μ$M$ purified bacterial thioredoxin. As the endogenous heat-stable-activating activity behaves like thioredoxin according to its size and NADPH requirement and as it can be replaced by a relatively low concentration of purified bacterial thioredoxin, we would propose that the heat-stable-activating factor is thioredoxin and that glucocorticoid receptors are maintained in the active steroid-binding state by thioredoxin-mediated sulfhydryl reduction (Grippo *et al.*, 1983).

## C. PROPERTIES OF THE ENDOGENOUS GLUCOCORTICOID RECEPTOR-STABILIZING FACTOR

The second endogenous heat-stable activity that affects glucocorticoid-binding capacity is a very small $M_r$ factor (less than 700 by Sephadex G-10 chromatography) that stabilizes reduced receptors (Leach *et al.*, 1982b). We have found that the stabilizing activity is most easily assayed in a rat liver cytosol system from which low $M_r$ components have been removed by washing and filtration. If the large $M_r$ components of rat liver cytosol are washed by diluting cytosol with buffer and concentrating it back to its original volume by filtration on an Amicon UM10 filter (the filter excludes material having an $M_r$ greater than approximately 10,000), the glucocorticoid-binding activity of the resulting washed cytosol is very labile. The binding activity of receptor in this washed cytosol is stabilized by addition of boiled cytosols prepared from a variety of rat tissues.

The receptor-stabilizing activity in unheated cytosol is largely bound to components of $M_r > 30,000$ and boiling apparently denatures these molecules, releasing the low $M_r$ stabilizing factor (Leach *et al.*, 1982b). Nothing is known about the composition of the factor. The stabilizing activity is not affected by incubation with a variety of hydrolytic enzymes, including proteases, nucleases, glycohydrolases, phospholipase A, lipase, and alkaline phosphatase. As it binds to Dowex 1, the factor appears to be negatively charged. It coelutes with inorganic phosphate on both Sephadex G-10 and Dowex-1 chromatography, but it has been shown that the stabilizing activity is not due to inorganic phosphate, nucleotides, cyclic nucleotides, or pyridoxal phosphate, all of which would elute in a similar manner.

In addition to inhibiting thermal inactivation of unoccupied glucocorticoid receptors, the heat-stable factor inhibits transformation of the steroid-bound receptor to the DNA-binding state (Leach *et al.*, 1982b). Steroid-bound receptors in cytosol washed free of low $M_r$ components are more rapidly transformed to the DNA-binding state on incubation at 15°C than receptors in normal cytosol. This rapid transformation is also inhibited by addition of boiled cytosol. We would suggest that inhibition of receptor inactivation and inhibition of receptor transformation may be due to the same heat-stable component of cytosol because both activities coelute from Sephadex G-10 and from Dowex-1 columns. Both activities have been copurified more than 200-fold with respect to Lowry-reactive material.

The endogenous stabilizing factor was first described by Cake *et al.* in 1976 when they found that removal of low $M_r$ components from rat liver cytosol by gel filtration promoted both inactivation of the unbound glucocorticoid receptor and transformation of the bound receptor. Litwack and his coworkers (Cake *et al.*, 1976; Goidl *et al.*, 1977) have suggested that this low $M_r$ component(s) maintains the glucocorticoid receptor in a conformational state that allows the binding of glucocorticoid and that it has to be removed from the steroid–receptor complex before binding to DNA can occur. Subsequently, it was suggested that this endogenous "modulator" of the glucocorticoid receptor might be pyridoxal phosphate (Cake *et al.*, 1978; DiSorbo *et al.*, 1980), but it is now clear that the endogenous factor inhibits receptor transformation whereas pyridoxal phosphate interacts with the transformed receptor and blocks binding to DNA (Sekula *et al.*, 1981). Bailly *et al.* (1977) have also described a similar low $M_r$ heat-stable inhibitor of glucocorticoid receptor transformation in rat liver cytosol, and Sakaue and Thompson (1977) have shown that the heat-stable fraction of cytosol inhibits glucocorticoid receptor transformation as defined by a shift to the low salt-eluting form on DEAE-cellulose chromatography. It seems likely that we are studying the same low $M_r$ heat-stable activity that was reported earlier by these other laboratories. The only discrepancy we have noted is that Bailly *et al.* (1977) found that the transformation-inhibiting activity is removed by a cation exchange resin and have suggested that it may be positively charged, whereas we have found (Leach *et al.*, 1982b) that it binds to Dowex 1, behaving as an anion at pH 7.35.

The receptor-stabilizing factor may not have a function that is unique to glucocorticoid receptors. Sato *et al.* (1980) have reported that transformation of both androgen and estrogen receptors is also inhibited by a low $M_r$ (dialyzable) factor (or factors) present in cytosol. We (Leach *et al.*, 1982b) have found that the glucocorticoid receptor-stabilizing activity and transformation-inhibiting activity are present in boiled cytosols prepared from primitive eukaryotes, like lobster and yeast, as well as in liver from amphibians, avians, and mammals (including man). As the activity is present in primitive systems that are lower on the evolutionary scale than the point at which glucocorticoid receptors emerged, it is reasonable to propose that the stabilizing factor(s) functions in cellular metabolism in processes that do not involve steroid receptors. Recently, we have begun to ask what kind of general activity the factor might possess.

As several compounds that are phosphatase inhibitors can slow the rate of inactivation of glucocorticoid receptors, we have tested the ability of the partially purified low $M_r$ factor to inhibit protein phosphatase activity. As shown in Fig. 8, this material inhibits rat liver phosphorylase phosphatase with the same concentration dependency at which it inhibits both inactivation and transformation of the glucocorticoid receptor in filtered rat liver cytosol. Although the relationship is intriguing, there is no convincing evidence that the three activities are due to the same small $M_r$ heat-stable entity. As with the inhibition of receptor inactivation and transformation, it is clear that inhibition of phosphorylase phosphatase is not due to inorganic phosphate present in the preparation. The receptor-stabilizing factor has proven to be difficult to purify beyond the Sephadex G-10 step but purification will be necessary in order to study its mechanism of action. The heat-stable factor preparation acts in some ways like molybdate in that it reversibly inhibits both receptor inactivation and transformation (Leach *et al.*, 1982a,b), but in contrast to the factor preparation, molybdate is a poor inhibitor of phosphorylase–phosphatase activity (Housley *et al.*, 1982).

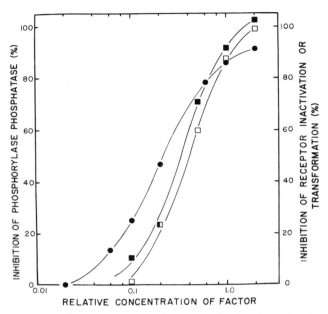

FIG. 8. Concentration dependency of inhibition of phosphorylase–phosphatase activity, glucocorticoid receptor inactivation, and receptor transformation by partially purified receptor-stabilizing factor. The low $M_r$ factor was purified approximately 200-fold from rat liver cytosol by boiling, Amicon filtration, and Sephadex G-10 chromatography as described by Leach *et al.* (1982b). Phosphorylase phosphatase was purified 20-fold from rat liver through the second ammonium sulfate step of Brandt *et al.* (1975) to a specific activity of 0.13 units/mg protein. Phosphorylase-*b* was converted to phosphorylase-*a* by incubation with $[\gamma\text{-}^{32}P]ATP$ and phosphorylase kinase by the method of Antoniw *et al.* (1979). Each incubation for the phosphatase assay (0.45 ml) contained 0.45 mg $[^{32}P]$phosphorylase-*a*, 0.2 units of the phosphorylase phosphatase preparation and the indicated amount of the partially purified heat-stable factor. Release of $^{32}P_i$ was assayed after precipitation with trichloroacetic acid using a modification of the procedure of Antoniw *et al.* (1979). (●), inhibition of phosphatase activity. Inhibition of glucocorticoid receptor inactivation (□) and inhibition of transformation (■) were assayed with the filtered liver cytosol system and the data are taken from Leach *et al.* (1982b). The concentration of factor is presented in normalized units of relative concentration as defined by Leach *et al.* (1982b).

# VI. POTENTIAL ROLE OF RECEPTOR PHOSPHATE IN STABILIZING SULFHYDRYL GROUPS ESSENTIAL FOR STEROID BINDING

We have exploited the observation that some phosphatase enzymes are not inhibited by molybdate in experiments designed to study the mechanism of molybdate-mediated stabilization and the role of receptor phosphate in maintaining steroid-binding capacity. We have found, for example, that 10 mM molybdate does not inhibit calf intestine alkaline–phosphatase activity assayed with p-nitrophenyl phosphate as substrate, and it does not prevent inactivation of glucocorticoid-binding capacity when this enzyme is added to rat liver cytosol (Leach *et al.*, 1983). In the experiment of Fig. 9, rat liver cytosol was first filtered and washed to remove low $M_r$ phosphorylated compounds and ions that might inhibit phosphatase activity, and the filtered cytosol preparation containing 10 mM sodium molybdate was then incubated at 20°C with calf intestinal alkaline phosphatase that had been purified to homogeneity. Glucocorticoid-binding capacity is inactivated, and if molybdate is present during the inactivation, the binding capacity can be reactivated by adding 10 mM dithiothreitol (Housley *et al.*, 1982). Molybdate must be present in order for reactivation with dithiothreitol to occur and dithiothreitol alone does not prevent receptor inactivation. The binding

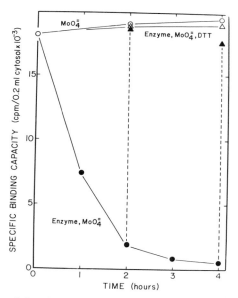

FIG. 9. Reactivation of phosphatase-treated receptors by dithiothreitol. Filtered cytosol containing molybdate was incubated alone (○), with purified calf intestine alkaline phosphatase at 20 μg/ml (●) or with alkaline phosphatase at 20 μg/ml plus 10 mM dithiothreitol (△). At the indicated times, 0.2 ml aliquots were removed and assayed for specific glucocorticoid-binding capacity. At 2 and 4 hours 0.2 ml aliquots were removed from the incubation mixture containing alkaline phosphatase alone, dithiothreitol was added to a final concentration of 10 mM, and the specific binding capacity assayed. The dithiothreitol-reactivated samples (▲) are connected to their corresponding phosphatase-inactivated samples by dashed lines. [From Housley *et al.* (1982).]

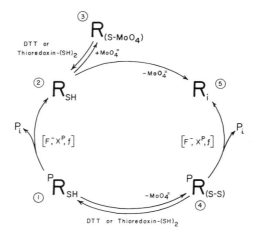

FIG. 10. Hypothetical model describing the different binding states of the receptor that have been observed in cytosol preparations. Receptor in states 1 and 2 binds steroid; states 3 and 4 are nonbinding but reversible by reduction; and state 5 is nonbinding and not reversible by reduction. It is proposed that fluoride ($F^-$), low $M_r$ phosphorylated compounds ($X^P$) and the endogenous low $M_r$ stabilizing factor ($f$) may be acting as phosphatase inhibitors (indicated by brackets). Molybdate ($MoO_4^=$) interacts directly with the receptor, possibly by interacting with sulfur groups. (See Section VI of the text for complete description.)

capacity can also be inactivated by highly purified rabbit muscle phosphoprotein phosphatase in the presence of molybdate and subsequently reactivated in a similar manner (Housley *et al.*, 1982).

In this type of experiment, the steroid-binding capacity of cytosol is clearly being inactivated by dephosphorylation and reactivated by reduction. We have inferred from this observation that dephosphorylation in some way promotes oxidation of sulfhydryl groups that are essential for steroid binding. Although it has not been directly demonstrated that inactivation is due to dephosphorylation of the receptor protein itself, we have made that assumption in constructing a model (Fig. 10) to represent the different binding states that have been observed in cytosol preparations. Three potential binding states exist in the experiment of Fig. 9. There is the untreated, active binding form, which is represented in the model by the phosphorylated and reduced receptor in state 1. Incubating cytosol with protein phosphatases in the presence of molybdate produces a nonbinding form of the receptor (state 3) that can be returned to a steroid-binding form (state 2) by addition of a reducing agent. As this reactivation occurs in the absence of ATP at 0°C, phosphorylation is not involved, and some kind of reduction must be occurring. If molybdate is not present, incubation with protein phosphatases results in a nonbinding state (state 5) that is not reactivated by reduction.

As shown in Fig. 7B, the binding capacity of thymocyte cytosol that has been inactivated by endogenous processes in the absence of molybdate or reducing agent can be reactivated with dithiothreitol to the level of binding that exists when the reducing agent is present during receptor inactivation. Thus, in this system, which has little endogenous reducing activity, receptor can be converted from a nonbinding form (state 4) to a steroid-binding form (state 1) by reduction in the absence of molybdate. The sulfhydryl group(s) required for binding may have formed a disulfide, and the binding capacity can be reactivated by reduction of this moiety, if other changes such as dephosphorylation have not occurred. If dephosphorylation occurs, as represented by the conversion of nonbinding state 4 to nonbinding state 5, then receptor cannot be reactivated by reduction alone. The partial reactivation of receptor we have observed on addition of ATP and molybdate to L cell cytosol (Fig. 6) may represent conversion of state 5 to state 4 with subsequent reduction to state 1. As we have not yet shown by direct means that phosphate from ATP is being transferred to the receptor protein in cytosol, we have not shown any phosphorylation reactions in the model, although it is clear that receptor phosphorylation occurs in the intact cell (Housley and Pratt, 1983).

We have found the model of Fig. 10 to be useful for several reasons. It allows one to envision how inhibitors of phosphatase action and possibly the low $M_r$ heat-stable factor could stabilize binding by inhibiting receptor dephosphorylation, whereas molybdate could produce a similar stabilizing effect via a direct interaction with the receptor. The model suggests a potential mechanism for both molybdate and phosphate stabilization. Molybdate clearly prevents some change that produces a form of the receptor that cannot be reactivated by dithiothreitol. It is possible that, as defined for some other molybdate–protein interactions (Weathers *et al.*, 1979), the transition metal oxyanion complexes with sulfur groups on the receptor. It is also possible that molybdate interacts elsewhere with the receptor to prevent conformational changes that lead to inactivation after oxidation of a sulfhydryl moiety(ies) that is required for steroid binding. As the molybdate-stabilized, phosphatase-inactivated receptor can be reactivated, it would seem that the phosphate moiety(ies) itself is not required for steroid binding. Rather, it would seem that phosphorylation of the receptor may ensure a conformation such that sulfhydryl oxidation does not readily occur. If fluoride or the low $M_r$ stabilizing factor are present during inactivation of the receptor by endogenous processes, the fraction of receptors that can be reactivated by reduction (state 4) is increased substantially (Leach *et al.*, 1982b). This leads us to suggest that receptor phosphate, like molybdate, may also inhibit conformational changes that lead to inactivation after sulfhydryl group oxidation. The model of Fig. 10 is presented here in the hope that it may stimulate the asking of new questions about the roles of phosphorylation and sulfur reduction in determining the active steroid-binding state of the receptor that is assayed in cytosol preparations.

## ACKNOWLEDGMENTS

The authors' studies on receptor phosphorylation are supported by Grant CA-28010 from the National Cancer Institute and studies on the endogenous steroid receptor-stabilizing and activating factors are supported by Grant AM31573 from the National Institute of Arthritis, Diabetes, Digestive and Kidney Diseases.

## REFERENCES

Abou-Issa, H., Foecking, M. K., and Minton, J. P. (1982). *Fed. Proc., Fed. Am. Soc. Exp. Biol.* **41**, 1164.

Anderson, K. M., Bonomi, P., Marogil, M., Hendricksen, C., and Economou, S. (1980). *Cancer Res.* **40**, 4127–4132.

Antoniw, J. F., Nimmo, H. G., Yeaman, S. J., and Cohen, P. (1979). *Biochem. J.* **162**, 423–433.

Auricchio, F., and Migliaccio, A. (1980). *FEBS Lett.* **117**, 224–226.

Auricchio, F., Migliaccio, A., and Castoria, G. (1981a). *Biochem. J.* **198**, 699–702.

Auricchio, F., Migliaccio, A., Castoria, G., Lastoria, S., and Schiavone, E. (1981b). *Biochem. Biophys. Res. Commun.* **101**, 1171–1178.

Auricchio, F., Migliaccio, A., and Rotondi, A. (1981c). *Biochem. J.* **194**, 569–574.

Bailly, A., Sallas, N., and Milgrom, E. (1977). *J. Biol. Chem.* **252**, 858–863.

Bell, P. A., and Munck, A. (1973). *Biochem. J.* **136**, 97–107.

Brandt, H., Capulong, Z. L., and Lee, E. Y. C. (1975). *J. Biol. Chem.* **250**, 8038–8044.

Cake, M. H., Goidl, J. A., Parchman, L. G., and Litwack, G. (1976). *Biochem. Biophys. Res. Commun.* **71**, 45–52.

Cake, M. H., DiSorbo, D. M., and Litwack, G. (1978). *J. Biol. Chem.* **253**, 4886–4891.

Cantley, L. C., Cantley, L. G., and Josephson, L. J. (1978). *J. Biol. Chem.* **253**, 7361–7368.

Chader, G. J. (1973). *J. Neurochem.* **21**, 1525–1532.

Dahmer, M. K., Quasney, M. W., Bissen, S. T., and Pratt, W. B. (1981) *J. Biol. Chem.* **256**, 9401–9405.

DiSorbo, D. M., Phelps, D. S., Ohl, V. S., and Litwack, G. (1980) *J. Biol. Chem.* **255**, 3866–3870.

Dougherty, J. J., Puri, R. K., and Toft, D. O. (1982). *J. Biol. Chem.,* **257**, 14226–14230.

Feldman, D., McCain, T. A., Hirst, M. A., Chen, T. L., and Colston, K. W. (1979). *J. Biol. Chem.* **254**, 10378–10384.

Giannopoulos, G. (1976). *J. Steroid Biochem.* **7**, 553–555.

Goidl, J. A., Cake, M. H., Dolan, K. P., Parchman, L. G., and Litwack, G. (1977). *Biochemistry* **16**, 2125–2130.

Granberg, J. P., and Ballard, P. L. (1977). *Endocrinology (Baltimore)* **100**, 1160–1168.

Grandics, P., and Litwack, G. (1982). *Fed. Proc.* **41**, 1163.

Grandics, P., Puri, R. K., and Toft, D. O. (1982). *Endocrinology (Baltimore)* **110**, 1055–1057.

Grippo, J. F., Dahmer, M. K., Housley, P. R., and Pratt, W. B. (1983). *J. Biol. Chem.,* in press.

Grody, W. W., Compton, J. G., Schrader, W. T., and O'Malley, B. W. (1980). *J. Steroid Biochem.* **12**, 115–120.

Hackney, J. F., Gross, S. R., Aronow, L., and Pratt, W. B. (1970). *Mol. Pharmacol.* **6**, 500–512.

Horwitz, K. B., and McGuire, W. L. (1978). *J. Biol. Chem.* **253**, 2223–2228.

Housley, P. R., and Pratt, W. B. (1983). *J. Biol. Chem.* **258**, 4630–4635.

Housley, P. R., Dahmer, M. K., and Pratt, W. B. (1982). *J. Biol. Chem.* **257**, 8615–8618.

Ishii, D. N., and Aronow, L. (1973). *J. Steroid Biochem.* **4**, 593–603.

Ishii, D. N., Pratt, W. B., and Aronow, L. (1972). *Biochemistry* **11**, 3896–3904.

Jungblut, P. W., Gaues, J., Huges, A., Kallweit, E., Sierralta, W., Szendro, P., and Wagner, R. K. (1976). *J. Steroid Biochem.* **7**, 1109–1116.

Kaine, J. L., Nielsen, C. J., and Pratt, W. B. (1975). *Mol. Pharmacol.* **11**, 578–587.

Karlish, S. J. D., Beauge, L. A., and Glynn, I. M. (1979). *Nature (London)* **282**, 333–335.

Kassis, J. A., and Gorski, J. (1981). *J. Biol. Chem.* **256**, 7378–7382.

Kirkpatrick, A. F., Kaiser, N., Milholland, R. J., and Rosen, F. (1972). *J. Biol. Chem.* **247**, 70–74.

Koblinsky, M., Beato, M., Kalimi, M., and Feigelson, P. (1972). *J. Biol. Chem.* **247**, 7897–7904.

Leach, K. L., Dahmer, M. K., Hammond, N. D., Sando, J. J., and Pratt, W. B. (1979). *J. Biol. Chem.* **254**, 11884–11890.

Leach, K. L., Erickson, R. P., and Pratt, W. B. (1982a). *J. Steroid Biochem.* **17**, 121–123.

Leach, K. L., Grippo, J. F., Housley, P. R., Dahmer, M. K., Salive, M. E., and Pratt, W. B. (1982b). *J. Biol. Chem.* **257**, 381–388.

Leach, K. L., Dahmer, M. K., and Pratt, W. B. (1983). *J. Steroid Biochem.* **18**, 105–107.

Lopez, V., Stevens, T., and Lindquist, R. N. (1976). *Arch. Biochem. Biophys.* **175**, 31–38.

McBlain, W. A., Toft, D. O., and Shyamala, G. (1981). *Biochemistry* **20**, 6790–6798.

Marver, D. (1980). *Endocrinology (Baltimore)* **106**, 611–618.

Mauck, L. A., Day, R. N., and Notides, A. C. (1982). *Biochemistry* **21**, 1788–1793.

Miller, L. K., Tuazon, F. B., Niu, E.-M., and Sherman, M. R. (1981). *Endocrinology (Baltimore)* **108**, 1369–1378.

Munck, A., and Brinck-Johnsen, T. (1968). *J. Biol. Chem.* **243**, 5556–5565.

Munck, A., and Foley, R. (1976). *J. Steroid Biochem.* **7**, 1117–1122.

Munck, A., and Leung, K. (1977). *In* "Receptors and Mechanism of Action of Steroid Hormones Part 2," (J. R. Pasqualini ed.) pp. 311–397. Dekker, New York.

Munck, A., Wira, C., Young, D. A., Mosher, K. M., Hallahan, C., and Bell, P. A. (1972). *J. Steroid Biochem.* **3**, 567–578.

Nielsen, C. J., Sando, J. J., and Pratt, W. B. (1977a). *Proc. Natl. Acad. Sic. U.S.A.* **74**, 1398–1402.

Nielsen, C. J., Sando, J. J., Vogel, W. M., and Pratt, W. B. (1977b). *J. Biol. Chem.* **252**, 7568–7578.

Nielsen, C. J., Vogel, W. M., and Pratt, W. B. (1977c). *Cancer Res.* **37**, 3420–3426.

Nishigori, H., and Toft, D. (1980). *Biochemistry* **19**, 77–83.

Noma, K., Nakao, K., Sato, B., Nishizawa, Y., Matsumoto, K., and Yamamura, Y. (1980). *Endocrinology (Baltimore)* **107**, 1205–1211.

Nordlie, R. C., and Arion, W. J. (1964). *J. Biol. Chem.* **239**, 1680–1685.

Paigen, K. (1958). *J. Biol. Chem.* **233**, 388–394.

Poietta, E., and Sands, H. (1978). *Biochim. Biophys. Acta* **282**, 121–132.

Pratt, W. B., and Ishii, D. N. (1972). *Biochemistry* **11**, 1401–1410.

Pratt, W. B., Kaine, J. L., and Pratt, D. V. (1975). *J. Biol. Chem.* **250**, 4584–4591.

Puri, R. K., Grandics, P., Dougherty, J. J., and Toft, D. O. (1982). *J. Biol. Chem.* **257**, 10831–10837.

Redeuilh, G., Secco, C., Baulieu, E.-E., and Richard-Foy, H. (1981). *J. Biol. Chem.* **256,** 11496–11502.

Rees, A. M., and Bell, P. A. (1975). *Biochim. Biophys. Acta* **411,** 121–132.

Richards, J. M., and Swislocki, N. I. (1979). *J. Biol. Chem.* **254,** 6857–6860.

Roberts, R. M., and Brazer, F. W. (1976). *Biochem. Biophys. Res. Commun.* **68,** 450–455.

Sakaue, Y., and Thompson, E. B. (1977). *Biochem. Biophys. Res. Commun.* **77,** 533–541.

Sando, J. J., Nielsen, C. J., and Pratt, W. B. (1977). *J. Biol. Chem.* **252,** 7579–7582.

Sando, J. J., Hammond, N. D., Stratford, C. A., and Pratt, W. B. (1979a). *J. Biol. Chem.* **254,** 4779–4789.

Sando, J. J., LaForest, A. C., and Pratt, W. B. (1979b). *J. Biol. Chem.* **254,** 4772–4778.

Sato, B., Noma, K., Nishizawa, Y., Nakao, K., Matsumoto, K., and Yamamura, Y. (1980). *Endocrinology (Baltimore)* **106,** 1142–1148.

Schaumburg, B. P. (1972). *Biochim. Biophys. Acta* **261,** 219–235.

Sekula, B. C., Schmidt, T. J., and Litwack, G. (1981). *J. Steroid Biochem.* **14,** 161–166.

Sherman, M. R., Tuazon, F. B., and Miller, L. K. (1980). *Endocrinology (Baltimore)* **106,** 1715–1727.

Shyamala, G., and Leonard, L. (1980). *J. Biol. Chem.* **255,** 6028–6031.

Simons, S. S., Jr., and Thompson, E. B. (1981). *Proc. Natl. Acad. Sci. U.S.A.* **78,** 3541–3545.

Simons, S. S., Jr., Pons, M., and Johnson, D. F. (1980). *J. Org. Chem.* **45,** 3084–3088.

Simons, T. J. B. (1979). *Nature (London)* **281,** 337–338.

Sloman, J. C., and Bell, P. A. (1976). *Biochim. Biophys. Acta* **428,** 403–413.

Toft, D., and Nishigori, H. (1979). *J. Steroid Biochem.* **11,** 413–416.

VanEtten, R. L., Waymack, P. P., and Rehkop, D. M. J. (1974). *J. Am. Chem. Soc.* **96,** 6782–6785.

Wallick, E. T., Lane, L. K., and Schwartz, A. (1979). *J. Biol. Chem.* **254,** 8107–8109.

Weathers, B. J., Grate, J. H., and Schrauzer, G. N. (1979). *J. Am. Chem. Soc.* **101,** 917–924.

Weigel, N. L., Tash, J. S., Means, A. R., Schrader, W. T., and O'Malley, B. W. (1981). *Biochem. Biophys. Res. Commun.* **102,** 513–519.

Wheeler, R. H., Leach, K. L., LaForest, A. C., O'Toole, T. E., Wagner, R., and Pratt, W. B. (1981). *J. Biol. Chem.* **256,** 434–441.

Yuh, K. M., and Keyes, P. L. (1981). *Proc. 63rd Annu. Meet. Endocrine Soc.,* p. 83 (Abstract).

# Index

# Contents of Previous Volumes

Volume VII